Second Edition

Williams
Obstetrics

A Study Guide

Second Edition

Williams Obstetrics
A Study Guide

Thomas M. Julian, M.D.
Associate Professor
Department of Obstetrics and Gynecology
Center for Health Sciences
University of Wisconsin–Madison

with a Foreword by
F. Gary Cunningham, M.D.
Paul C. MacDonald, M.D.
Norman F. Gant, M.D.
Authors, *Williams Obstetrics, Eighteenth Edition*

DR UmoLu

APPLETON & LANGE
Norwalk, Connecticut/San Mateo, California

Notice: The author and publisher of this volume have taken care that
the information and recommendations contained herein are accurate and
compatible with the standards generally accepted at the time of publication.

Copyright © 1989 by Appleton & Lange; © 1985 by Appleton-Century-Crofts
A Publishing Division of Prentice Hall

89 90 91 92 93 / 10 9 8 7 6 5 4 3 2 1

Prentice Hall International (UK) Limited, *London*
Prentice Hall of Australia Pty. Limited, *Sydney*
Prentice Hall Canada, Inc., *Toronto*
Prentice Hall Hispanoamericana, S.A., *Mexico*
Prentice Hall of India Private Limited, *New Delhi*
Prentice Hall of Japan, Inc., *Tokyo*
Simon & Schuster Asia Pte. Ltd., *Singapore*
Editora Prentice Hall do Brasil Ltda., *Rio de Janeiro*
Prentice Hall, Inc., *Englewood Cliffs, New Jersey*

Library of Congress Cataloging-in-Publication Data

Julian, Thomas M.
    Williams obstetrics, a study guide. — 2nd ed./Thomas M. Julian;
with a foreword by F. Gary Cunningham.
    p.   cm.
    Rev. ed. of: Williams obstetrics, a study guide/Charles R.B.
Beckmann, Barbara M. Barzanksy, Frank W. Ling. 1st ed. 1985.
    Companion v. to: Williams obstetrics. 18th ed.
    Includes index.
    ISBN 0-8385-9726-2
    1. Obstetrics — Examinations, questions, etc.   I. Beckmann,
Charles R.B. Williams obstetrics, a study guide.   II. Williams, J.
Whitridge (John Whitridge), 1866–1931. Obstetrics.   III. Title.
    [DNLM: 1. Obstetrics — examination questions.   WQ 100 W724W
Suppl.]
RG532.B44   1989
618.2′0076 — dc20
DNLM/DLC
for Library of Congress   89-6657
                                                              CIP

Editor: R. Craig Percy
Production Editor: John Williams
Designer: Steven Byrum

PRINTED IN THE UNITED STATES OF AMERICA

Contents

Foreword

The easiest and surest way of acquiring facts is to learn them in groups, in systems and systematized knowledge is science. You can very often carry two facts fastened together more easily than one by itself, as a housemaid can carry two pails of water with a hoop more easily than one without it.——Oliver Wendell Holmes, *Scholastic and Beside Teaching*

This quote from Oliver Wendell Holmes was cited in the foreword for the Study Guide assembled to accompany the Seventeenth Edition of *Willams Obstetrics*. The wisdom of this quote holds true today as it did when written more than one hundred years ago. With the influx of seemingly endless new information, which may or may not withstand the light of truth or the test of time, the student of medicine is inundated today as never before with choices for the correct source of information. Most of us—medical students, house officers, and practitioners—remain true to our professions and actively seek new information that is grouped into ''systems'' and ''systematized'' into textbooks.

The correct choice of an obstetrical textbook allows the beginning or continuing student to pursue new information that is added to established knowledge gained through the scientific method or, in many cases, through years of clinical experience.

Thus, never-ending new information must be shifted, condensed, updated, and presented in understandable written and graphic form in textbooks. Simultaneously, outdated dogma, misinformation, or simply misapplied information must be deleted and previous errors in understanding acknowledged and corrected. Most good textbooks have all of these characteristics and we believe that the Eighteenth Edition of *Williams Obstetrics* is such a textbook.

Before learning begins, the correct sources of information must be grouped together and presented in concise and palatable forms such as in *Williams Obstetrics*. Then, as in the Holmes analogy, ''this pail of water'' can be more easily managed by combining it with a second ''pail'' that is not heavier or less manageable, but may balance the first and make it easier to carry. This Study Guide is such a balancing factor. It is designed and written to be the companion of the Eighteenth Edition of *Williams Obstetrics*. It is not intended to be an added weight but rather to balance and augment the process of learning, and we believe that it accomplishes these objectives.

F. Gary Cunningham, M.D.
Paul C. MacDonald, M.D.
Norman F. Gant, M.D.

Preface

For decades *Williams Obstetrics* has been the standard against which medical students, residents, and practicing physicians have measured their knowledge of obstetrics. The task of acquiring this knowledge is increasingly formidable as the body and complexity of information concerning obstetrics increases.

Williams Obstetrics: A Study Guide is designed to help by providing study questions organized both by chapter and by concept-area or topic. The questions are written in simple formats (short answer, multiple choice, matching, true/false) so that the reader's efforts may be specifically directed toward learning and understanding the information in *Williams Obstetrics*.

Each question is referenced to a page (or pages) in *Williams Obstetrics* and cross-referenced to related concepts.

We believe that the use of *Williams Obstetrics: A Study Guide* will ease and speed the reader's understanding and retention of the vital information provided in this classic textbook of obstetrics.

This edition is based on the First Edition of *Williams Obstetrics: A Study Guide*, as formulated and authored by Charles R. B. Beckmann, Frank W. Ling, and Barbara Barzansky.

Thomas M. Julian, M.D.

Instructions for Use

This book is designed to help you master the information contained in the Eighteenth Edition of *Williams Obstetrics*. Use of the Study Guide should help you efficiently organize and direct your learning, whatever the level of knowledge and experience that you possess.

ORGANIZATION OF THE STUDY GUIDE

The Study Guide is a companion volume to *Williams Obstetrics*. No new information is presented beyond that found in the recent edition of the text. The chapters in the Study Guide are numbered identically to the chapters in *Williams Obstetrics*. The Study Guide is divided into three basic sections:

- The first section contains questions based on the content of each chapter in *Williams Obstetrics*. The questions are designed to emphasize and synthesize the major points covered in the chapter.
- The second section consists of the answers to the questions from each chapter. For each question, the page references to *Williams Obstetrics* where the information to answer the question may be found are included. In addition, the specific content areas (topics) relevant to the question are listed. The topics come from an analysis of both the subject matter of the question and the way that the subject matter is applied in practice (e.g., the topics listed for a question on cesarean delivery for a fetus in the breech position may include ''breech presentation'' as well as ''cesarean delivery'').

- The third section of the Study Guide is a ''topics list'' that serves as an index. For all the topics named in the second section, it enumerates the questions (by number) that include that topic.

QUESTION FORMATS

There are four basic types of questions used in the Study Guide: multiple choice, true–false, matching, and short answer. For the multiple choice items, one, more than one, or none of the options may be correct.

USE OF THE STUDY GUIDE

Based on the reader's level of expertise, there are several ways in which the Study Guide may be used. The beginning student in a clerkship in OB-Gyn should probably read the chapter in *Williams Obstetrics* and then attempt to answer the questions in the Study Guide. For those questions that are incorrectly answered, the student should re-read the relevant pages and attempt to correct any misunderstanding before proceeding to the next chapter. The junior house officer might attempt to answer the questions in the Study Guide first, and then read the text to specifically correct any problem areas that are identified. For a senior house officer or a practitioner, it might be most appropriate to answer all the questions related to a topic of interest (e.g., fetal distress, prostaglandins, cesarean delivery). This approach will help the experienced individual synthesize the content in a given area that is presented throughout *Williams Obstetrics*.

Second Edition

Williams
Obstetrics
A Study Guide

Questions

PART I HUMAN PREGNANCY

1. OBSTETRICS IN BROAD PERSPECTIVE

1-1. Obstetrics is defined as the study of labor and delivery, both normal and abnormal.

    a. True
    b. False

1-2. The fertility rate is defined as the number of

    a. Births per 1,000 population
    b. Births per 1,000 women aged 15 to 44
    c. Live births per 1,000 women aged 15 to 44
    d. Births per 100,000 women aged 15 to 44

1-3. The birth rate is defined as the number of

    a. Births/1,000 population
    b. Births/10,000 population
    c. Births/100,000 population
    d. Live births/10,000 population
    e. Live births/1,000 women

Instructions for Items 1-4 to 1-6: Match the term with the appropriate definition.

    a. Abortus
    b. Stillbirth
    c. Live birth

1-4. When the infant at birth or sometime after birth breathes spontaneously or shows another sign of life

1-5. A fetus removed or expelled from the uterus at 20 weeks or less of gestation

1-6. An infant who at birth shows no signs of life nor breathes spontaneously

1-7. Which of the following is a criterion for a live birth?

    a. Presence of a heart beat
    b. Presence of voluntary muscle movements
    c. Spontaneous breathing
    d. Weight at birth greater than 2,500 g

1-8. The perinatal mortality rate is defined as _____ .

1-9. The stillbirth rate is synonymous with the

    a. Neonatal mortality rate
    b. Perinatal mortality rate
    c. Fetal death rate
    d. Reproductive mortality rate

Instructions for Items 1-10 to 1-13: Match the term with the appropriate description.

    a. Abortus
    b. Preterm or premature infant
    c. Term infant
    d. Postterm infant
    e. Low-birthweight infant

1-10. An infant born any time after the 42nd week

1-11. An infant with a first recorded weight of less than 2500 g

1-12. An infant born before 38 completed weeks of gestation

1-13. An infant born no earlier than 38 completed weeks and no later than 42 completed weeks of gestation

1-14. A woman dies from complications of mitral stenosis during the course of her pregnancy. This would be defined as

    a. A direct maternal death
    b. An indirect maternal death
    c. A nonmaternal death

Answers begin on page 191

1-15. The maternal death rate is defined as the number of maternal deaths per

    a. 1,000 pregnancies
    b. 100,000 pregnancies
    c. 1,000 live births
    d. 100,000 live births
    e. 1,000 births
    f. 100,000 births

1-16. Reproductive mortality is defined as _____ .

1-17. Which of the following factors is directly related to the maternal mortality rate?

    a. Age
    b. Race
    c. Parity
    d. Socioeconomic status

1-18. Which of the following is a common cause of maternal mortality?

    a. Hypertension
    b. Diabetes
    c. Infection
    d. Hemorrhage

1-19. The most useful statistical index of the quality of obstetric care is the

    a. Birth rate
    b. Stillbirth rate
    c. Neonatal mortality rate
    d. Perinatal mortality rate
    e. Maternal mortality rate

1-20. Which of the following statements about neonatal deaths is correct?

    a. Currently there are more fetal deaths than neonatal deaths.
    b. Most neonatal deaths occur during the second to the sixth months of life.
    c. Neonatal death is more common in low-birthweight infants.
    d. Central nervous system injury is a significant cause of neonatal death.

1-21. Birth certificates serve to

    a. Provide evidence of age
    b. Provide evidence of citizenship
    c. Provide evidence of family relationships
    d. Provide vital statistics for health care planning

2.   HUMAN PREGNANCY: OVERVIEW, ORGANIZATION, AND DIAGNOSIS

2-1. In populations of women in whom early marriage was the rule and in whom contraception was not practiced, menstruation was relatively uncommon.

    a. True
    b. False

2-2. Which of the following statements regarding estrogen is true?

    a. Estrogen effect on bone is beneficial in women.
    b. There is no mechanism by which breast, uterus, bone, or vaginal tissues provide feedback for estrogen regulation.
    c. The ovary and pituitary–brain both have mechanisms for estrogen regulation.
    d. In the ovary, estrogen production is confined largely to one ovary at a time.

2-3. Regarding ovarian function, which of the following statements is true?

    a. During the first and last days of each ovarian cycle, there is very little estradiol-17 β formed in the ovarian follicle.
    b. Most estrogens at the extremes of the menstrual cycle are produced by extraglandular formation of estrogens from molecules containing C_{19}-androgens.
    c. Aromatization of C_{19}-steroids cannot occur in peripheral tissues of the body.
    d. Estrogen production in the ovary is dependent on follicle formation.

2-4. Regarding progesterone production in the human female, which of the following is true?

    a. The majority of progesterone is produced by the corpus luteum.
    b. Progesterone is generally thought to be essential to the maintenance of pregnancy in most mammalian species.
    c. Destruction of the corpus luteum before 16 weeks' gestation in the human will result in abortion.
    d. The endocrine events of the menstrual cycle are an investment made almost singularly toward the achievement of normal function of bone, skin, mucosa, and breast development in the human.

2-5. Regarding the reproductive physiology of women, which statements is true?

    a. The function of the fallopian tube is mainly the transport of egg and sperm.
    b. The likely source of uterotropins is in the decidua.
    c. The most intricate and complex function of the ovary is estrogen production.
    d. Ovulation is independent of brain, pituitary, or ovarian action.

2-6. Regarding the ''communication system'' of pregnancy, which of the following statements is true?

  a. It would appear that a biomolecular communication system exists between the developing human and the mother from nidation through parturition.
  b. The blastocyst is the dynamic force in the process of implantation.
  c. It is the paracrine arm of the communication system that provides for pregnancy maintenance, the semiallogenic fetal graft.
  d. The placental arm of the communication system provides for direct communication of the maternal and fetal circulations.

2-7. The role of the fetus in pregnancy is that of a

  a. More or less passive passenger
  b. Symbiont
  c. Dynamic force, producing bioactive agents essential to pregnancy
  d. Producer of progesterone

2-8. Fertilization of the human ovum by a spermatozoan occurs most often in the

  a. Cervical mucus
  b. Uterine cavity
  c. Fallopian tube
  d. Peritoneal cavity

2-9. Which statement regarding the fetus during pregnancy is UNTRUE?

  a. The role of the fetus in pregnancy is similar to that of a rapidly growing neoplasm in many ways.
  b. The fetus may benefit from transplacental passage of maternal antibodies.
  c. The fetal demands are sacrificed in most instances when the maternal organism is in any way stressed.
  d. Fetal membranes also play an important role in the endocrinology of pregnancy.

2-10. In human pregnancy there is evidence of a luteolytic agent produced in women that causes ''murder of the corpus luteum'' and is responsible for the beginning of a new menstrual cycle.

  a. True
  b. False

2-11. Almost without exception the endocrine changes of pregnancy are a consequence of

  a. Maternal ovarian function
  b. Uterine hormone production
  c. Production of amniotic fluid hormones
  d. Fetal placental function

Instructions for Items 2-12 to 2-14: Match the lettered item with the appropriate descriptive phrase.

  a. Estrogen
  b. Oxytocin
  c. Progesterone
  d. Inhibin

2-12. Acts on the myoepithelial cells of the breast ducts to cause milk letdown

2-13. Withdrawal promptly after delivery commences lactogenesis

2-14. Responsible for growth of breast ducts

2-15. Regarding the diagnosis of pregnancy, which of the following statements is true?

  a. Knowledge of the existence of pregnancy is crucial to the proper diagnosis and treatment of all disease processes in women.
  b. Failure to diagnose pregnancy is a frequent cause in professional liability cases.
  c. The diagnosis of pregnancy is always easy to establish.
  d. Mistakes in the diagnosis of pregnancy are most commonly made in the second trimester secondary to decreased human chorionic gonadotropin (hCG) levels.

2-16. Of the following which may be used in making the diagnosis of pregnancy?

  a. The subjective impression of the patient
  b. Symptoms elicited on history taking
  c. Physical signs during examination
  d. Laboratory tests

2-17. Which of the following is a positive sign of pregnancy?

  a. Softening of the lower uterine segment
  b. Uterine enlargement
  c. Fetal heart tone identification
  d. Perception of fetal movement by the examiner
  e. Ultrasonographic/radiographic identification of fetus

2-18. The normal fetal heart rate ranges from _____ .

2-19. Fetal heart activity can be identified by 8 weeks' gestation using which of the following?

  a. Auscultation with a stethoscope
  b. Instruments employing the Doppler principle
  c. Real time sonography
  d. Flat plate of the abdomen

2-20. Which of the following may interfere significantly with correct identification of fetal heart action?

  a. Maternal tachycardia
  b. Fetal tachycardia
  c. Maternal bradycardia
  d. Fetal bradycardia
  e. Funic souffle
  f. Uterine souffle

Instructions for Items 2–21 to 2–28: Match the sounds heard on auscultation of the abdomen with the appropriate descriptions.

    a. Funic (umbilical souffle)
    b. Uterine souffle
    c. Intrauterine fetal movement
    d. Intestinal peristalsis or gas/fluid movement

2–21. Soft blowing sound synchronous with maternal pulse
2–22. Sharp whistling sound synchronous with fetal pulse
2–23. Gurgling sound
2–24. Irregular, sharp sound not synchronous with maternal or fetal pulse
2–25. Caused by rush of blood through umbilical arteries
2–26. Produced by blood rushing through dilated uterine vessels
2–27. Heard in 15 percent of pregnancies
2–28. May be heard in women with leiomyoma uteri

2–29. Which of the following statements about fetal movement is correct?

    a. Fetal movement can be felt by an examiner throughout the second trimester.
    b. Fetal movement may vary in intensity.
    c. Fetal movement may be visible through the maternal abdominal wall.
    d. Fetal movement may be simulated by muscular contractions of the maternal abdominal wall.
    e. Fetal movement may be simulated by maternal intestinal peristalsis.

2–30. Which of the following statements about the ultrasonographic evaluation of pregnancy is correct?

    a. By 4 to 5 weeks from the LMP, a normal intrauterine pregnancy may often be detected.
    b. By 6 weeks from the LMP, a small white gestational ring may be seen, but its absence this early in pregnancy does not raise doubts about the pregnancy.
    c. By 8 weeks from the LMP, the embryo (fetal pole) may usually be identified.
    d. By 11 weeks from the LMP, fetal heart motion can usually be identified by real time ultrasonography.
    e. By the 11th week, the fetal head and thorax can be identified.

2–31. Which of the following is characteristic of gestations in which there is a blighted ovum?

    a. Spontaneous abortion will ultimately occur.
    b. Ultrasonography shows an unusually small gestational sac.
    c. Ultrasonography shows a loss of definition of the gestational sac.
    d. Ultrasonography shows strong echoes emanating from the fetus after 8 weeks' gestation.

2–32. Which of the following may be determined using ultrasonography at some time during pregnancy?

    a. Gestational age of fetus
    b. Number of fetuses
    c. Presenting part
    d. Some fetal anomalies
    e. Presence of hydramnios
    f. Rate of fetal growth

2–33. To date, no adverse effects on the human fetus have been identified from exposure to energies comparable to those used for clinical ultrasonographic examinations.

    a. True
    b. False

2–34. Positive identification of pregnancy, based on visualization of the fetal skeleton by x-ray, cannot be made until about _____ weeks of gestation.

Instructions for Items 2–35 to 2–38: Match the description of the abdomen with the types of pregnancy with which it is most often associated.

    a. Nulliparous
    b. Multiparous

2–35. Uterus usually palpable abdominally by 12 weeks of gestation
2–36. Abdominal enlargement pronounced due to loss of muscle tone
2–37. Presence of a pendulous abdomen
2–38. Significant changes in abdominal shape due to body position.

2–39. Which of the following statements about changes in the uterus and the cervix during pregnancy is correct?

    a. During the first few weeks of pregnancy, the increase in size is limited to the anteroposterior diameter.
    b. At about 4 weeks after the LMP, Hegar's sign becomes manifest.
    c. Hegar's sign is not diagnostic of pregnancy.
    d. The cervix normally remains firm and closed until labor ensues.
    e. In certain inflammatory conditions, the cervix may soften during pregnancy.
    f. Oral contraceptive use may cause softening and congestion of the cervix.

2–40. Which of the following is not characteristic of Braxton Hicks contractions?

    a. Palpable
    b. Painless
    c. Irregular
    d. Enhanced by massage
    e. Confined to the third trimester

2-41. Near midpregnancy, sudden pressure exerted on the uterus may cause the fetus to sink in the amnionic fluid. The rebound, which may be felt by the examiner, is termed _____ .

2-42. Outlining ''a fetus'' by palpation through the maternal abdominal wall is not a positive sign of pregnancy because _____ .

2-43. Hormonal tests commonly used in the clinical laboratory absolutely identify the presence or absence of pregnancy.

    a. True
    b. False

2-44. Most chemical tests for the detection of pregnancy involve the identification of _____ in blood or urine.

2-45. Which of the following statements about pregnancy tests is correct?

    a. Radioreceptor assays, using bovine corpus luteum plasma membranes, are specific for hCG.
    b. Antibodies against the entire hCG molecule do not recognize LH.
    c. In immunoassay procedures, the principle of hemagglutination inhibition of erythrocytes may be employed.
    d. In radioassays, the results are based on the competition between radiolabeled hCG and hCG in the sample to be tested.

2-46. In early pregnancy, the concentration of hCG in maternal plasma doubles about every _____ days.

    a. 0.5
    b. 1.5
    c. 3
    d. 5
    e. 7

2-47. Human chorionic gonadotropin can be first detected by radioimmunoassay _____ the embryo can first be visualized by ultrasonography.

    a. Earlier than
    b. At the same time as
    c. Later than

2-48. Enzyme-linked immunoabsorbent assays (ELISA) will often have a sensitivity of _____ miU/mL of hCG.

    a. 10
    b. 50
    c. 500
    d. 1000

2-49. In home pregnancy tests, the false-negative rate is _____ the false-positive rate.

    a. Lower than
    b. The same as
    c. Higher than

2-50. Which of the following statements about progesterone or synthetic progestin-induced withdrawal bleeding is correct?

    a. It is able to specifically differentiate pregnancy from other etiologies of amenorrhea.
    b. It requires an estrogen-primed endometrium.
    c. It requires high levels of endogenous progesterone production.
    d. It is a safe procedure with no potentially harmful fetal effects.

2-51. Which of the following statements about hCG levels in ectopic pregnancy is correct?

    a. Sensitive assays for hCG show positive results in at least 80 percent of cases.
    b. Normal levels of hCG are never found in ectopic pregnancy.
    c. A doubling of plasma hCG concentration every 2 days is associated with an ectopic pregnancy in about 20 percent of cases.
    d. Falling levels of hCG over time distinguish impending spontaneous abortion from ectopic pregnancy.

2-52. Due to the half-life of hCG, if postabortion monitoring for hCG is indicated, how long after the procedure should this be conducted?

    a. 1 to 2 days
    b. 3 to 4 days
    c. 5 to 7 days
    d. 2 to 3 weeks
    e. 4 to 6 weeks

2-53. Which of the following constitutes presumptive evidence of pregnancy?

    a. Cessation of menses
    b. Discoloration of vaginal mucosa
    c. Breast changes
    d. Skin changes
    e. Self-awareness of being pregnant
    f. Nausea and vomiting
    g. Perception of fetal movement
    h. Constipation
    i. Fatigue
    j. Urinary disturbance
    k. Poor libido

2-54. Which of the following statements about pregnancy, menstruation, and vaginal bleeding is correct?

   a. In a woman with spontaneous, cyclic, predictable menstruation, a delay in the onset of menstruation greater than 3 days is strongly suggestive of pregnancy.
   b. Gestation must be preceded by menstruation.
   c. Macroscopic vaginal bleeding may occur in pregnancies with normal outcomes.
   d. Bleeding during pregnancy is more common in primaparas than in multiparas.
   e. Bleeding per vagina during pregnancy should be regarded as abnormal.

2-55. Breast changes similar to those seen in pregnancy may occasionally be found in which of the following situations?

   a. Tranquilizer ingestion
   b. Prolactin-secreting pituitary tumor
   c. Pseudocyesis
   d. Repeated breast stimulation

2-56. Increased skin pigmentation and the appearance of abdominal striae, common to pregnancy, may also be seen in users of oral steroidal contraceptives.

   a. True
   b. False

2-57. Which of the following statements about the symptoms of pregnancy is correct?

   a. ''Morning sickness'' usually begins before the first missed period.
   b. ''Morning sickness'' usually lasts 6 to 12 weeks.
   c. Increased frequency of urination, unassociated with urinary tract infection, is more common at the beginning and end of pregnancy.
   d. Easy fatigability is a characteristic of late pregnancy.
   e. Sensations of fetal movement usually begin around 20 weeks after the LMP.

2-58. Which of the following conditions simulates the menstrual pattern of pregnancy?

   a. Adenomyosis
   b. Hematometra
   c. Leiomyomata
   d. Pelvic extrauterine mass

2-59. Which of the following statements about pseudocyesis (spurious pregnancy) is correct?

   a. It is more common in women with an intense desire for children and in women nearing menopause.
   b. Patients often experience morning sickness.
   c. Abdominal distention may be present.
   d. An enlarged, soft uterus may be present.
   e. There may be a perception of fetal movement.
   f. Irregular menses or amenorrhea may be present.

Instructions for Items 2-60 to 2-64: Match the physical finding with its most typical appearance in nulliparous and/or multiparous women.

   a. Nulliparous
   b. Multiparous

2-60. Pink abdominal striae present
2-61. Labia majora in close apposition
2-62. Abdominal wall lax or pendulous
2-63. Myrtiform caruncles present
2-64. Vagina narrow with well-developed rugae

2-65. Which of the following statements about fetal death is correct?

   a. In the early months of pregnancy, hCG level is the most sensitive test for fetal death.
   b. Fetal death may be suspected when the uterus fails to increase in size or begins to decrease in size.
   c. The absence of fetal heart tones in auscultation with a stethoscope is positive proof of fetal demise.
   d. Real time ultrasonographic examination can serve to accurately identify the presence of fetal heart action.

2-66. Which of the following is *not* a radiologic sign characteristic of fetal death?

   a. Hyperextension of neck
   b. Skull bone overlap
   c. Exaggerated spinal curve
   d. Gas in fetus
   e. Transverse lie

3.   THE ENDOMETRIUM AND UTERINE DECIDUA

3-1. In terms of the endometrium, which of the following statements are true?

   a. The endometrium is the lining of the uterine cavity.
   b. With menses two thirds of the lining of the uterine cavity is shed.
   c. The average woman undergoes menses about 400 times during her life.
   d. During an entire lifetime a woman will have lost from 10 to 20 liters of blood due to menstruation.

3-2. Decidua is the

   a. Endometrium after ovulation
   b. Submucosal layer of the endometrium
   c. Specialized endometrium of pregnancy
   d. Membranous covering of the placenta

3-3. Current hypotheses seem to indicate that the most important role of the decidua may be in the

  a. Protection of the fetus from teratogens
  b. Early production of progesterone in gestation
  c. Initiation of parturition
  d. Suppression of fetal antigenicity

3-4. Which of the following statements about estradiol-17β is correct?

  a. It is a potent natural estrogen.
  b. It enters the endometrial cell by simple diffusion.
  c. It is involved in the synthesis of receptor molecules for progesterone.
  d. It is involved in the synthesis of receptor molecules for estradiol-17β.

3-5. Progesterone negates the effects of estrogen by

  a. Bringing about a decrease in the production of estradiol-17β receptors
  b. Causing a decrease in intracellular estradiol-17β concentration
  c. Increasing the sulfurylation of estrogen
  d. Competitively occupying estrogen receptors

3-6. The absence of progesterone receptors in a breast tumor indicates that the tumor is more likely to be responsive to endocrine ablation procedures.

  a. True
  b. False

3-7. Menstruation is ultimately due to

  a. Estrogen withdrawal
  b. Estrogen stimulation
  c. Progesterone withdrawal
  d. Progesterone stimulation

3-8. Ovarian cycle events occur _____ the corresponding menstrual cycle events.

  a. Before
  b. Coincident with
  c. After

Instructions for Items 3-9 to 3-11: Match the phase of the ovulatory ovarian cycle with the characteristics of the endometrium.

  a. Early follicular
  b. Late follicular
  c. Luteal

3-9. Significant gland mitoses, no visible secretion in gland lumena, little stromal edema, considerable stromal mitoses

3-10. Increasing numbers of gland mitoses, no visible secretion in gland lumena, some stromal edema, low level of stromal mitoses

3-11. Sharply decreasing number of gland mitoses, considerable secretion in gland lumena, significant stromal edema, decreasing stromal mitoses

3-12. The follicular phase of the menstrual cycle is commonly synonymous with the

  a. Preovulatory phase of the ovarian cycle
  b. Postovulatory phase of the ovarian cycle
  c. Proliferative phase of the endometrial cycle
  d. Secretory phase of the endometrial cycle

Instructions for Items 3-13 to 3-16: Match the phase of the menstrual/endometrial cycle with the appropriate histologic description.

  a. Secretory phase
  b. Proliferative phase
  c. Premenstrual phase

3-13. Development of coiled or spiral arterioles
3-14. Basal, compact, and spongy zones of endometrium become well defined
3-15. "Dating" of endometrium not possible
3-16. Infiltration of the stroma by polymorphonuclear leucocytes occurring

Instructions for Items 3-17 to 3-21: Match the stage of the endometrial cycle with its histologic characteristics.

  a. Early proliferative
  b. Late proliferative
  c. Early secretory
  d. Late secretory
  e. Premenstrual

3-17. Extremely vascular, rich in glycogen, stromal cells undergoing hypertrophic changes, spiral arterioles become highly tortuous
3-18. Glands narrow and tubular, glandular epithelium low columnar, deep stromal cells densely packed
3-19. Three zones (basal, spongy, and compact) become well defined, stromal edema prominent
3-20. Infiltration of stroma by polymorphonuclear or mononuclear leucocytes
3-21. Glandular epithelium becomes taller and pseudostratified, glands of deeper zone become crowded and tortuous

3-22. The menstrual phase of the normal menstrual cycle is

a. Preceded by corpus luteum regression
b. Preceded by falling levels of progesterone and estrogen
c. Preceded first by spiral arteriole vasoconstriction and slowed circulation and then by vasodilation and increased blood flow
d. Characterized by predominantly venous bleeding

3-23. The decidua (the specialized endometrium of pregnancy)

a. May be the source of amnionic fluid prolactin
b. Serves as an allograft model
c. Has high levels of phospholipase A_2 activity
d. Contains a low concentration of arachidonic acid

3-24. Which of the following statements about the synthesis and action of prostaglandins is correct?

a. They cannot be synthesized from the esterified form of arachidonic acid.
b. Their synthesis is dependent on the action of phospholipase A_2.
c. They can precipitate the initiation of menstruation in nonpregnant women.
d. They can cause symptoms of dysmenorrhea when administered in large doses.

3-25. Which of the following are potentially normal events during the menstrual cycle?

a. The follicular phase may vary in length from 1 to 3 weeks.
b. There may be bleeding during anovulatory cycles.
c. Bleeding ("placental sign") may result from the implantation of the fertilized ovum.

3-26. A 26-year-old woman who has been using oral contraceptives for 3 years has been menstruating regularly. This woman is most probably ovulating normally.

a. True
b. False
c. Cannot be determined from the data available

3-27. Which of the following statements concerning cervical mucus secretion is correct?

a. Secretion is maximal at the time of ovulation.
b. Spinnbarkeit is minimal at the time of ovulation.
c. Cervical mucus secretion is the result of estrogenic stimulation.
d. Maximal secretion of cervical mucus coincides with the maximal secretion of the endometrial glands.

3-28. In which of the following situations is a well-developed "fern pattern" likely to be seen when cervical mucus is spread on a glass slide?

a. During pregnancy
b. When the sodium chloride concentration is less than 1 percent
c. During the late secretory portion of the menstrual cycle
d. When estrogen, but not progesterone, is being produced

Instructions for Items 3-29 and 3-30: Match the hormone with its effect on the sodium chloride concentration of cervical mucus.

a. Estrogen
b. Progesterone

3-29. Results in raised sodium chloride concentration
3-30. Results in lowered sodium chloride concentration

Instructions for Items 3-31 to 3-34: Match the stage of the menstrual cycle with the cellular characteristics of the vagina.

a. Follicular phase
b. Luteal phase

3-31. Leukopenia
3-32. Increased number of basophilic cells
3-33. Enlarged, flattened superficial cells
3-34. Increased number of leucocytes

3-35. Which of the following statements regarding menarche is correct?

a. Menarche always occurs between the ages of 11 and 14.
b. Menarche is a sign of puberty.
c. Menarche occurs at an earlier age now than 30 years ago.
d. Menarche is indicative of sexual maturity.

Instructions for Items 3-36 to 3-39: Match the term with its definition.

a. Menarche
b. Puberty
c. Menopause
d. Climacteric

3-36. Cessation of menses
3-37. Transition between childhood and maturity
3-38. Onset of first menstruation
3-39. "Change of life"

3-40. Which of the following statements about the normal menstrual cycle is correct?

    a. There is marked variation among women in the length of the menstrual cycle.
    b. There is often considerable variation in the length of a given woman's menstrual cycles.
    c. There is considerable variation among women in the duration of menstrual flow.
    d. There is usually considerable variation in the duration of a given woman's menstrual flow.

3-41. A marked irregularity in the length of a patient's menstrual cycles usually means that she is sterile.

    a. True
    b. False

3-42. The normal menstrual cycle is usually characterized by

    a. A highly coagulable menstrual discharge
    b. A usual flow duration of 4 to 6 days
    c. An average weight gain of 1 to 2 pounds
    d. A yearly iron loss of 150 to 400 mg

3-43. A premenstrual weight gain of 3 to 5 pounds is a common physiologic phenomenon.

    a. True
    b. False

4. THE PLACENTA AND FETAL MEMBRANES

4-1. Place the following developmental stages into the correct chronologic sequence.

    a. Fetus
    b. Morula
    c. Blastomere
    d. Embryo
    e. Zygote
    f. Blastocyst

4-2. Which of the following statements about implantation is correct?

    a. The fertilized ovum undergoes cleavage for 3 days in the fallopian tube.
    b. After entering the uterine cavity, the blastocyst remains free (i.e., does not implant) for 1 or 2 days.
    c. The zona pellucida disappears before implantation occurs.
    d. The pole of the blastocyst with the inner cell mass implants first.

4-3. Which of the following statements about the inner cell mass is correct?

    a. It forms the embryo.
    b. It develops into the cytotrophoblast.
    c. It induces a decidual reaction in surrounding maternal tissues.
    d. It gives rise to extraembryonic mesoderm.

4-4. Development of syncytiotrophoblast is required for

    a. Formation of new cytotrophoblast cells
    b. Successful invasion of the endometrium
    c. Elicitation of a decidual response
    d. Formation of the amnion

Instructions for Items 4-5 to 4-12: Refer to Figure 1.
Match the letter with the appropriate structure.

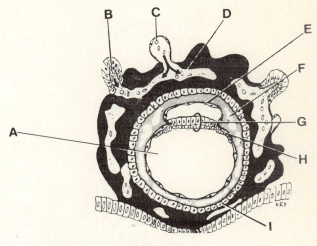

FIGURE 1

4-5. Embryonic disc
4-6. Amnionic cavity
4-7. Maternal blood in lacunar network
4-8. Extraembryonic endoderm
4-9. Cytotrophoblast
4-10. Lacunar network
4-11. Primitive yolk sac
4-12. Extraembryonic coelom developing in extraembryonic mesoderm

Instructions for Items 4–13 to 4–19: Match the germ layer with the structures derived from it.

    a. Ectoderm
    b. Mesoderm
    c. Endoderm

4–13. Epidermis
4–14. Lining of the GI tract
4–15. Nervous system
4–16. Vascular system
4–17. Skeletal muscle
4–18. Liver
4–19. Dermis

4–20. Which of the following statements about the notochord is correct?

    a. It arises as a forward extension of the primitive streak.
    b. It constitutes the primordial supporting structure of vertebrates.
    c. It disappears early in embryonic life.
    d. Remnants of notochord persist in the adult as the nucleus pulposus of the intervertebral discs.

4–21. Differentiation of the embryo proceeds from the cephalic end to the caudal end.

    a. True
    b. False

4–22. Somites

    a. Are derived from lateral mesoderm
    b. Give rise to skeletal and connective tissues
    c. Begin at the level of the developing neck

4–23. Primary placental villi become secondary villi when _____ and tertiary villi after _____ .
    (1)   (2)

    a. Solid trophoblastic columns are formed
    b. Angiogenesis occurs in situ
    c. The solid trophoblast is invaded by a mesenchymal cord, presumably from the cytotrophoblast

Instructions for Items 4–24 to 4–26: Match the event with the time after fertilization when it occurs.

    a. 7 days
    b. 10 days
    c. 12 days
    d. 14 days
    e. 17 days

4–24. Placental circulation established
4–25. Maternal arterial blood enters intervillous spaces
4–26. Villi distinguishable in the placenta

4–27. Which of the following statements about chorionic villi is correct?

    a. Chorionic villi are not recognizable until about 4 weeks after fertilization.
    b. Incomplete or absent angiogenesis may present as hydatidiform mole.
    c. Villi in contact with the decidua basalis proliferate to form the chorion frondosum.
    d. An extension of the syncytiotrophoblast anchors the villi to the decidua at the basal plate.

Instructions for Items 4–28 and 4–29: Match the component with its correct location.

    a. Cytotrophoblast cells
    b. Decidua of basal plate
    c. Trophectoderm
    d. Chorionic plate

4–28. Floor of intervillous space
4–29. Roof of intervillous space

4–30. At 19 days postfertilization, which of the following does *not* describe human embryonic development?

    a. The embryo is at the primitive streak stage.
    b. The decidua basalis is present.
    c. The decidua capsularis is present.
    d. The embryo is trilaminar.
    e. A choriovitelline placenta has formed.

Instructions for Items 4–31 and 4–32: Match the descriptions of components of the chorion at 3 weeks after fertilization.

    a. Cuboidal cells
    b. Clear cytoplasm
    c. Light, vesicular nuclei
    d. Dark nuclei
    e. Granular cytoplasm

4–31. Cytotrophoblast
4–32. Syncytiotrophoblast

4–33. The chorionic villi in contact with the decidua basalis proliferate to form the _____ , whereas the villi in contact with the decidua capsularis degenerate, which results in the _____ .
    (1)   (2)

    a. Chorion laeve
    b. Chorion frondosum

4-34. Which of the following statements about the chorion is correct?

   a. Villi are distributed over the entire periphery of the chorionic membrane throughout pregnancy.
   b. The chorion laeve comprises only a small portion of the chorion.
   c. Prostaglandin synthesis at parturition is associated with the amniochorion.
   d. The amniochorion in the human is formed from the amnion and the chorion frondosum.
   e. The amniochorion is not formed until near the end of the third trimester.

4-35. The amniochorion functions in transfer and metabolic activity

   a. True
   b. False

4-36. A placental cotyledon is formed from _____ .

4-37. Which of the following changes is seen in the placenta as pregnancy advances?

   a. Volume of cytotrophoblast cells decreases
   b. Syncytium thickens
   c. Syncytium forms knots
   d. Stroma becomes denser
   e. Number of Hofbauer cells increases

4-38. Which of the following statements about the decidua is correct?

   a. The decidua is the endometrium of pregnancy.
   b. The decidual reaction occurs in response to estrogen.
   c. The decidual reaction occurs in response to human placental lactogen.
   d. The decidual reaction is completed before nidation.
   e. Decidual cells arise from stromal cells of the endometrium.

4-39. Which of the following occurs in the decidua as pregnancy progresses?

   a. The decidua thickens to a depth of 2 cm or more.
   b. The decidua basalis overlies the developing embryo and separates it from the rest of the uterine cavity.
   c. The decidua capsularis is formed directly beneath the site of implantation.
   d. The uterine cavity is obliterated after the fusion of the decidua capsularis and parietalis (vera).

Instructions for Items 4-40 to 4-44: Refer to Figure 2.
Match the letter with the appropriate description.

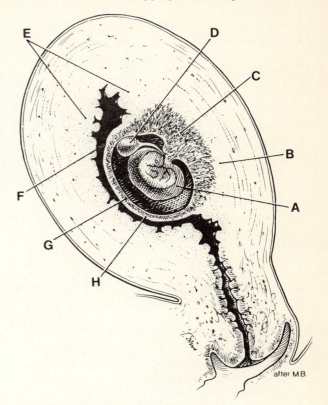

FIGURE 2

4-40. Decidua vera
4-41. Decidua capsularis
4-42. Decidua basalis
4-43. Chorion frondosum
4-44. Chorion laeve

4-45. The correct sequence of layers, starting from the surface, in the decidua vera and the decidua basalis is

   a. Compacta, spongiosa, basalis
   b. Compacta, basalis, spongiosa
   c. Spongiosa, compacta, basalis
   d. Spongiosa, basalis, compacta
   e. Basalis, compacta, spongiosa
   f. Basalis, spongiosa, compacta

4-46. After delivery, which of the following portions of the decidua remains to give rise to the new endometrium?

   a. Zona compacta
   b. Zona spongiosa
   c. Zona functionalis
   d. Zona basalis

Instructions for Items 4–47 and 4–48: Match the decidual zone with the appropriate histologic description.

    a. Zona compacta
    b. Zona spongiosa
    c. Zona basalis

4–47. Large distended glands, minimal stroma
4–48. Large closely-packed polygonal cells, numerous small round cells

4–49. Which of the following distinguishes the decidua vera from the decidua basalis?

    a. The decidua vera enters into the formation of the placental basal plate.
    b. The decidua basalis contains a large number of trophoblastic giant cells.
    c. By term, the glands of the zona spongiosa in the decidua basalis have largely disappeared.
    d. The zona spongiosa of the decidua vera consists mainly of arteries and widely dilated veins.

4–50. The zone of fibrinoid degeneration where trophoblasts invade the decidua is called the _____ .

4–51. Which of the following statements about the decidua is correct?

    a. Nitabuch layer is usually absent in placenta accreta.
    b. Some necrotic decidua may be found in a placental specimen taken at any stage of gestation.
    c. Necrotic decidua always indicate threatened or actual abortion.

4–52. The presence of necrotic decidua during the first trimester is compatible with which of the following possibilities?

    a. Threatened abortion
    b. Incomplete abortion
    c. Septic abortion
    d. Completed abortion
    e. Normal pregnancy

4–53. Which of the following statements about prolactin and the decidua is correct?

    a. Prolactin occurs in high concentration in amnionic fluid.
    b. Amnionic fluid prolactin concentration is decreased when a pregnant woman is treated with bromocriptine.
    c. Dopamine increases decidual prolactin secretion.
    d. Thyrotropin-releasing hormone decreases decidual prolactin secretion.
    e. Arachidonic acid decreases decidual prolactin secretion.
    f. Pituitary and decidual prolactin are immunologically and biologically distinguishable.

4–54. Which of the following statements about the biochemistry of the decidua is correct?

    a. Relaxin is produced in the decidua.
    b. 1,25-dihydroxyvitamin D_3 is produced in the decidua.
    c. Throughout pregnancy, there are elevated levels of polyamines in maternal fluids.
    d. The enzyme ornithine carboxylase has been identified in the decidua of women.
    e. Diamine oxidase levels rise significantly in mid-pregnancy.

4–55. Which of the following describes the typical human placenta at term?

    a. Discoid shape
    b. 20 cm diameter
    c. 10 cm thickness
    d. 500 g weight
    e. Succenturiate lobe

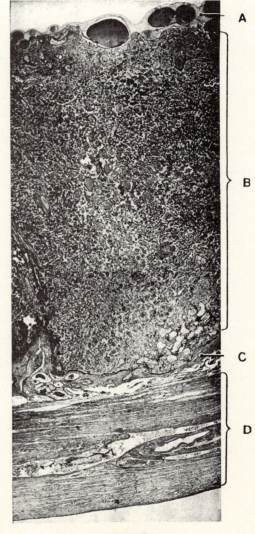

FIGURE 3

Instructions for Items 4-56 to 4-59: Refer to Figure 3. Match the letter with the appropriate part of the placenta and uterus.

4-56. Myometrium
4-57. Chorionic plate with fetal blood vessels
4-58. Placental villi
4-59. Decidua basalis

4-60. Which fetal vessel carries blood with the highest oxygen content?

   a. Umbilical artery
   b. Aorta
   c. Umbilical vein
   d. Pulmonary artery
   e. Pulmonary vein

4-61. Which of the following statements about placental circulation is correct?

   a. Maternal blood enters the intervillous space via spiral arteries (arterioles).
   b. Maternal blood traverses the placenta in preformed channels.
   c. Maternal blood traverses the placenta as a result of the negative pressure of the maternal venous system relative to that of the maternal arterial system.
   d. The arterial entrances and the venous exits are scattered at random over the entire base of the placenta.
   e. The spiral arteries (arterioles) are generally perpendicular and the placental veins parallel to the uterine wall.
   f. Countercurrent flow plays an important part in the mechanism of placental circulation.

4-62. Which of the following statements about the effect of uterine contractions on placental circulation is correct?

   a. The arrangement of spiral arterioles and placental veins facilitates maternal blood loss from the placenta during contractions.
   b. Drainage through veins is decreased during contractions.
   c. The amount of blood entering the intervillous space is decreased during contractions.
   d. Distention of the placenta with blood during contractions results in an increase in the dimensions of the placenta.

4-63. The regulation of blood flow in the intervillous space is dependent on which of the following factors?

   a. Arterial blood pressure
   b. Countercurrent flow
   c. Intrauterine pressure
   d. Uterine contraction pattern

4-64. Which of the following progressive changes in uteroplacental circulation occurs during gestation?

   a. There is an intra-arterial accumulation of trophoblasts.
   b. There is a decrease in the number of arterial openings into the intervillous space.
   c. There is an extension of trophoblasts proximally from the terminal portions of uteroplacental arteries.
   d. The normal muscular and elastic tissue of the wall of spiral vessels is replaced by fibrous tissue and fibrinoid.
   e. A prominent venous plexus develops between the decidua basalis and the myometrium.

4-65. The ability of the placenta and fetus to ''defy the laws'' of transplantation immunology has been adequately explained by which of the following?

   a. The placenta's ability to absolutely separate the maternal and fetal circulations.
   b. The antigenic immaturity of the fetus.
   c. The presence of a diminished maternal immune response.

4-66. Which of the following statements about placental immunology is correct?

   a. Blood group antigens are lacking in human trophoblast.
   b. Class II MHC antigen expression protects trophoblast immunologically.
   c. Lack of blood supply is the major protection of the placenta immunologically.
   d. Interferon may moderate antigen expression in the human trophoblast.

4-67. Which of the following statements about the amnion is correct?

   a. Near the end of the first trimester, the amnion physically unites with the chorion to produce a single membrane, the amniochorion.
   b. The amnion is highly innervated.
   c. The number of blood vessels in the amnion increases as gestation proceeds.
   d. Amnionic caruncles represent sites of incomplete attachment of the amnion to the chorion.
   e. The amnion contains glycerophospholipids rich in arachidonic acid and the enzyme phospholipase A_2.

4-68. Which vessels are normally found in the umbilical cord at term?

   a. Right umbilical artery
   b. Left umbilical artery
   c. Right umbilical vein
   d. Left umbilical vein

4-69. When the intra-abdominal portion of the duct of the umbilical vesicle remains patent it is called _____ .

4-70. The most common vascular anomaly in humans is the absence of one umbilical artery.

    a. True
    b. False

4-71. The average length of the umbilical cord in humans is

    a. 15 cm
    b. 25 cm
    c. 35 cm
    d. 45 cm
    e. 55 cm
    f. 65 cm

4-72. Which of the following statements about the umbilical cord is correct?

    a. False knots (nodulations on the surface of the cord) are the result of folding and tortuosity of the umbilical vessels.
    b. The matrix of the cord consist of Wharton jelly.
    c. The umbilical artery has a smaller diameter than the umbilical vein.
    d. The umbilical vein empties directly into the inferior vena cava.

5. THE PLACENTAL HORMONES

5-1. The species producing the largest amounts of hCG are:

    a. Humans
    b. Dogs
    c. Mice
    d. Whales

5-2. Which of the following statements about the biochemistry of hCG is correct?

    a. It is a glycoprotein with a high carbohydrate content.
    b. It is composed of two similar subunits, designated alpha and beta.
    c. The two subunits are covalently linked.
    d. The molecular weight of hCG is approximately 37,000.
    e. The syntheses of the alpha and beta chains of hCG are regulated by separate mRNAs.
    f. Biologic activity of hCG requires the bonding of the alpha and beta subunits, neither of which is active alone.

5-3. Which of the following glycoprotein hormones has an alpha subunit significantly different from the others?

    a. hCG
    b. hLH
    c. hFSH
    d. hTSH

5-4. The beta subunit of hCG is most similar to the beta subunit of

    a. hLH
    b. hTSH
    c. hFSH

5-5. The beta subunit of glycoprotein hormones confers their characteristic biologic activity.

    a. True
    b. False

5-6. Which of the following statements about the synthesis of hCG is correct?

    a. Human chorionic gonadotropin is produced principally by cells in the cytotrophoblast.
    b. The greatest concentration of hCG in the plasma of pregnant women is found at 8 to 10 weeks' gestation.
    c. The alpha and beta subunits of hCG are synthesized as larger presubunits.
    d. The synthesis of the alpha subunit is the rate-limiting step in the synthesis of hCG.

5-7. Which of the following statements about the secretion of hCG is correct?

    a. The amounts of alpha and beta subunits in the placenta and plasma of pregnant women are essentially equal.
    b. The alpha and beta subunits are secreted separately and also as the hCG hormone.
    c. The rate of secretion of hCG may be subject to trophic regulation.

5-8. The most apparent function of hCG is _____ .

5-9. Which of the following statements about the activity of hCG is correct?

    a. The half-life of hCG is approximately 24 hours.
    b. The half-life of hCG is long compared with that of LH.
    c. The high concentration of hCG at 8 to 10 weeks' gestation may ultimately result in down regulation of the hCG/LH receptors in the corpus luteum resulting in decreased progesterone secretion.
    d. In the human ovary primed by FSH, hCG can be used as an LH surrogate to induce ovulation.
    e. The life span of a corpus luteum induced by LH and one induced by hCG are approximately equal.
    f. A role for hCG in the provision of immunologic privilege to the trophoblast has been suggested.

5-10. Which of the following is relevant in the use of bioassays and immunoassays for hCG in pregnancy testing?

   a. Cross-reactivity of the alpha subunits of glycoprotein hormones causes a lack of specificity in immunoassays for hCG.
   b. The present specificity of immunologic pregnancy tests is primarily a result of the development of antibodies to the beta subunit of hCG.
   c. Antibodies to the beta subunit of hCG cross-react significantly with the beta subunit of LH.

5-11. Which of the following statements about hCG levels in urine is correct?

   a. Urinary excretion of hCG is maximal between the 60th and 70th day of gestation.
   b. A nadir in urinary excretion is reached between the 100th and 130th days.
   c. The level of urinary excretion rises about the 200th day and maintains a high level throughout the rest of pregnancy.
   d. Women at the same phase of gestation excrete similar amounts of hCG.

5-12. Which of the following statements about hCG levels is correct?

   a. The concentrations of the alpha and beta subunits of hCG rise steadily until about 30 weeks' gestation and remain at a plateau for the remainder of pregnancy.
   b. Significantly higher levels of hCG are found in multiple gestations.
   c. Levels of hCG are lower in an Rh-sensitized pregnancy.
   d. Levels of hCG are higher in women with hydatidiform mole.

5-13. The renal clearance of hCG as the native molecule accounts for _____ percent of the total metabolic clearance rate (MCR), the remainder being metabolized by pathways other than renal excretion.

   a. 10
   b. 30
   c. 50
   d. 70
   e. 90

5-14. Human chorionic gonadotropin can act on the fetal testes as an LH surrogate to promote male sexual differentiation and testosterone synthesis and secretion.

   a. True
   b. False

5-15. Which of the following statements about the synthesis of human placental lactogen (hPL) is correct?

   a. It is concentrated in the syncytiotrophoblast.
   b. It consists of a single polypeptide chain with a molecular weight of about 22,000.
   c. It is immunochemically similar to human growth hormone.
   d. The synthesis of hPL is stimulated by cAMP and insulin.
   e. The secretion of hPL is stimulated by PGE_2 and $PGF_{2\alpha}$.
   f. The production rate of hPL near term is the greatest of any known hormone.

5-16. Human placental lactogen

   a. Can be detected in the serum of pregnant women about 4 weeks after fertilization
   b. Has a plasma level in maternal blood that is proportional to placental mass
   c. Has a plasma concentration that is lower than the concentration in amnionic fluid
   d. Is found in high levels in the fetal circulation
   e. Is found in low levels in maternal urine
   f. Is concentrated in fetal tissues, where its main metabolic effects are manifest

5-17. The highest level of hPL is found in the

   a. Cord blood
   b. Maternal urine
   c. Maternal blood
   d. Fetal urine
   e. Amnionic fluid

5-18. Possible actions of hPL include

   a. Increasing the levels of circulating free fatty acids
   b. Inhibiting both the uptake of glucose and gluconeogenesis in the mother
   c. Decreasing the maternal levels of insulin
   d. Ensuring a mobilizable source of amino acids for transport to the fetus

5-19. Human placental lactogen has been demonstrated to be a requirement for a normal pregnancy outcome.

   a. True
   b. False

5-20. The plasma levels of ACTH in pregnant women before labor are significantly higher than in nonpregnant women.

   a. True
   b. False

5-21. There is evidence that the placenta is a source of which of the following hormones?

   a. ACTH
   b. LHRH
   c. TRH
   d. CRF

5-22. Which of the following statements about pregnancy ''specific'' proteins is correct?

   a. These proteins were identified by use of antibodies developed in animals against the serum of pregnant women.
   b. Approximately five of these proteins have been discovered.
   c. The functions of these proteins have not as yet been well defined.

5-23. The mechanisms of estrogen synthesis in the normal pregnant woman are essentially the same as those in the normal premenopausal nonpregnant woman.

   a. True
   b. False

5-24. Which of the following statements about the production of estrogen in pregnancy is correct?

   a. Pregnancy is a normo-estrogenic state relative to the nonpregnant state.
   b. The placenta is the site of origin of estrogens during pregnancy.
   c. The prehormones used to synthesize estrogens are produced by cytotrophoblast cells.
   d. Maternal urinary estriol originates by conversion of fetal products.
   e. Estriol is formed primarily by the conversion of estrone and estradiol-17β.

5-25. Bilateral oophorectomy performed in the second trimester will result in spontaneous loss of the pregnancy due to the lack of circulating estrogens produced by the ovary.

   a. True
   b. False

5-26. Which of the following statements is the *principal* reason for the increase in urinary estriol during pregnancy?

   a. Alteration in the fractional conversion of estrone and estradiol-17β to estriol in the mother.
   b. Alteration in the fractional conversion of estrone and estradiol-17β to estriol in the fetus.
   c. Placental formation of estrone and estradiol from C_{19}-steroids
   d. De novo synthesis of estriol from acetate and cholesterol.

5-27. In the placenta, the synthesis of estrogen from acetate or cholesterol is not possible because _____ .

Instructions for Items 5-28 to 5-31: Match the hormone with its predominant site of origin.

   a. Estradiol-17β
   b. Estrone
   c. Estriol
   d. Dehydroisoandrosterone sulfate

5-28. Placenta
5-29. Extraglandular origin, nonpregnant
5-30. Ovary, nonpregnant
5-31. Fetal adrenal cortex

5-32. Which of the following is a potential precursor of estrogens produced by the placenta?

   a. Dehydroisoandrosterone sulfate
   b. Dehydroisoandrosterone
   c. Testosterone
   d. Androstenedione

5-33. The *principal* circulating precursor of placental estrone and estradiol-17β is

   a. Dehydroisoandrosterone sulfate
   b. Dehydroisoandrosterone
   c. Testosterone
   d. Androstenedione

5-34. Which of the following statements about dehydroisoandrosterone sulfate (DS) and its metabolism is correct?

   a. In pregnancy, DS is derived primarily from the fetal adrenal cortex.
   b. The rich supply of placental sulfatase allows the use of DS in estrogen production.
   c. The concentration of DS in the plasma of pregnant women increases as pregnancy progresses.
   d. The increased clearance of DS in pregnancy is attributable to its conversion to estradiol-17β and its metabolism by increased 16α-hydroxylation in the maternal compartment.
   e. The placental clearance of maternal DS is decreased in women who will develop pregnancy-induced hypertension.

5-35. The estriol in the urine of pregnant women can be accounted for by the metabolism of estrone and estradiol-17β.

   a. True
   b. False

5–36. Which of the following occurs when a woman is pregnant with an anencephalic fetus?

   a. The rate of formation of placental estriol is lower than in a normal pregnancy.
   b. Production of estrogens can almost totally be accounted for by placental utilization of maternal dehydroisoandrosterone sulfate.
   c. Administration of ACTH results in decreased urinary estriol levels.
   d. Administraton of a potent glucocorticosteriod results in decreased placental production of estrogens.

5–37. In a pregnant woman with Addison's disease, there is an equivalent decrease in all types of estrogens excreted in the urine.

   a. True
   b. False

5–38. In a woman with an androgen-secreting ovarian tumor, a female fetus is only rarely virilized because _____.

5–39. Which of the following statements about the fetal adrenal gland is correct?

   a. A large portion of the gland is occupied by the fetal zone.
   b. The weight of the gland at term approximates the weight of an adult adrenal gland.
   c. There is a rapid involution of fetal adrenal cortex after birth.
   d. Fetal adrenal growth and steroid secretion is controlled by a single trophic stimulus similar to that which is present in the adult.

Instructions for Items 5–40 to 5–42: Match the structure with the appropriate function.

   a. Fetal adrenal cortex
   b. Maternal adrenal cortex

5–40. Site of origin of placental estrogen precursors
5–41. Important in fetal lung maturation
5–42. Important in the initiation of labor

5–43. Administration of glucocorticoids to the mother can result in decreased levels of

   a. Fetal pituitary ACTH
   b. Fetal cortisol
   c. Progesterone

5–44. The primary pathway for production of fetal cortisol is _____.

5–45. Which of the following statements about the biosynthetic activities of the fetal adrenal gland is correct?

   a. LDL-cholesterol is a primary source of precursors for fetal adrenal steroidogenesis.
   b. Cortisol biosynthesis from cholesterol and pregnenolone is enhanced.
   c. The output of steroids from the fetal adrenal gland greatly exceeds that in the adult.
   d. The majority of cholesterol used for fetal steroidogenesis is transferred from the mother.
   e. The fetal adrenal gland secretes large amounts of dehydroisoandrosterone sulfate.

5–46. Which of the following substances probably has an important trophic influence upon the fetal adrenal gland?

   a. Chorionic ACTH
   b. Progesterone
   c. LDL-cholesterol
   d. Fetal pituitary prolactin
   e. Urinary estriol

5–47. The fetus is the source of 90 percent of the estriol precursor formed in the placenta at term.

   a. True
   b. False

5–48. Which of the following statements about the use of estriol levels as a test of fetal well-being is correct?

   a. Fetal death is accompanied by a reduction in the levels of urinary estrogens.
   b. Plasma estriol levels correlate well with urinary estriol levels.
   c. The use of plasma estriol levels has the advantage of ease and reliability of sample collection.
   d. Estriol levels have been proven to be a reliable indicator of placental functions.

5–49. A single measurement of urinary estriol that falls outside the normal range is a reliable indicator of fetal jeopardy or death.

   a. True
   b. False

5–50. The usefulness of maternal estriol levels as a test of fetal well-being must be interpreted in light of which of the following?

   a. There is a narrow range of normal values in serum and urine.
   b. Single measurements outside the "normal" range are very reliable.
   c. Estriol production can be independent of placental function.
   d. Estriol levels may be lowered due to drug ingestion.
   e. Lower estriol levels may be due to lack of placental sulfatase activity.
   f. Elevated estriol levels may be seen in multiple gestations.

Instructions for Items 5–51 to 5–55: Match the cause of altered estriol levels with the appropriate result.

    a. Decreased estriol levels
    b. Increased estriol levels

5–51. Maternal ingestion of aspirin
5–52. Acute pyelonephritis
5–53. Fetal anencephaly
5–54. Rh sensitized mother with an erythroblastic fetus
5–55. Maternal ingestion of glucocorticosteroids

5–56. Lack of placental sulfatase activity is associated with pregnancies resulting in male infants who develop the skin disorder _____ .

5–57. Which of the following statements about estetrol is correct?

    a. Estetrol is 15α-hydroxyestriol.
    b. Estetrol is derived principally from estriol by the utilization of fetal precursors.
    c. Estetrol is produced almost exclusively by the fetus.
    d. The measurement of estetrol has not, so far, proved advantageous over that of estriol in the evaluation of fetal well-being.

5–58. Maternal urinary estriol levels provide clinically indispensable insight into the fetal condition in high-risk pregnancies.

    a. True
    b. False

5–59. Which of the following statements about progesterone synthesis in pregnancy is correct?

    a. It occurs in cytotrophoblast cells.
    b. The principal precursor is maternal plasma cholesterol.
    c. The fetus produces little or no precursor to progesterone.
    d. The rate of progesterone secretion is dependent on uteroplacental blood flow.
    e. Immediately after fetal death there is a significant decrease in plasma levels of progesterone.

5–60. The vast majority of which of the following placental steroids enters the maternal circulation?

    a. Estradiol-17β
    b. Estriol
    c. Estrone
    d. Progesterone

Instructions for Items 5–61 to 5–65: Match the appropriate letter describing the amount of hormone production present in a normal singleton pregnancy at term with the hormone it describes.

    a. 250–600 mg/day
    b. 50–150 mg/day
    c. 1 g/day
    d. 10–20 mg/day
    e. nearly 0

5–61. Human placental lactogen
5–62. Estriol
5–63. Cortisol
5–64. Progesterone
5–65. Free β subunit of human chorionic gonadotropin

PART II PHYSIOLOGY OF PREGNANCY

6. THE MORPHOLOGICAL AND FUNCTIONAL DEVELOPMENT OF THE FETUS

6–1. Gestational age is calculated from the

    a. Time of ovulation
    b. Time of fertilization
    c. First day of the last menstrual period
    d. Last day of the last menstrual period

6–2. Which of the following terms are synonymous?

    a. Gestational age
    b. Ovulation age
    c. Fertilization age
    d. Menstrual age

6-3. In a woman with a 28-day menstrual cycle, implantation usually occurs _____ weeks after the first day of the last menstrual period (LMP)?

    a. 1
    b. 2
    c. 3
    d. 4

6-4. Place the following developmental events in correct chronologic sequence.

    a. Ovulation
    b. Implantation
    c. Blastocyst formation
    d. Fertilization
    e. Primitive villi formation

6-5. After which of the following events is the fertilized ovum referred to as an embryo?

    a. Entrance into the uterus
    b. Formation of a blastocyst
    c. Implantation
    d. Development of chorionic villi

6-6. Which of the following statements about the beginning of the 5th week after the onset of the LMP is correct?

    a. Most pregnant women will have a positive pregnancy test at this time.
    b. The embryonic disc is well defined.
    c. The body stalk has differentiated.
    d. Chorionic villi have formed.
    e. The intervillous space contains maternal blood.

6-7. Most body structures have been formed by the end of the embryonic period.

    a. True
    b. False

Instructions for Items 6-8 to 6-12: Match the time after the last menstrual period with the developmental events that have occurred (menstrual age considering a normal 28-day cycle).

    a. Week 8
    b. Week 12
    c. Week 16
    d. Week 20
    e. Week 24
    f. Week 28

6-8. Crown–rump length 6 to 7 cm
6-9. Less than 4 cm long
6-10. Fetal sex can be determined by examination of the external genitalia.
6-11. Eyebrows and eyelashes present
6-12. Some scalp hair

6-13. The average crown–rump length of the fetus at term is approximately _____$_{(1)}$ cm and the average fetal term weight is approximately _____$_{(2)}$ g.

6-14. Which of the following statements about fetal measurement is correct?

    a. Sitting height is synonymous with crown–rump length.
    b. Standing height is a more accurate measurement than sitting height.
    c. Length is a more accurate criterion of fetal age than weight.
    d. Length and weight increase linearly throughout gestation.

6-15. Which of the following statements about fetal weight is correct?

    a. Male birth weights tend to be higher than female birth weights.
    b. Socioeconomic factors affect fetal growth rate.
    c. Size of parents is unrelated to birth weight.
    d. Parity of the mother affects birth weight.

6-16. Which of the following statements about the fetal head is correct?

    a. A large proportion of the head at term is represented by the face.
    b. The irregular spaces where sutures meet are protected by a cartilage roof.
    c. The bones of the fetal skull are rigidly united.
    d. All bones of the skull are paired.
    e. As a rule, the infants of multiparas have larger heads than those of nulliparas.

6-17. Which of the following sutures is midline?

    a. Lambdoidal
    b. Sagittal
    c. Frontal
    d. Coronal
    e. Temporal

6-18. With a vertex presentation, all sutures are palpable during labor except the

    a. Frontal
    b. Sagittal
    c. Coronal
    d. Lambdoid
    e. Temporal

Instructions for Items 6–19 to 6–22: Match the fontanel with the appropriate description.

    a. Anterior (greater)
    b. Posterior (lesser)
    c. Temporal (Casserian)

6–19. Situated at the intersection of the sagittal and lambdoid sutures

6–20. Situated at the junction of the lambdoid and temporal sutures

6–21. Situated at the junction of the sagittal and coronal sutures

6–22. May be readily felt during labor

Instructions for Items 6–23 to 6–25: Match the diameter of the infant's head with the appropriate description.

    a. Occipitofrontal
    b. Biparietal
    c. Bitemporal
    d. Occipitomental
    e. Suboccipitobregmatic

6–23. The greatest transverse diameter of the head

6–24. Measured from the chin to the most prominent portion of the occiput

6–25. Measured from the root of the nose to the most prominent portion of the occipital bone

6–26. The greatest circumference of the head corresponds to the plane of the _____ diameter and the smallest circumference corresponds to the plane of the _____ diameter.
<small>(1)</small>   <small>(2)</small>

6–27. All fetal heads at the same gestational age are equally able to adapt to the maternal pelvis by molding.

    a. True
    b. False

6–28. Fetal age can be accurately determined from the external appearance of the brain.

    a. True
    b. False

6–29. Which of the following statements about placental transfer is correct?

    a. The placenta supplies materials for fetal growth and removes the products of fetal catabolism.
    b. There is continuous direct communication between fetal blood in chorionic villi vessels and maternal blood in the intervillous space.
    c. The escape of fetal erythrocytes into the maternal circulation is the mechanism by which Rh sensitization occurs.
    d. A large number of maternal erythrocytes can be found in the fetal circulation.

6–30. Which of the following variables influences the effectiveness of the human placenta as an organ of transfer?

    a. The plasma concentration of a substance
    b. The rate of maternal blood flow in the intervillous space
    c. The area available for exchange across the villous epithelium
    d. The characteristics of the tissue barrier between the intervillous space and the fetal capillaries
    e. The placental capacity for active transfer
    f. The amount of placental metabolism of the transferred substance
    g. The area available for exchange across the fetal capillaries in the placenta
    h. The concentration of the substance in fetal blood
    i. The rate of fetal blood flow through villous capillaries

6–31. Which of the following statements about blood flow in the intervillous space is correct?

    a. The intervillous space combines functions of the lung, gastrointestinal tract, and kidney.
    b. Most of the 1600 cc/min of uteroplacental blood flow goes through the intervillous space.
    c. Blood flow through the intervillous space is decreased during contractions in proportion to the contraction intensity.
    d. Blood pressure within the intervillous space is less than uterine arterial pressure but greater than uterine venous pressure.
    e. Maternal posture affects pressure in the intervillous space.
    f. During normal labor, the rise in fetal blood pressure parallels the pressure in the intervillous space.

6–32. Substances passing from maternal blood in the intervillous space to fetal blood must cross the

    a. Maternal capillary wall
    b. Trophoblast
    c. Stroma
    d. Fetal capillary wall

6–33. Which of the following changes affecting placental permeability occurs as pregnancy progresses?

    a. The syncytiotrophoblast disappears.
    b. The number of cytotrophoblast cells decreases
    c. The walls of villous capillaries become thinner
    d. The relative number of fetal vessels increases in relation to the villous connective tissue

6-34. Which of the following statements about diffusion through the placenta is correct?

    a. Substances with molecular weights under 1500 daltons readily diffuse through placental tissue.
    b. Diffusion is the only mechanism of transport for low molecular weight substances.
    c. Oxygen and water are transferred by diffusion.
    d. Anesthetic gases apparently cross the placenta by simple diffusion.

6-35. No substance of very high molecular weight ($>150,000$ daltons) can traverse the placenta.

    a. True
    b. False

6-36. Which of the following statements about oxygen transfer to the fetus is correct?

    a. The oxygen saturation of maternal blood in the intervillous space resembles that in maternal capillaries.
    b. The oxygen saturation of maternal blood in the intervillous space is less than that of maternal arterial blood.
    c. The average oxygen saturation of intervillous space blood is approximately 90 percent.
    d. The partial pressure of intervillous space blood is 65 to 75 mm Hg.

6-37. Mechanisms which compensate for the relatively low PO_2 of umbilical vein blood include

    a. Increased fetal cardiac output
    b. Higher fetal hemoglobin concentration
    c. Increased oxygen-carrying capacity of fetal hemoglobin
    d. A larger fetal heart in proportion to the body than in the adult

6-38. Which of the following statements about the transfer of carbon dioxide is correct?

    a. Carbon dioxide traverses the chorionic villus more rapidly than does oxygen.
    b. Fetal blood has more affinity for carbon dioxide than does maternal blood.
    c. Maternal hyperventilation favors carbon dioxide transfer from the fetus to the mother.
    d. Carbon dioxide traverses the placenta by selective transport.

6-39. Which of the following support the concept of selective transfer by the placenta?

    a. Different rates of transfer for the two histidine isomers
    b. Different ascorbic acid concentrations in mother and fetus
    c. Unidirectional iron transfer
    d. Metastatic malignant melanomas of maternal origin in the fetus
    e. Intrauterine infections

6-40. Which of the following statements about fetal nutrition and metabolism is correct?

    a. Due to the relatively large amount of yolk in the human ovum, the fetus is independent of the mother for nutrition until the second month of gestation.
    b. Stored maternal glycogen is the main source of glucose for maternal and fetal needs during pregnancy.
    c. Glucose transfer across the placenta appears to be carrier mediated.
    d. The uptake of amino acids by the placenta is solely a result of diffusion.
    e. Placental lactogen acts to block the maternal peripheral uptake and utilization of free fatty acids.
    f. Glycerol and neutral fats cross the placenta by active transport.

6-41. The plasma levels of glucose in pregnant women are relatively constant.

    a. True
    b. False

6-42. Which of the following conditions is significantly associated with small for gestational age or growth-retarded infants?

    a. Maternal diabetes
    b. Severe maternal vascular disease
    c. Inadequate maternal nutrition
    d. Decreased uteroplacental blood flow
    e. Rh isoimmunization
    f. Impaired placental transport mechanisms

6-43. Regarding fetal physiology, which of the following statements is untrue?

    a. Glycerol crosses the placenta.
    b. Amino acids are concentrated by trophoblast.
    c. Iodine transport across the placenta is actively carrier-mediated.
    d. The concentration of vitamin A is greater in fetal than in maternal plasma.
    e. The levels of vitamin D metabolites are greater in the fetus than in the mother.

6-44. Blood ejected from the right ventricle into the pulmonary trunk is shunted to the descending aorta through the

6-45. Place the following fetal vessels in order from lowest to highest oxygen concentration.

a. Blood in inferior vena cava
b. Blood in umbilical vein
c. Blood in superior vena cava
d. Blood in umbilical artery

6-46. Which of the following characterizes fetal circulation?

a. Pulmonary vascular resistance high
b. Pulmonary blood flow high
c. Ductus arteriosus resistance high
d. Umbilicoplacental resistance low

6-47. Which of the following factors plays a role in regulating blood flow through the ductus arteriosus?

a. Difference in pressure between the pulmonary vein and aorta
b. Difference in pressure between the pulmonary artery and aorta
c. Oxygen tension of blood passing through the ductus arteriosus
d. pH of blood passing through the ductus arteriosus
e. Effect of prostaglandins on the ductus arteriosus

6-48. Inhibitors of prostaglandin synthetase may be used postnatally to induce closure of a patent ductus arteriosus.

a. True
b. False

6-49. Which of the following takes place as a result of lung expansion at birth?

a. Pressure in the right ventricle decreases.
b. Pressure in the pulmonary artery decreases.
c. Foramen ovale immediately closes.
d. There is a temporary reflux blood flow from the right ventricle to the right atrium.

Instructions for Items 6-50 to 6-52: Match the fetal vessel with its remnant in the adult.

a. Umbilical vein
b. Ductus venosus
c. Umbilical artery
d. Ductus arteriosus

6-50. Umbilical ligament
6-51. Ligamentum teres
6-52. Ligamentum venosum

6-53. Which of the following statements about fetal blood is correct?

a. Sites of hematopoiesis include the yolk sac, liver, and bone marrow.
b. All fetal erythrocytes are nucleated.
c. The hematocrit at term is slightly less than that of the adult male.
d. The reticulocyte count decreases as pregnancy progresses.
e. The life span of fetal erythrocytes is shorter than erythrocytes in the adult.

Instructions for Items 6-54 to 6-58: Match the type of hemoglobin with its composition.

a. Hemoglobin A_2
b. Hemoglobin A
c. Gower-2
d. Hemoglobin F
e. Gower-1

6-54. $\epsilon,\epsilon,\epsilon,\epsilon$
6-55. $\alpha,\alpha,\epsilon,\epsilon$
6-56. $\alpha,\alpha,\gamma,\gamma$
6-57. $\alpha,\alpha,\beta,\beta$
6-58. $\alpha,\alpha,\delta,\delta$

6-59. Hemoglobin A, the main adult hemoglobin, is present in the fetus after what week of pregnancy?

a. 5
b. 11
c. 16
d. 21

6-60. Fetal hypoxia can be intensified as a result of maternal hyperthermia because _____ .

6-61. Which of the following statements about the fetal hematopoietic process is correct?

a. At term, the fetal hemoglobin concentration is higher than the maternal concentration.
b. The higher viscosity of fetal erythrocytes is offset by their increased deformability.
c. The fetoplacental blood volume at term is approximately 125 cc/kg.
d. The increased oxygen affinity of the fetal erythrocyte compared with the maternal erythrocyte is a result of decreased 2,3-diphosphoglycerate binding.
e. The concentration of hemoglobin F falls steadily during pregnancy to about 10 percent of the total at term.
f. The fetus is able to respond to anemia with increased production of erythropoietin.

6-62. Which fetal organ appears to be an important source of erythropoietin?

    a. Liver
    b. Kidney
    c. Adrenal gland
    d. Pituitary gland

Instructions for Items 6-63 to 6-67: Match the level of blood coagulation factors at the time of birth compared with a few weeks after birth.

    a. Increased
    b. Decreased
    c. Unchanged

6-63. Factor II
6-64. Factor VII
6-65. Factor IX
6-66. Factor XIII
6-67. Fibrinogen

6-68. Platelet counts in cord blood are in the normal range for a nonpregnant adult.

    a. True
    b. False

6-69. Thrombin time (time for conversion of plasma fibrinogen to fibrin clot when thrombin is added) in the neonate is _____ as compared with older children and adults.

    a. Prolonged
    b. The same
    c. Shortened

6-70. The measurement of Factor _____ coagulation activity in cord blood is of value for making a diagnosis of hemophilia.

6-71. Which immunoglobulins are found in lower concentrations in cord sera than in maternal sera?

    a. IgA
    b. IgG
    c. IgM

6-72. IgM levels are increased in the fetus when _____ .

6-73. Which of the following statements about the fetal immune system is true?

    a. B lymphocytes appear in the liver by 9 weeks' gestation.
    b. Transfer of some IgG antibodies from mother to fetus may be harmful.
    c. The fetus is immunologically incompetent.
    d. All components of human complement are produced at an early stage of fetal development.

6-74. Regarding the fetal nervous system and sensory organs, which of the following statements is true?

    a. There is synaptic function by the eighth week of gestation.
    b. Fetal movement can be observed as early as 10 weeks' gestation.
    c. By 7 lunar months the fetal eye is sensitive to light.
    d. The fetus can hear by the 24th week of gestation.

6-75. Which of the following statements about the fetal digestive system is correct?

    a. By the 11th week of gestation, the small intestine undergoes peristalsis.
    b. Fetal swallowing is developed in the fourth month.
    c. Late in pregnancy, the volume of amnionic fluid is affected by fetal swallowing.
    d. The amnionic fluid swallowed supplies most of the caloric requirements of the fetus.

6-76. Which of the following statements about meconium is correct?

    a. Meconium consists of undigested debris from amnionic fluid and the products of secretion, excretion, and desquamation from the gastrointestinal tract.
    b. The color of meconium is partially due to biliverdin.
    c. Fetal hypoxia is associated with the release of meconium into the amnionic fluid.

6-77. Which of the following statements about bilirubin is correct?

    a. The more immature the fetus, the more deficient the system to conjugate bilirubin.
    b. Relatively more bilirubin is produced in the fetus than in the mother.
    c. The fetal liver has a considerable ability to conjugate bilirubin.
    d. Transfer of unconjugated bilirubin across the placenta is unidirectional from the fetus to the mother.
    e. Conjugated bilirubin is not exchanged to any significant degree between the fetus and the mother.

6-78. Which of the following statements about fetal insulin is correct?

    a. Plasma insulin is detectable by 8 weeks of gestation.
    b. Insulin containing granules can be identified in the fetal pancreas by 9 weeks of gestation.
    c. The fetal pancreas responds to hyperglycemia by increasing plasma insulin levels.
    d. Serum insulin levels are high in infants of diabetic mothers.
    e. Fetal insulin helps meet the requirements of a diabetic mother.

6-79. The lack of fetal pancreatic α-cell response to hypogly-cemia is a consequence of inadequate hormone production.

   a. True
   b. False

6-80. Which of the following statements about the fetal urinary system is correct?

   a. Failure of the pronephros or mesonephros to develop properly may result in anomolous development of the urinary system.
   b. The kidneys are functionally mature by 28 weeks of gestation.
   c. The fetus at term produces about 650 ml of urine per day.
   d. A diuretic administered to the mother has no effect on fetal urine formation.
   e. Fetal glomerular filtration rates are reduced in growth-retarded infants.
   f. Fetal glomerular filtration rates are reduced in cases of polyhydramnios.

6-81. Normal fetal kidney function is essential for survival in utero.

   a. True
   b. False

6-82. Which of the following is a function of amnionic fluid?

   a. Medium for fetal movement
   b. Cushions fetus against injury
   c. Assists in maintaining constant temperature
   d. Dilates cervical canal during labor

6-83. Prolonged pregnancies result in hydramnios.

   a. True
   b. False

6-84. Which of the following changes occur in amnionic fluid as pregnancy progresses?

   a. Phospholipids accumulate
   b. Osmolarity increases
   c. Particulate matter increases
   d. Urea, creatinine, and uric acid concentrations increase

6-85. The fetal organ systems that affect amnionic fluid composition and volume are the _____ .

Instructions for Items 6-86 to 6-88: Match the amount of amnionic fluid with the condition with which it is associated.

   a. Oligohydramnios
   b. Hydramnios

6-86. Fetal esophageal atresia
6-87. Fetal renal agenesis
6-88. Early and prolonged rupture of the membranes

6-89. Which of the following statements about the development of the fetal respiratory system is correct?

   a. The forces that promote deflation or collapse of the air-containing lung result from surface tension at the alveolar air–tissue interface.
   b. The surface active components of the alveoli are attributable primarily to the properties of surfactant.
   c. The principal surface active component of surfactant is the lecithin, dipalmityl phosphatidylcholine.
   d. Respiratory distress syndrome is caused by a deficiency in surfactant production.
   e. Surfactant is formed primarily in type II pneumocytes.

6-90. Phosphatidylcholines (lecithin) comprise what percent of surfactant glycerophospholipids?

   a. 20
   b. 40
   c. 60
   d. 80

6-91. Infants born before the appearance of _____ in surfactant are at increased risk for the development of respiratory distress syndrome, even when their lecithin levels are normal for mature lungs.

6-92. An increasing ratio of _____ relative to that of _____ is an index of fetal lung maturation.
(1) (2)

6-93. Phosphatidic acid forms the backbone for which of the following?

   a. Phosphatidylglycerol
   b. Phosphatidylcholine
   c. Phosphatidylinositol
   d. Dipalmityl phosphatidylcholine

6-94. There is considerable evidence that the enzyme _____ occupies a central regulatory role in the biosynthesis of the glycerophospholipids of surfactant.

6-95. As the fetal lung matures, the concentration of phosphatidylinositol in surfactant _____ and the concentration of phosphatidylglycerol _____ .
(1) (2)

   a. Decreases
   b. Remains the same
   c. Increases

6-96. Infants of diabetic mothers can be at greater risk for development of respiratory distress syndrome because their surfactant is rich in _____ and deficient in _____ .
(1) (2)

6-97. Which of the following statements about the control of surfactant production is correct?

a. Glucocorticosteroids, administered in large doses to women at any stage of pregnancy, will cause an increased production of surfactant.
b. Glucocorticosteroids, administered in large doses to mothers during the 29th to 33rd week of gestation result in a reduced incidence of respiratory distress syndrome.
c. Respiratory distress syndrome is always present in infants whose capacity to secrete cortisol is limited.
d. Increased surfactant synthesis in the third trimester may be causally linked to prolactin production.
e. Infants of mothers treated with bromocriptine while pregnant will suffer iatrogenic respiratory distress syndrome.
f. Infants whose mothers are heroin addicts demonstrate an increased incidence of respiratory distress syndrome.

6-98. Regarding fetal lung maturation, which of the following statements are true?

a. A consistent temporal relationship exists between administration of cortisol to the mother and the maturation of the fetal lung.
b. Infants with impaired adrenal function (anencephaly, adrenal hypoplasia, congenital adrenal hyperplasia) are seldom born with mature lungs.
c. It is doubtful that prolactin plays a role in lung maturation.
d. Type II pneumocytes produce surfactant.

6-99. Which of the following statements about fetal respiration is correct?

a. Fetal respiratory movements sufficiently intense to cause movement of amnionic fluid into and out of the lungs occur by the fourth month in utero.
b. The normal human fetus demonstrates irregular breathing movements in utero, typically with a frequency from 30 to 70 per minute.
c. Asphyxia in utero results in the initiation of gasping fetal respiratory efforts.
d. Crying in utero is a common phenomenon.
e. Fetal hiccuping in utero has been identified.

6-100. Which of the following have been identified in the fetal pituitary gland by 10 weeks of gestation?

a. Growth hormone
b. ACTH
c. Prolactin
d. LH
e. FSH

6-101. Fetal growth hormone has been shown to be required for normal fetal growth and development.

a. True
b. False

6-102. Which of the following statements about fetal thyroid function is correct?

a. Until midpregnancy, secretion of thyroid-stimulating hormone and thyroid hormones is low.
b. Maternal thyrotropin readily crosses the placenta.
c. Long-acting thyroid stimulators (LATS) cross from mother to fetus when the maternal concentration is high.
d. The fetal thyroid concentrates iodine more avidly than the maternal thyroid.
e. Maternal thyroid secretion can compensate for inadequate fetal synthesis.
f. Thyrotropin secretion increases markedly after birth.

6-103. Fetal parathyroid glands begin to elaborate parathormone by what time in gestation?

a. End of the first trimester
b. End of the second trimester
c. Middle of the third trimester
d. End of the third trimester

6-104. The lack of urine-concentrating ability in the newborn is felt to be due to the lack of fetal production of

_____ .

6-105. The fetal testis is capable of synthesizing testosterone by _____ weeks of gestation?

a. 5
b. 10
c. 20
d. 28
e. 36

6-106. Both the primary and secondary sex ratios in humans are unity.

a. True
b. False

6-107. A fetus with an XY chromosome complement and with no testis will develop as a

a. Male
b. Female

6-108. Which of the following statements about fetal sex differentiation is correct?

a. Genetic sex is determined at the time of fertilization.
b. The Y chromosome directs testicular differentiation.
c. Müllerian duct regression factor is synthesized by the fetal testis.
d. Müllerian duct regression factor acts locally.
e. Virilization of the external genitalia is brought about by 5α-dihydrotestosterone.

6-109. Ambiguous genitalia are caused by an abnormal in utero concentration of _____ .

Instructions for Items 6-110 to 6-116: Match the category of abnormal sexual differentiation with the appropriate description.

    a. Female pseudohermaphroditism (category 1)
    b. Male pseudohermaphroditism (category 2)
    c. Dysgenetic gonads and true hermaphroditism (category 3)

6-110. Müllerian duct regression factor is not produced
6-111. Müllerian duct regression factor is produced
6-112. Karyotype is 46,XX
6-113. Uterus, fallopian tubes, and upper vagina present
6-114. Testis may be present
6-115. Ovaries are present
6-116. No gonads are present

6-117. In female pseudohermaphroditism androgenic excess most commonly occurs due to oversecretion by what gland?

6-118. The female fetus is usually protected from virilization by maternal androgen excess because of the _____ .

6-119. With appropriate therapy, all patients with female pseudohermaphroditism can be normal, fertile women.

    a. True
    b. False

6-120. Diminished masculinization may be caused by

    a. Inadequate production of testosterone
    b. Diminished responsiveness to normal quantities of androgen
    c. Increased production of estrogen
    d. Increased responsiveness to normal levels of estrogen

6-121. Which of the following are characteristic of testicular feminization?

    a. Female phenotype
    b. No Wolffian duct structures
    c. Rise of testosterone levels at the time of puberty
    d. Virilization occurs after puberty
    e. Increased estrogen secretion by the testis

6-122. Reifenstein's syndrome is _____ .

6-123. Turner syndrome is an example of what category of sexual differentiation abnormalities?

    a. Female pseudohermaphroditism
    b. Male pseudohermaphroditism
    c. Dysgenetic gonads and true hermaphroditism

6-124. At birth, if a uterus is present in an infant with genital ambiguity, a possible diagnosis is

    a. True hermaphroditism
    b. Female pseudohermaphroditism
    c. Male pseudohermaphroditism
    d. Gonadal dysgenesis

6-125. If the urethra opens onto the perineum, the infant should be designated

    a. Male
    b. Female

7.   MATERNAL ADAPTATIONS TO PREGNANCY

7-1. Myometrial enlargement during pregnancy is primarily the result of smooth muscle

    a. Hyperplasia
    b. Hypertrophy

7-2. Which of the following statements about the uterus in pregnancy is correct?

    a. There is an accumulation of fibrous tissue, particularly in the external muscle layer.
    b. The amount of elastic tissue is increased.
    c. There is a relative decrease in the size and the number of lymphatics in the uterus.
    d. Hypertrophy of the nerve supply of the uterus occurs.
    e. There is an increase in the size and the number of blood vessels in the uterus.

7-3. Hypertrophy of the uterus in the first 2 months of pregnancy results mainly from mechanical pressure caused by the products of conception.

    a. True
    b. False

7-4. Polyamine levels in the urine of normal pregnant women are maximal at _____ weeks of gestation.

    a. 6 to 8
    b. 13 to 14
    c. 18 to 20
    d. 28 to 30

7-5. Uterine enlargement in pregnancy is most marked in the

    a. Cervix
    b. Lower uterine segment
    c. Fundus
    d. Uterine cornua

7–6. The portion of the uterus surrounding the placental site enlarges more rapidly than does the myometrium distal to the site of implantation.

    a. True
    b. False

7–7. In what ways does the uterus and its anatomic relationships change as pregnancy progresses?

    a. With the pregnant woman standing, the abdominal wall supports the uterus.
    b. With the pregnant woman supine, the uterus rests on the vertebral column and adjacent great vessels.
    c. The uterus usually undergoes levorotation due to pressure from the inferior vena cava.
    d. As the uterus enlarges, it displaces the intestines laterally and superiorly.

7–8. Which of the following statements about uterine contractions is correct?

    a. Uterine contractions begin in the first trimester.
    b. Uterine contractions first become palpable on physical examination during the third trimester.
    c. Braxton Hicks contractions increase in frequency during the last 2 weeks of pregnancy.
    d. Late in pregnancy, Braxton Hicks contractions can cause discomfort.
    e. Late in pregnancy, Braxton Hicks contractions may assume some rhythmicity.

7–9. Uteroplacental blood flow near term is approximately _____ cc/min.

    a. 100
    b. 300
    c. 500
    d. 700
    e. 900

7–10. Uterine contractions cause a decrease in uterine blood flow roughly proportional to the intensity of the contraction.

    a. True
    b. False

7–11. Which of the following statements about uteroplacental blood flow in animal models is correct?

    a. The majority of uterine blood flow is directed to the endometrium and placenta.
    b. Reduction in uteroplacental blood flow leads to fetal acidosis.
    c. Estrogen stimulation can increase placental blood flow.
    d. Epinephrine and norepinephrine can induce an increase in placental perfusion.
    e. Similar to humans, pregnant sheep are relatively refractory to the pressor effects of angiotensin II.

7–12. Increased vascularity and edema of the cervix bring about what two early signs of pregnancy?

7–13. Which of the following statements about the cervical mucosa in pregnancy is correct?

    a. Cervical glands undergo both hypertrophy and hyperplasia.
    b. Proliferation of glands and endocervical epithelium commonly extends to the portio vaginalis.
    c. Eversions of the cervix are usually an inflammatory response.
    d. Ferning of cervical mucus usually heralds a poor pregnancy outcome.
    e. The mucus plug that obstructs the cervical canal usually first appears during the second trimester.

7–14. Which of the following statements about ovarian function during pregnancy is correct?

    a. Maturation of new follicles continues during pregnancy.
    b. The corpus luteum of pregnancy functions maximally for about 7 weeks after the last menstrual period.
    c. Usually only a single corpus luteum of pregnancy is found in the ovaries of pregnant women.
    d. Ovulation continues throughout pregnancy.

7–15. Relaxin

    a. Is a protein hormone secreted by the corpus luteum during pregnancy
    b. Is synthesized in the largest amounts by the decidua
    c. Is secreted throughout pregnancy
    d. The pattern of secretion is similar to human chorionic gonadotropin.

7–16. The luteoma of pregnancy.

    a. Is a true neoplasm
    b. Generally regresses after delivery
    c. May give rise to maternal virilization
    d. May give rise to fetal virilization

7–17. A decidual reaction on or within the ovary or uterine serosa is common in pregnancy.

    a. True
    b. False

7–18. Which of the following changes occurs in the oviduct during pregnancy?

    a. The musculature undergoes marked hypertrophy.
    b. The epithelium proliferates significantly.
    c. Decidual cells may develop in the stroma of the endosalpinx.
    d. A continuous decidual membrane is formed.

7–19. Which of the following changes in the vagina occurs during pregnancy?

   a. There is an increased vascularity, presenting as Chadwick's sign, a violet color of the mucosa.
   b. The vaginal mucosa thins.
   c. There is smooth muscle hypertrophy.
   d. The length of the vaginal wall increases.

7–20. Hyperreaction luteinalis is

   a. A benign lesion of the ovary in pregnancy
   b. A cause of virilization in pregnancy
   c. Similar in cellular pattern to a luteoma of pregnancy
   d. Associated with high levels of human chorionic gonadotropin

7–21. Which of the following statements about vaginal secretions in pregnancy is correct?

   a. The pH ranges from 3.5 to 6.0.
   b. The pH predisposes to bacterial infection of the vagina.
   c. Lactic acid is produced from glycogen by the action of *Lactobacillus acidophilus*.
   d. There is an increase in both cervical and vaginal secretions.

7–22. Striae gravidarum

   a. Occur in all pregnant women
   b. Appear as reddish slightly depressed streaks
   c. From previous pregnancies appear as glistening, silvery lines
   d. Rarely occur in nulliparous women

7–23. The separation of the rectus muscles in the midline during pregnancy is termed _____ .

Instructions for Items 7–24 to 7–26: Match the skin change in pregnancy with the appropriate description.

   a. Linea nigra
   b. Chloasma

7–24. Abdominal skin markedly pigmented at the midline
7–25. Irregular brownish patches of varying size on face and neck
7–26. May be stimulated by the use of oral contraceptives

Instructions for Items 7–27 to 7–30: Match the cutaneous vascular change in pregnancy with the appropriate description.

   a. Vascular spiders
   b. Palmar erythema

7–27. More frequent in white women than in black women
7–28. Probably due to the hyperestrogenemia of pregnancy

7–29. Usually disappears shortly after the termination of pregnancy
7–30. Also designated as nevus or telangiectasis

7–31. Which of the following is a common sign or symptom related to the breasts that occurs at some time during pregnancy?

   a. Tenderness
   b. Tingling
   c. Nipples larger, darker, more erectile
   d. Colostrum expressed
   e. Striations

7–32. The hypertrophic sebaceous glands scattered through the areolae of the breasts during pregnancy are termed the

_____ .

7–33. The average weight gain in pregnancy is probably about _____ pounds.

7–34. Which of the following statements about water metabolism in pregnancy is correct?

   a. Increased retention of water is normal in pregnancy and is mediated by a change in osmotic thresholds and vasopressin secretion.
   b. Demonstrable pitting edema of the ankles at the end of the day is abnormal and pathologic.
   c. It is not unusual for a woman to retain 6.5 liters of extra fluid in a normal pregnancy.
   d. Weight loss during the first 10 days after delivery in normal primiparas averages 5 pounds.

7–35. The fetus and placenta account for about 90 percent of the total protein increase normally induced by pregnancy.

   a. True
   b. False

7–36. Daily requirements for protein in pregnancy are increased appreciably from the nonpregnant requirements.

   a. True
   b. False

7–37. Both fasting plasma glucose and plasma free fatty acids are decreased in pregnancy.

   a. True
   b. False

7-38. Which of the following statements about carbohydrate metabolism in pregnancy is correct?

a. Pregnancy is potentially diabetogenic.
b. Human placental lactogen promotes lipolysis and opposes the action of insulin.
c. Progesterone and estrogen produce an increased plasma insulin response to glucose.
d. "Accelerated starvation" is a term used to refer to the switch from glucose to lipids in pregnancy.
e. Both pancreatic β-cell and α-cell sensitivity to a glucose challenge is significantly increased during pregnancy.

7-39. Which plasma lipids increase appreciably during pregnancy relative to the nonpregnant state?

a. Free fatty acids
b. Serum phospholipids
c. Esterified cholesterol
d. Total cholesterol

7-40. Which of the following statements about fat metabolism in pregnancy is correct?

a. Starvation causes more intense ketonemia in pregnant women than in nonpregnant women.
b. Plasma lipids increase appreciably in pregnancy.
c. Fat is deposited more peripherally than centrally.
d. Progesterone may act to reset a hypothalamic "lipostat."
e. Breast feeding significantly alters the rate at which plasma lipids decrease postpartum.

7-41. Which of the following factors affects the acid-base equilibrium of the pregnant woman?

a. There is normally a maternal respiratory alkalosis due to hyperventilation.
b. There is a moderate reduction in plasma bicarbonate.
c. The affinity of maternal hemoglobin for oxygen is increased (Bohr effect).
d. An increase in 2, 3-diphosphoglycerate in maternal erythrocytes facilitates oxygen release to the fetus.

Instructions for Items 7-42 to 7-46: Indicate how serum levels of the following are altered during pregnancy as compared with the nonpregnant state.

a. Increased
b. Decreased
c. Unchanged

7-42. Copper
7-43. Sodium
7-44. Magnesium
7-45. Phosphorus
7-46. Potassium

7-47. Which of the following statements about maternal blood volume in pregnancy is correct?

a. A fetus is essential for the development of hypervolemia.
b. Blood volume increases an average of 50 percent above nonpregnant levels.
c. Maternal blood volume increases linearly throughout pregnancy.
d. The increase in blood volume results from an increase in both plasma and erythrocytes.

7-48. The increase in the volume of circulating erythrocytes in pregnancy occurs _____ the increase in plasma volume.

a. Before
b. At the same time as
c. After

7-49. The increase in the volume of circulating erythrocytes is approximately _____ percent.

7-50. Which of the following statements about erythrocytes in pregnancy is correct?

a. The increase in the volume of circulating erythrocytes is due to prolongation of erythrocyte life span.
b. The cell volume is increased.
c. Erythroid hyperplasia is present in the bone marrow.
d. The reticulocyte count is elevated in pregnancy.
e. Erythropoietin levels are decreased in pregnancy.

7-51. Regarding atrial natriuretic peptide and plasma volume, which of the following statements is true?

a. Atrial natriuretic peptides are secreted by atrial myocytes.
b. These peptides produce significant diuresis.
c. These peptides reduce the basal release of aldosterone.
d. The mechanisms of secretion of atrial natriuretic peptides explain well all the volume changes associated with pregnancy.

7-52. The total iron requirement during a normal singleton pregnancy is approximately

a. 0.1 g
b. 1 g
c. 10 g
d. 100 g

7-53. Approximately half the iron required in a normal pregnancy is used in the production of maternal erythrocytes.

a. True
b. False

7-54. Which of the following statements about iron requirements in pregnancy is correct?

a. In a normal pregnancy, exogenous iron is not usually required.
b. Iron absorption from the intestine is increased in pregnancy.
c. Hemoglobin production in the fetus is impaired if the mother is iron deficient.
d. In the absence of added exogenous iron, the maternal hemoglobin concentration falls during the second half of pregnancy.

7-55. The average blood loss during and after vaginal delivery of a single fetus is approximately

a. 200 mL
b. 400 mL
c. 600 mL
d. 800 mL
e. 1000 mL

7-56. The average blood loss associated with cesarean section is _____ the blood loss associated with vaginal delivery of twins.

a. Less than
b. The same as
c. Greater than

7-57. Which of the following statements about changes in maternal blood volume near the time of delivery is correct?

a. Some hemoconcentration occurs during labor.
b. Blood volume is reduced during and soon after labor.
c. Excess circulating hemoglobin yields iron for storage through accelerated erythrocyte destruction.
d. Blood volume returns to the nonpregnant level by 5 days postpartum.

7-58. During labor and the early puerperium, the blood leukocyte count is _____ the leukocyte count during pregnancy.

a. Less than
b. The same as
c. Greater than

7-59. Alpha interferon is present in almost all fetal tissues but absent in the gravida.

a. True
b. False

Instructions for Items 7-60 to 7-67: Match the blood coagulation factor with its activity in pregnancy relative to the nonpregnant state.

a. Increased
b. Decreased
c. Unchanged

7-60. Factor I (plasma fibrinogen)
7-61. Factor II (prothrombin)
7-62. Factor VII (proconvertin)
7-63. Factor VIII (antihemophiliac globulin)
7-64. Factor IX (Christmas factor)
7-65. Factor X (Stuart factor)
7-66. Factor XI (plasma thromboplastin antecedent)
7-67. Factor XIII (fibrin-stabilizing factor)

Instructions for Items 7-68 to 7-71: Match the procedure with its rate in pregnancy as compared to the nonpregnant state.

a. Increased
b. Decreased
c. Unchanged

7-68. Sedimentation rate
7-69. Quick one-stage prothrombin time
7-70. Partial thromboplastin time
7-71. Clotting time of whole blood in a plain glass tube

7-72. Which of the following statements about coagulation in pregnancy is correct?

a. There is a decrease in platelets per unit volume.
b. High molecular weight soluble fibrin-fibrinogen complexes circulate in normal pregnancy.
c. Antithrombin III levels are higher in pregnancy.
d. There is a decreased capacity for neutralizing heparin.
e. All of the pregnancy-induced changes in levels of coagulation factors can be duplicated in nonpregnant women by administration of estrogen-progestin oral contraceptives.

7-73. Which of the following statements about fibrinolytic activity in pregnancy is correct?

a. During normal pregnancy, the level of maternal plasminogen (profibrinolysin) in plasma is increased.
b. An increase in profibrinolysin can be induced by estrogen treatment.
c. The measured time for clotted plasma to dissolve is decreased compared with the normal nonpregnant state.
d. Plasma fibrinolytic activity increases after delivery.
e. Fibrin degradation products usually rise after delivery.

7-74. During pregnancy, the heart is

a. Displaced to the right
b. Displaced upward
c. Slightly rotated in its long axis
d. Displaced due to the progressive elevation of the diaphragm

7-75. During pregnancy, it is easier to identify moderate degrees of cardiomegaly by physical examination or by simple radiographic studies than it is to identify this condition in the nonpregnant state.

a. True
b. False

Instructions for Items 7-76 to 7-80: Match the effect of pregnancy on the following.

a. Increased
b. Decreased
c. Unchanged

7-76. Cardiac volume
7-77. Ventricular wall mass
7-78. Stroke volume
7-79. Inotropic state of the myocardium
7-80. Heart rate

7-81. Which of the following changes in cardiac sounds may be present in a normal pregnancy?

a. Split first heart sound
b. Split second heart sound
c. Loud third heart sound
d. Systolic murmur
e. Loud, persistent diastolic murmur
f. Continuous murmurs

7-82. Factors controlling vascular reactivity in pregnancy include which of the following?

a. Reactivity to angiotensin II increases in hypertensive women.
b. Hypertension does not develop in women who maintain refractory to angiotensin II.
c. The renin-angiotensin-aldosterone system does not change remarkably in pregnant women.
d. Calcium channel blockers may be associated with fetal acidosis.
e. Aspirin may reduce vascular reactivity and, therefore, be a possible treatment agent in preeclampsia.

7-83. Which of the following statements about cardiac output in pregnancy is correct?

a. Cardiac output increases in the first trimester and remains elevated throughout pregnancy.
b. In late pregnancy, cardiac output is greater if a woman is supine than if she is in the lateral recumbent position.
c. In response to physical activity, cardiac output is greater late in pregnancy than in the nonpregnant woman.
d. Cardiac output progressively increases in the first and second stages of labor.

7-84. Blood pressure in the brachial artery is highest when the gravida is in the _____ position.

a. Lateral recumbent
b. Supine
c. Sitting

7-85. During pregnancy, arterial blood pressure decreases to a nadir during the second trimester or early third trimester and rises thereafter.

a. True
b. False

7-86. Which of the following statements about venous pressure in pregnancy is correct?

a. The antecubital venous pressure increases progressively during pregnancy.
b. The femoral venous pressure measured in the supine position remains unchanged.
c. Except in the lateral recumbent position, blood flow in the legs is retarded.
d. The enlarged uterus may occlude the pelvic veins and inferior vena cava.

7-87. Retarded blood flow and increased venous pressure contribute to which of the following conditions?

a. Preeclampsia
b. Dependent edema
c. Varicose veins
d. Hemorrhoids
e. Striae

7-88. Potential effects of a pregnant woman lying in the supine position near term include

a. Decreased venous return
b. Decreased cardiac output
c. Aortic compression
d. Arterial hypotension

7-89. In the pregnant woman, brachial artery pressure provides a reliable estimate of uterine artery pressure.

a. True
b. False

7-90. Compared with a woman in the supine position, a woman in the lateral recumbent position has

a. A lower blood pressure in the brachial artery
b. A higher cardiac output
c. An increased blood flow in the veins of the legs
d. An increased venous pressure in the legs

7-91. In pregnancy, the blood flow to the skin is

a. Increased
b. Decreased

7-92. Which of the following anatomic changes occurs during pregnancy?

   a. The transverse diameter of the thoracic cage increases.
   b. The thoracic circumference increases.
   c. The level of the diaphragm rises.
   d. The diaphragm is "splinted."

Instructions for Items 7-93 to 7-99: How does pregnancy affect the following pulmonary functions?

   a. Increased
   b. Decreased
   c. Unchanged

7-93. Maternal arteriovenous oxygen difference
7-94. Maximum breathing capacity
7-95. Functional residual capacity
7-96. Lung compliance
7-97. Airway conductance
7-98. Tidal volume
7-99. Total pulmonary resistance

7-100. The increased respiratory effort in pregnancy is mostly induced by _____ .

7-101. Which of the following statements about the urinary system in pregnancy is correct?

   a. The kidney increases in size.
   b. The increases in glomerular filtration rate and renal plasma flow persist to term.
   c. Water and sodium excretion are affected by posture late in pregnancy.
   d. Amino acids and water-soluble vitamins are excreted in the urine of pregnant women in much higher amounts than in the urine of nonpregnant women.

7-102. The most useful measure of renal function during pregnancy is

   a. Plasma urea concentration
   b. Plasma creatinine concentration
   c. Creatinine clearance
   d. Urine concentration tests
   e. Dye excretion tests

7-103. During pregnancy, urine concentration tests may give misleading results because _____ .

7-104. Which of the following statements about glucosuria in pregnancy is correct?

   a. It is caused by increased glomerular filtration.
   b. It is caused by decreased renal tubular absorption.
   c. The possibility of diabetes mellitus can be ignored in patient with minimal glucosuria.

7-105. Proteinuria is a fairly common, normal occurrence during pregnancy.

   a. True
   b. False

7-106. Which of the following statements about the urinary collecting system is correct?

   a. The ureters are compressed at the pelvic brim by the uterus after it has risen out of the pelvis.
   b. Ureteral dilation is usually greater on the right.
   c. Progesterone may play a role in the development of a hydroureter.
   d. The ureters are elongated during pregnancy.
   e. After delivery, the urinary tract does not usually return to prepregnancy dimensions.

7-107. Which of the following statements about the bladder in pregnancy is correct?

   a. Most anatomic changes occur in the first half of pregnancy.
   b. The trigone becomes deeper and wider.
   c. Late in pregnancy, the bladder becomes edematous and probably more prone to infection.
   d. Urethral pressure and length are increased in all pregnancies.

7-108. Which of the following changes occurs in the gastro-intestinal tract during pregnancy?

   a. Tone is decreased.
   b. Motility is decreased.
   c. Gastric-emptying time is increased.
   d. Intraesophageal pressures are higher than in nonpregnant women.

7-109. During pregnancy, the appendix is progressively displaced _____ .

7-110. In human pregnancy, the liver both increases in size and changes in histologic appearance.

   a. True
   b. False

Instructions for Items 7-111 to 7-114: How does pregnancy affect the following?

   a. Increased
   b. Decreased
   c. Unchanged

7-111. Total serum alkaline phosphatase activity
7-112. Plasma albumin concentration
7-113. Plasma cholinesterase activity
7-114. Serum leucine aminopeptidase activity

7-115. For which conditions does pregnancy serve as a pre-disposing factor?

   a. Hemorrhoids
   b. Tooth decay
   c. Heartburn (pyrosis)
   d. Swelling of gums
   e. Gallstones

7-116. In normal pregnancy, the pituitary enlarges enough to significantly reduce the visual fields.

   a. True
   b. False

7-117. Which of the following statements about the pituitary gland in pregnancy is correct?

   a. Pituitary microadenomas may enlarge significantly during pregnancy.
   b. The maternal pituitary gland is essential for the maintenance of pregnancy.
   c. The level of growth hormone is decreased in pregnancy and remains low after delivery for quite some time.
   d. The prolactin level at term may be ten times the nonpregnant level.
   e. Plasma prolactin decreases immediately postpartum except in the lactating woman.

7-118. Prolactin levels in both fetal plasma and amnionic fluid peak at 20 weeks' gestation.

   a. True
   b. False

7-119. Which of the following statements about β-endorphins in pregnancy is correct?

   a. β-endorphin is a fragment of β-lipotrophin.
   b. Maternal plasma levels of β-endorphin, β-lipotrophin, and γ-lipotrophin steadily increase in pregnancy.
   c. The level of β-endorphin is lower in women who receive no analgesics than in women who have epidural anesthesia.
   d. β-endorphin levels may be pathologically raised by fetal acidosis.

7-120. Which of the following statements about the thyroid in pregnancy is correct?

   a. The thyroid enlarges through hyperplasia in pregnancy.
   b. Goiter is a normal occurrence in pregnancy.
   c. Abortion is frequently the result of a lack of increase of thyroxine early in pregnancy.
   d. Increased thyroid activity in women with hydatidiform mole is due to the action of chronic gonadotropin.

7-121. Complete the following table by filling in whether the value is *increased* or *not increased*.

TEST	NORMAL PREGNANCY	ESTROGEN ADMINIS-TRATION	HYPER-THYROIDISM
Basal metabolic rate	(a)	(b)	(c)
Total thyroxine	(d)	(e)	(f)
Thyoxine-binding globulin	(g)	(h)	(i)
Free thyroxine	(j)	(k)	(l)
Free triiodothy-ronine	(m)	(n)	(o)

7-122. Thyroxine, thyroxine-binding capacity, and triiodothyronine resin uptake values in cord serum are _____[(1)] those in maternal serum, and _____[(2)] levels in non-pregnant adults.

   a. Less than
   b. The same as
   c. Greater than

7-123. Which of the following are clearly elevated in pregnancy?

   a. Parathyroid hormone
   b. Plasma-ionized calcium
   c. Calcitonin
   d. Plasma 1,25-dihydroxyvitamin D

7-124. Which of the following statements related to the adrenal gland in pregnancy is correct?

   a. Adrenal secretion of cortisol is doubled in pregnancy.
   b. The levels of ACTH are high initially, then gradually decrease as pregnancy progresses.
   c. Renin and angiotensin are normally elevated, especially in the latter half of pregnancy.
   d. Deoxycorticosterone markedly increases in maternal plasma during the third trimester.

7-125. Which of the following statements about the musculoskeletal system in pregnancy is correct?

   a. There is a progressive maternal lordosis.
   b. Traction on the ulnar and median nerves increases.
   c. There is increased mobility of the sacroiliac and sacrococcygeal joints.
   d. There is decreased mobility of the pubic joints.

7-126. Musculoskeletal disorders of pregnancy are due solely to hormonal changes in the mother.

   a. True
   b. False

7-127. True precocious puberty is becoming much more frequent as the average age of menarche is decreasing.

    a. True
    b. False

7-128. Maternal and fetal complications in women over 40 years of age are _____ in patients less than 40.

    a. More frequent than
    b. As frequent as
    c. Less frequent than

PART III SPONTANEOUS LABOR AND DELIVERY

8.   THE NORMAL PELVIS

8-1. The mechanisms of labor are essentially processes of _____ of the fetus to the bony passage through which it must pass.

8-2. The _____ demarcates the false pelvis from the true pelvis.

Instructions for Items 8-3 to 8-6: Match the anatomic site with the appropriate boundary of the false pelvis.

    a. Anterior
    b. Inferior
    c. Posterior
    d. Lateral

8-3. Lumbar vertebrae
8-4. Linea terminalis
8-5. Abdominal wall
8-6. Iliac fossae

8-7. Complete the following table by listing the boundaries of the true pelvis.

BOUNDARY	ANATOMIC CONSTITUENTS
Anterior	_____ (a)
Posterior	_____ (b)
Lateral	_____ (c)
Superior	_____ (d)
Inferior	_____ (e)

8-8. Which of the following statements about the true pelvis is correct?

    a. The true pelvis is shaped like a truncated oblique cylinder.
    b. The anterior and posterior walls of the true pelvis are almost always of equal height.
    c. The walls of the true pelvis are partly ligamentous.
    d. With a woman in the upright position, the upper portion of the pelvic canal is directed downward and forward and the lower portion directed downward and backward.
    e. Normally, the side walls of the true pelvis converge slightly.
    f. The angle of the pubic arch is usually 90 to 100 degrees.
    g. The distance between the ischial spines is usually the smallest diameter of the pelvic cavity.

8-9. Which of the following statements about the sacrum is correct?

    a. It forms the posterior wall of the pelvis.
    b. The upper anterior margin of the sacrum (the first sacral vertebra) is called the promontory.
    c. Normally, the sacrum is flat.
    d. The sacrum has no relevance in clinical pelvimetry.

8-10. Which of the following statements about the pelvic inlet is correct?

    a. Typically, the pelvic inlet is ovoid in shape.
    b. The obstetric conjugate is the shortest distance from the sacral promontory to the symphysis pubis.
    c. The obstetric conjugate is the same as the true conjugate.
    d. The oblique diameters of the pelvic inlet average about 10 cm each.

8-11. The obstetric conjugate can be measured directly.

    a. True
    b. False

8-12. How is the length of the obstetric conjugate determined?

8-13. It is the measurement of the anteroposterior diameter of the plane of greatest pelvic dimensions that determines the ability of the fetus to pass through the birth canal.

a. True
b. False

8-14. Fill in the following chart describing the boundaries and diameters of some of the planes of the pelvis.

BOUNDARIES	PELVIC INLET	PELVIC OUTLET
Anterior	(a)	(b)
Lateral	(c)	(d)
Posterior	(e)	(f)
Anterior-posterior diameter	(g)	(h)
Transverse diameter	(i)	(j)

Instructions for Items 8-15 to 8-18: Refer to Figure 4.
Match the letter with the correct anteroposterior diameter of the pelvis.

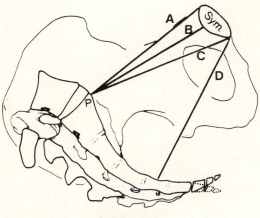

FIGURE 4

8-15. Anteroposterior diameter of midpelvis
8-16. Obstetric conjugate
8-17. True conjugate
8-18. Diagonal conjugate

8-19. Which term is not synonymous with the others?

a. Interspinous diameter
b. Plane of least pelvic dimensions
c. Transverse diameter of midplane
d. Plane of greatest pelvic dimensions

8-20. Placing which *two* of the following landmarks in a vertical plane reproduces the normal position of the pelvis in an erect woman?

a. Anterior superior spines of ilium
b. Ischial tuberosities
c. Sacral promontory
d. Ischial spines
e. Pubic tubercles

8-21. Which of the following is *not* involved in the anterior junction of the pelvic bones?

a. Inferior pubic ligament
b. Superior pubic ligament
c. Arcuate ligament
d. Symphysis pubis
e. Sacroiliac joint

8-22. Hazards of diagnostic radiation include:

a. The increased potential for mutation or malignancy.
b. Acne
c. Resultant osteopenia
d. Hypothyroidism in the infant

8-23. Regarding x-ray examinations, it may be stated that:

a. Radiation exposure of less than 5 rads represents no measureable risk to the embryo.
b. There is no "safe" time during the menstrual cycle for x-ray examination.
c. Computed tomography can image the pelvis using less radiation than conventional x-ray methods.
d. Ultrasound is the best tool available for pelvic bony imaging.

8-24. Which of the following statements concerning the Caldwell-Moloy classification of pelvic shapes is correct?

a. The shape of the posterior and anterior segments of the pelvic inlet are important determinants.
b. Anterior and posterior segments are divided by a line through the greatest transverse diameter of the inlet.
c. The anterior segment determines the type of pelvis.

Instructions for Items 8-25 to 8-28: Match the Caldwell-Moloy classification of pelvic shape with appropriate description.

a. Gynecoid
b. Android
c. Anthropoid
d. Platypelloid

8-25. Round shape, transverse and anterior-posterior diameters of inlet about equal
8-26. Flattened oval shape, transverse diameter of inlet greater than anterior-posterior diameter
8-27. Heart shape, anterior-posterior diameter of inlet greater than transverse diameter

8-28. Oval shape, anterior-posterior diameter of inlet greater than transverse diameter

Instructions for Items 8-29 to 8-32: Match the pure Caldwell-Moloy type with its frequency in a population of white women.

   a. Gynecoid
   b. Android
   c. Anthropoid
   d. Platypelloid

8-29. 25 percent
8-30. 50 percent
8-31. 33 percent
8-32. Less than 3 percent

8-33. In nonwhite women, which are the *two* most frequent pelvic types?

   a. Gynecoid
   b. Android
   c. Anthropoid
   d. Platypelloid

8-34. Most pelves are pure Caldwell-Moloy types.

   a. True
   b. False

8-35. Which pure pelvic shape (Caldwell-Moloy classification) has the poorest prognosis for vaginal delivery?

   a. Gynecoid
   b. Android
   c. Anthropoid
   d. Platypelloid

8-36. Which of the following statements concerning clinical measurement of the anteroposterior diameter of the pelvic inlet is correct?

   a. Palpation of the entire anterior sacral surface is easily accomplished.
   b. Evaluation of mobility of the coccyx is considered a part of the routine evaluation.
   c. To reach the sacral promontory, it is commonly necessary for the examiner to depress his/her elbow and to thereby exert enough pressure to forcibly indent the perineum.
   d. The procedure described in answer (c) commonly causes discomfort to the patient.

8-37. If the diagonal conjugate is greater than 11.5 cm, it is usually justifiable to assume that the pelvic inlet is adequate for vaginal delivery.

   a. True
   b. False

8-38. Engagement is defined as _____ .

8-39. What type of examination can ascertain engagement?

   a. Abdominal palpation
   b. Rectal examination
   c. Vaginal examination

8-40. Fixation of the fetal head is synonomous with engagement.

   a. True
   b. False

8-41. Which of the following statements relating to engagement is correct?

   a. If the lowest part of the occiput is at or below the level of the ischial spine, the head is usually but not always engaged.
   b. Absence of engagement at the onset of labor indicates pelvic contraction.
   c. Engagement commonly occurs prior to the onset of labor.
   d. Engagement is conclusive evidence of an adequate pelvic inlet for this fetus.

8-42. Which of the following terms are synonymous?

   a. Transverse diameter of the outlet
   b. Biischial diameter
   c. Intertuberous diameter
   d. Plane of least pelvic dimensions

8-43. The diameter between the ischial tuberosities should be at least _____ cm to be considered normal.

   a. 4
   b. 6
   c. 8
   d. 10

8-44. Midpelvic capacity may be precisely determined by

   a. The clinical measurement of ischial spine prominence
   b. The clinical measurement of side wall convergence
   c. The clinical measurement of sacral concavity
   d. Imaging studies

8-45. Which of the following factors important for the outcome of labor is amenable to reasonably precise radiographic measurement?

   a. Size and shape of bony pelvis
   b. Size of fetal head
   c. Presentation of fetus
   d. Position of fetus
   e. Moldability of fetal head

8-46. Which of the following pelvic diameters is *only* obtainable by x-ray pelvimetry?

a. Transverse diameter of the pelvic inlet
b. Obstetric conjugate
c. True conjugate
d. Transverse diameter of midpelvis
e. Interischial spinous diameter

8-47. X-ray pelvimetry may be indicated in which of the following circumstances?

a. Previous injury to bony pelvis
b. Breech presentations where vaginal delivery is considered
c. Failure to progress in labor (cephalopelvic disproportion)
d. All anticipated cesarean sections

9. ATTITUDE, LIE, PRESENTATION, AND POSITION OF THE FETUS

9-1. The position which a fetus assumes in late pregnancy is called its _____ .

9-2. Which of the following is a description of typical fetal posture in late pregnancy?

a. The back is convex.
b. The head is extended.
c. The thighs are flexed.
d. The legs are bent at the knee.
e. The arms are crossed over the thorax.

9-3. The characteristic fetal posture in late pregnancy results solely from a process of accommodation to the uterine cavity.

a. True
b. False

9-4. The lie of the fetus is defined as the _____ .

9-5. Which of the following fetal lies is most unstable?

a. Longitudinal
b. Oblique
c. Transverse

9-6. What percentage of fetal lies are longitudinal?

a. 50 percent
b. 75 percent
c. 99 percent

9-7. In longitudinal lies, the presenting part can be the

a. Head
b. Breech
c. Shoulder

Instructions for Items 9-8 to 9-11: Refer to Figure 5. Match the letter with the appropriate type of cephalic presentation.

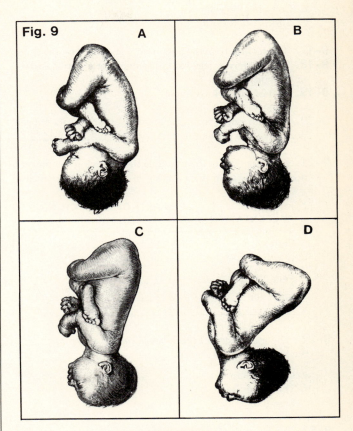

FIGURE 5

9-8. Vertex
9-9. Face
9-10. Sinciput
9-11. Brow

Instructions for Items 9-12 to 9-15: Match the type of cephalic presentation with the appropriate description.

a. Face presentation
b. Vertex presentation
c. Brow presentation
d. Sinciput presentation

9-12. Occipital fontanel presenting
9-13. Head in extreme extension
9-14. Head in partial extension
9-15. Anterior fontanel presenting

9-16. Sinciput and brow presentations almost always convert to face or vertex presentations during labor.

a. True
b. False

Instructions for Items 9–17 to 9–19: Match the type of breech presentation with the appropriate description.

   a. Frank breech
   b. Complete breech
   c. Incomplete (footling) breech

9–17. Thighs flexed on the abdomen, legs flexed on the thigh
9–18. Thighs flexed, legs extended over the anterior surface of the body
9–19. Feet or knees lowermost

9–20. Position refers to the relation of an arbitrarily chosen portion of the presenting fetal part to _____ .

9–21. Complete the following table by supplying the percent occurrence of each presentation in singleton pregnancies.

PRESENTATION	PERCENT OF SINGLETON PREGNANCIES
Vertex	(a)
Breech	(b)
Face	(c)
Shoulder	(d)

9–22. The incidence of breech presentation at term is _____ the incidence at 34 weeks.

   a. Greater than
   b. The same as
   c. Less than

9–23. Which of the following statements related to fetal presentation is correct?

   a. The podalic pole of the fetus is bulkier than the cephalic pole.
   b. At 32 weeks, the fetus starts becoming less crowded by the uterine walls.
   c. At about 32 weeks, the fetal lie becomes more dependent upon the piriform shape of the uterus.
   d. Fetal attitude may prevent it from turning in utero.
   e. The cephalic pole in hydrocephalic fetuses is larger than the podalic pole.

9–24. Which of the following methods may be used to determine the position and presentation of the fetus?

   a. Ultrasonography
   b. X-ray
   c. Abdominal palpation
   d. Vaginal palpation
   e. Auscultation

Instructions for Items 9–25 to 9–28: Match the maneuver of Leopold with its proper description.

   a. First maneuver
   b. Second maneuver
   c. Third maneuver
   d. Fourth maneuver

9–25. Examiner faces patient's head, determines engagement, lie, position
9–26. Examiner faces patient's head, determines position/orientation
9–27. Examiner faces patient's head, determines fetal pole, lie, presentation
9–28. Examiner faces patient's feet, determines engagement, presentation

9–29. What information can be obtained using the maneuvers of Leopold?

   a. Fetal descent
   b. Fetal position
   c. Fetal presentation
   d. Estimation of fetal size

9–30. The fetal cephalic suture felt during vaginal examination that provides information of primary importance is the _____ .

9–31. Which statements about auscultation in relation to fetal position and presentation is correct?

   a. Auscultation by itself provides very reliable information about fetal position.
   b. Fetal heart sounds are heard best through the fetal thorax in a face presentation.
   c. In a cephalic presentation, fetal heart sounds are best heard midway between the maternal umbilicus and the anterior superior spine of the ilium.
   d. In the occiput anterior position, heart sounds are best heard in the maternal flank.

9–32. In light of the safety of ultrasonography, there is no indication for the use of diagnostic x-rays in determining fetal position or presentation.

   a. True
   b. False

10. PARTURITION: BIOMOLECULAR AND PHYSIOLOGIC PROCESSES

10-1. From the biomolecular and physiologic perspective it is more convenient to consider the parturitional process as encompassing those final events of pregnancy when

a. Distinctive morphological and biochemical changes in uterine tissues preparatory for coordinated, forceful contractions begin
b. Labor brings forth the delivery of the fetus, placenta, and membranes
c. The morphological and biochemical identity of the uterus is returned to what is characteristic of the nonpregnant state
d. Only the events surrounding conception and the prevention of delivery preterm

10-2. Phase or parturition consist of which of the following?

a. The time of conception and implantation
b. The time of uterine preparedness for labor
c. The time of forceful contractions of active labor and delivery
d. The time of puerperal contraction and involution of the uterus

Instructions for Items 10-3 to 10-7: Match the substance with the best descriptor.

a. Uterotropin
b. Uterotonin

10-3. Substances that act to cause myometrial contractions.
10-4. An agent that causes uterine preparedness for labor.
10-5. Prostaglandins and oxytocin
10-6. Responsible for cervical softening and ripening
10-7. Increases the number of myometrial receptors in the endometrium

10-8. The mammal used as the ''gold standard'' in the study in parturition models has been the

a. Chimpanzee
b. Rat
c. Sheep
d. Dolphin

10-9. Regarding the mechanism of progesterone withdrawal as the inciting event in the initiation of labor, which of the following statements are true?

a. In some species progesterone production dramatically decreases just before the onset of labor.
b. Progesterone withdrawal is responsible for preterm labor in humans.
c. In humans there is no reduction of progesterone before labor commences.
d. Estrogen must surge in humans before progesterone withdrawal to initiate labor.

10-10. Which of the following statements are true?

a. The life span of the corpus luteum of a nonpregnant woman is about 12 to 14 days.
b. Human chorionic gonadotropin produced in the trophoblast acts to ''rescue'' the corpus luteum by stimulating continued progesterone production by this organ within an organ.
c. Fetal trophoblast takes over progesterone production about 2 weeks after fertilization.
d. Progesterone production plateaus in human pregnancy at about 32 to 34 weeks after having risen steadily before that time.

10-11. Oxytocin

a. Serves an active role in the initiation of labor
b. Is important in placental expulsion
c. Has an increased number of myometrical receptors just before the onset of labor
d. Causes postpartum contraction of the uterus
e. May act to effect milk letdown in lactating women

10-12. Prostaglandins

a. In amniotic fluid, maternal blood, and uterine tissues increase strikingly during labor
b. PGE_2 and $PGF_{2\alpha}$ administered at any stage of pregnancy will evoke myometrical contractions
c. Will only initiate labor when administered intravenously or per vagina
d. Are formed in tissue from the substrate arachidonic acid

10-13. Which of the following statements about labor in sheep is correct?

a. The sheep is the experimental animal in which the biomolecular events of parturition have been defined most clearly.
b. The signal for the initiation of labor clearly comes from the fetus.
c. Intact fetal hypothalamus or pituitary glands are not necessary for the initiation of labor.
d. The earliest trigger for labor is a sharp increase in fetal cortisol production.
e. Infusion of ACTH causes prematurre parturition.

10-14. Which of the following statements about prostaglandins and labor is correct?

a. Prostaglandins induce cervical softening and effacement.
b. Ingestion of prostaglandin synthetase inhibitors by pregnant women lengthens the time between induction and abortion in pregnancies terminated by hypertonic saline instillation.
c. Inhibitors of prostaglandin synthetase can suppress preterm labor.
d. Prostaglandin levels in amnionic fluid and maternal plasma are significantly increased during labor.

10-15. Which of the following statements is true?

a. The PGF₂ produced in human labor arises in the decidua.
b. Tumor necrosis factor alpha (TNR-a) is found in amniotic fluid of some pregnancies complicated by bacterial toxin-induced preterm labor.
c. Decidua is capable of producing high quantities of interleukin-1 beta.
d. The major site of prostaglandin synthesis is the fetal membranes.

10-16. Preterm labor

a. Occurs to about 250,000 fetuses per year
b. Is the greatest single cause of neonatal morbidity and mortality
c. May be due in part to "silent infection"
d. Is unaffected by bioactive microbial products

10-17. Which of the following statements related to the Organ Communication System model is correct?

a. The fetus is in communication with the mother by means of the fetal membranes.
b. Premature onset of labor may be initiated by rupture, stripping, or infection of the fetal membranes.
c. Prostaglandin biosynthesis and metabolism in the fetal membranes is similar to that in other fetal tissues.
d. The only prostaglandin synthesized in the uterine decidua vera is PGE₂.

Instructions for Items 10-18 and 10-19. Match the state of the uterus with the appropriate event involving calcium.

a. Uterine contraction
b. Uterine relaxation

10-18. Release of calcium from sarcoplasmic reticulum
10-19. ATP-dependent translocation of calcium to a stored form

10-20. What is the function of the myometrial extracellular matrix?

10-21. The function of gap junctions is to _____ .

10-22. Which of the following statements about myometrial gap junctions is correct?

a. Gap junctions are present in the myometrium throughout pregnancy.
b. The number of gap junctions increases during labor.
c. Gap junctions persist for 4 to 6 weeks postpartum.
d. Gap junctions are not present if labor is induced or premature.
e. Progesterone prevents the formation of gap junctions.
f. All prostanoids stimulate gap junction formation.
g. Estrogen promotes the formation of gap junctions.

10-23. Which of the following statements about uterine smooth muscle contraction is correct?

a. The protein of primary importance in muscle contraction is myosin.
b. The "head" portion of the myosin molecule controls its interaction with actin.
c. Calcium ion is required for muscle contraction.
d. The interaction of actin and myosin requires the dephosphorylation of myosin light chains.
e. Contraction is initiated through the interaction of phosphorylated myosin and actin.

10-24. The association of the calcium-dependent regulatory protein _____ with myosin light chain kinase is mandatory for enzyme activity.

10-25. Cervical ripening is associated with which of the following events?

a. Collagen breakdown
b. Smooth muscle hypertrophy
c. Alteration in the relative amounts of glycosaminoglycans
d. Randomization of smooth muscle bundles
e. Altered capacity of the tissue to retain water

10-26. Which of the following prostanoids act to induce the maturational changes of cervical ripening?

a. PGE₂
b. PGF₂α
c. Prostacyclin

10-27. The hormone that appears to be most closely related to accelerated prostaglandin synthesis is

a. Estrogen
b. Progesterone
c. Relaxin

10-28. Complete the following table which describes the stages of labor.

STAGE	BEGINS WHEN:	ENDS WHEN:
First	(a)	(b)
Second	(c)	(d)
Third	(e)	(f)

Instructions for Items 10-29 and 10-30: Match the stage of labor with the appropriate events.

a. Prelabor
b. Latent phase

10-29. Infrequent, irregular uterine contractions; precedes labor by several hours.
10-30. Increased uterine activity; precedes labor by several weeks

10-31. The time immediately after delivery of the placenta when uterine contractions are assisting hemostasis by contracting about the spiral arteries (arterioles) beneath the placental bed is defined as the _____ .

10-32. Ripening of the cervix occurs during the _____ of labor.

a. Prelabor phase
b. First stage
c. Second stage
d. Third stage
e. Fourth stage

10-33. Which of the following statements about "lightening" is correct?

a. Change in abdominal shape may occur several weeks before the onset of labor.
b. Fundal height decreases at this time.
c. It is described by the mother as "the baby dropped."
d. It is due to fetal descent and development of the lower uterine segment.
e. It is due to an increase in the volume of amnionic fluid.

Instructions for Items 10-34 and 10-35: Match the type of labor with the appropriate description.

a. True labor
b. False labor

10-34. Discomfort mostly in lower abdomen and groin
10-35. Discomfort begins in the fundal region and radiates to the lower back

10-36. False labor

a. Is more common in nulliparous women
b. May proceed directly to true labor
c. May occur at any time during pregnancy
d. Contributes to cervical dilation
e. Is the only time infrequent, short-lived, yet uncomfortable contractions occur

10-37. Discharge of a small amount of blood-tinged mucus from the vagina prior to labor is called _____ .

10-38. Which of the following statements about uterine contractions is correct?

a. The cause of the pain of uterine contractions during labor is unclear.
b. Uterine contractions are involuntary.
c. Uterine contractions are unaffected by epidural anesthesia.
d. Uterine contractions in paraplegic women are painless.
e. Pacemaker sites for contractions appear to be in the lower uterine segment.

10-39. Enhancement of myometrial activity by manual stretching of the cervix is referred to as the _____ .

10-40. Uterine contractions

a. Are enhanced by cervical stretching
b. Occur about 1 minute apart during the second stage of labor
c. Average about 1 minute in length during the active phase of labor
d. Vary in intensity

10-41. Periods of uterine relaxation between contractions are necessary to prevent development of fetal hypoxia.

a. True
b. False

10-42. During labor, the upper uterine segment _____ and the lower uterine segment _____ .
(1)
(2)

a. Thins
b. Thickens

Instructions for Items 10-43 to 10-50: Match the segment of the uterus with the appropriate characteristics.

a. Upper uterine segment
b. Lower uterine segment

10-43. Develops gradually during pregnancy
10-44. Actively contracts
10-45. Retracts during labor
10-46. Distends during labor
10-47. Myometrial fibers progressively shorten during labor
10-48. Myometrial fibers progressively lengthen during labor
10-49. Uterine corpus
10-50. Uterine isthmus

10-51. In cases of obstructed labor, the ring marking the boundary between the upper and lower uterine segments becomes very prominent. In extreme cases it is termed the _____ .

10-52. In normal labor, the uterine contractions in the lower uterine segment are shorter and less intense than the contractions in the upper uterine segment.

a. True
b. False

10-53. During early labor, each contraction _____ the horizontal diameter of the uterus and _____ the uterine length.
(1)
(2)

a. Increases
b. Decreases

10-54. A voluntary increase in intraabdominal pressure—"pushing"—is useful during which stage of labor?

a. First stage
b. Second stage
c. Third stage
d. Fourth stage

10-55. The work involved in labor is close to the functional capacity of the normal woman.

a. True
b. False

10-56. The process by which the cervical canal shortens and the internal os is drawn up to become part of the lower uterine segment is known as _____ .

10-57. Which of the following statements about labor is correct?

a. The cervix must dilate to 10 cm to allow the head of the average term fetus to pass.
b. Early rupture of the fetal membranes invariably retards cervical dilation.
c. More fetal descent occurs during cervical effacement than during dilation.
d. During the second stage of labor, descent of the fetal presenting part may be very rapid in multiparas.

10-58. What two elements are considered by Friedman to be most useful in assessing the progression of labor?

Instructions for Items 10-59 to 10-62: Match the phase of cervical dilation with the appropriate statement.

a. Latent phase
b. Active phase

10-59. May be prolonged by sedation
10-60. Subdivided into an acceleration phase, phase of maximum slope, and deceleration phase
10-61. Duration has little bearing on the subsequent course of labor
10-62. Cervical dilation completed

10-63. According to Friedman, the acceleration phase is related to _____ , the maximum slope is related to _____ , and the deceleration phase is related to _____ .
₍₁₎ ₍₂₎ ₍₃₎

a. Fetopelvic relationships
b. The outcome of labor
c. The "efficiency of the machine"

10-64. Engagement always precedes the onset of labor.

a. True
b. False

Instructions for Items 10-65 to 10-69: Match the functional division of labor according to Friedman with the appropriate description.

a. Preparatory
b. Dilational
c. Pelvic

10-65. Changes occur in ground substance of the cervix
10-66. Dilation is at most rapid rate
10-67. Sensitive to sedation and anesthesia
10-68. Begins with deceleration phase of cervical dilation
10-69. Includes cardinal movements of labor

10-70. If the fetal membranes remain intact until the completion of delivery, the portion covering the head of the newborn is referred to as the _____ .

10-71. Place the components of the pelvic floor in correct order (from the inside proceeding outward).

a. Internal pelvic fascia
b. Subcutaneous tissue
c. Skin
d. Levator ani and coccygeus muscles
e. Subperitoneal connective tissue
f. Peritoneum
g. Superficial muscles and fascia
h. External pelvic fascia

10-72. Which of the following statements about the levator ani and its upper and lower fascial coverings is correct?

a. It fills the entire pelvic floor.
b. It consists of pelvic and iliac portions.
c. It encircles both the rectum and vagina.
d. It remains unchanged in pregnancy.
e. Contraction of the muscle acts to close the vagina.

10-73. Which of the following structures are part of the urogenital diaphragm?

a. Three fascial layers
b. Pubic vessels and nerves
c. Sphincter ani
d. Rami of clitoris
e. Bulbocavernosus muscle
f. Ischiocavernosus muscle

10-74. What is the principal change in the pelvic floor as a result of labor?

10-75. Placental separation occurs as a result of _____ .

10–76. Which of the following statements about placental separation is correct?

   a. The formation of a hematoma is usually the cause of placental separation.
   b. The entire decidua is cast off with the placenta.
   c. The membranes usually remain in situ until the separation of the placenta is nearly complete.
   d. Women frequently cannot expel the placenta spontaneously.

Instructions for Items 10–77 to 10–80: Match the mechanism of placental extrusion with the appropriate statement.

   a. Mechanism of Schultze (central placental expulsion)
   b. Mechanism of Duncan (peripheral placental expulsion)

10–77. Most common type of placental separation
10–78. Maternal surface appears first
10–79. Fetal surface appears first
10–80. Blood does not escape externally until after placental extrusion

11. MECHANISMS OF NORMAL LABOR IN OCCIPUT PRESENTATION

11–1. Occiput (vertex) presentations occur in about _____ percent of all labors.

11–2. Which of the following statements about the diagnosis of occiput presentation is correct?

   a. Presentation is usually first determined by abdominal examination and confirmed by vaginal exam.
   b. The vertex usually enters the pelvis with the sagittal suture in the anteroposterior pelvic diameter.
   c. With the fetus in the left occiput transverse (LOT) position, the fetal back is palpable in the maternal left flank.
   d. In the LOT position, the anterior fontanel is in the maternal right.
   e. In the LOT position, the fetal heart tones are best heard on the maternal right.

11–3. In the occiput anterior positions (LOA or ROA), the mechanism of labor is usually similar to that in the transverse positions (LOT or ROT).

   a. True
   b. False

11–4. Which of the following statements about the occiput posterior positions is correct?

   a. Occiput posterior positions occur in approximately 40 percent of pregnancies.
   b. The right occiput posterior position (ROP) is more common than the left (LOP).
   c. Posterior positions are associated with a narrow forepelvis.
   d. In the ROP position, the small fontanel is felt opposite the right sacroiliac synchondrosis.

11–5. Place the following cardinal movements of labor in their proper chronologic sequence.

   a. Extension
   b. Internal rotation
   c. Flexion
   d. Descent
   e. Engagement
   f. External rotation
   g. Expulsion

11–6. Which of the following statements about the cardinal movements of labor in the occiput presentation is correct?

   a. The cardinal movements of labor occur as the fetal head adapts and accommodates to the diameters of the maternal pelvis during labor.
   b. The cardinal movements of labor occur separately and independently in chronologic sequence.
   c. The cardinal movements of labor are independent of descent of the presenting part.
   d. The cardinal movements of labor occur concomitantly with modification of the habitus of the fetus under the influence of uterine contractions.
   e. As part of labor, the fetus straightens.
   f. As labor progresses, the extremities become more closely applied to the body.

11–7. In most multiparous women, engagement of the fetal head usually takes place after the start of labor.

   a. True
   b. False

11–8. Lateral deflection of the fetal head, where the sagittal suture is deflected either posteriorly or anteriorly, is termed _____ .

11–9. If the sagittal suture approaches the sacral promontory, it is termed _____ asynclitism.

   a. Anterior
   b. Posterior

11–10. Moderate degrees of asynclitism are common in normal labor.

   a. True
   b. False

11-11. Descent is brought about by which of the following forces?

    a. Pressure of the amnionic fluid
    b. Direct pressure of the fundus upon the breech
    c. Contraction of the abdominal muscles
    d. Extension and straightening of the fetal body

11-12. As flexion occurs, the shorter suboccipitobregmatic diameter is substituted for the longer _____ diameter.

11-13. Internal rotation is usually not accomplished until the head has reached the level of the _____ .

11-14. Which of the following statements about the cardinal movements of labor in the occiput anterior position is correct?

    a. Extension brings the base of the occiput into direct contact with the inferior margin of the symphysis pubis.
    b. Immediately after its birth, the head drops downward.
    c. The delivered head returns to the oblique position.
    d. Restitution is followed by completion of external rotation to the transverse position.
    e. The posterior shoulder is delivered before the anterior shoulder.

11-15. Transverse arrest and persistent occiput posterior position represent deviations from the normal mechanism of labor.

    a. True
    b. False

11-16. Which of the following statements about changes in the shape of the fetal head is correct?

    a. Swelling of the fetal scalp that develops during labor is known as caput succedaneum.
    b. Caput may be extensive enough to prevent differentiation of anatomic landmarks on the fetal head.
    c. In molding, the margins of the occipital bone may be pushed under those of the parietal bone.
    d. Molding may account for a diminution in the biparietal diameter.

12.   THE NEWBORN INFANT

12-1. Except for cases of hypoxic stress in utero, the infant makes its first respiratory efforts after delivery.

    a. True
    b. False

12-2. Which of the following statements about the initiation of air breathing is correct?

    a. Soon after birth, the infant changes from an initial shallow-breathing pattern to a pattern of deeper, regular inhalations.
    b. The initial breaths are especially difficult because they involve the inflation of a collapsed structure.
    c. Residual alveolar fluid is cleared primarily by the pulmonary circulation and lymphatics.
    d. Transient tachypnea of the newborn results from a delay in the removal of amnionic fluid from lung alveoli.
    e. High negative intrathoracic pressures are required to bring about the initial entry of air into the fluid-filled alveoli.

12-3. By about the _____ breath, the pressure-volume changes with each respiration in the normal mature infant are similar to those of the normal adult.

12-4. Closure of the ductus arteriosus is associated with the _____ in pulmonary arterial pressure after birth.

    a. Fall
    b. Rise

12-5. What condition develops if there is a lack of sufficient pulmonary surfactant at the time of delivery?

12-6. Which of the following may stimulate the infant to initiate respiration?

    a. Physical stimulation
    b. Compression of the fetal thorax incident to delivery
    c. Oxygen deprivation
    d. Carbon dioxide accumulation

12-7. Babies born by cesarean section tend to have _____ fluid in their lungs than babies born by vaginal delivery.

    a. More
    b. Less

12-8. Steps in the immediate care of the newborn infant include

    a. Wiping the face
    b. Suctioning the mouth and nares
    c. Clamping and cutting the cord
    d. Giving a sponge bath
    e. Placing in an incubator with the head elevated

12-9. Which of the following are determinants of fetal well-being that should be considered before and during delivery?

   a. Maternal health
   b. Gestational age
   c. Duration of labor
   d. Duration of rupture of membranes
   e. Analgesia administered to the mother
   f. Duration and kind of maternal anesthesia
   g. Difficulties encountered in delivery

12-10. What two methods are best utilized to determine the newborn's heart rate?

12-11. What is the minimal acceptable heart rate in the newborn?

   a. 60
   b. 80
   c. 100
   d. 120

12-12. Suctioning of the mouth and pharynx of the newborn should be performed in cases of bradycardia or infrequent respirations.

   a. True
   b. False

12-13. Which of the following is an effective method to stimulate breathing in the newborn?

   a. Tubbing
   b. Jackknifing
   c. Rubbing of back
   d. Slapping the soles of the feet
   e. Dilation of sphincters

12-14. Which of the following may be causes of failure to establish effective respirations?

   a. Fetal hypoxemia
   b. Drugs given to the mother
   c. Fetal immaturity
   d. Upper airway obstruction
   e. Pneumothorax
   f. Lung abnormalities
   g. Meconium aspiration
   h. CNS injury

12-15. List the five signs that are used to determine the Apgar score.

12-16. Regarding the use and misuse of the Apgar score, which of the following statements is true?

   a. The score is used as a quick method for assessing the state of the newborn infant.
   b. The Apgar score is low solely because of asphyxia and predicts future neurologic outcome.
   c. A low 5-minute Apgar score almost always insures cerebral palsy will develop in the infant.
   d. Low Apgar scores at 10, 15, and 20 minutes have no more long-term significance than the 1- and 5-minute scores.

12-17. An infant whose heart rate is 90, whose respiratory efforts are slow and irregular, who moves actively, grimaces when stimulated, and is completely pink in color would receive an Apgar score of _____ .

12-18. The Apgar score of an infant who is defined as mildly to moderately depressed would be _____ .

12-19. List the seven common errors in the resuscitation of the newborn.

12-20. List the four critically important components to successful newborn resuscitation.

12-21. It is not necessary to equip the site of every delivery for resuscitation as long as the necessary equipment and personnel are available within 5 minutes.

   a. True
   b. False

12-22. Which of the following statements is true regarding umbilical cord blood acid-base and blood gas measurements?

   a. Acidemia is defined as an umbilical artery pH of less than 7.2.
   b. These measurements bear no relationship to fetal metabolic status.
   c. These measures predict only long-term changes from the fetal environment and do not reflect changes induced by labor.
   d. Umbilical acidemia could be expected in 40 percent of neonates who have had moderate to severe bradycardia in labor.

12–23. Which of the following statements about the process of endotracheal intubation is correct?

   a. The infant should be supine with the head level.
   b. The laryngoscope is introduced through the left side of the mouth.
   c. Elevation of the laryngoscope tip will expose the vocal cords.
   d. The endotracheal tube is inserted through the vocal cords until the shoulder of the tube reaches the glottis.
   e. The laryngoscope should be left in place as long as the endotracheal tube is being utilized.

12–24. The sources of oxygen that should be used with an endotracheal tube are _____ and _____ .

Instructions for Items 12–25 to 12–27: Match the complications of endotracheal intubation with the appropriate cause.

   a. Excessive positive pressure
   b. Esophageal placement of endotracheal tube

12–25. Pneumothorax
12–26. Stomach expansion
12–27. Pneumomediastinum

12–28. Which of the following statements about the use of sodium bicarbonate in infant resuscitation is correct?

   a. The correct dose is 1 mEq/kg.
   b. Sodium bicarbonate is administered through the umbilical vein.
   c. It should be used in cases of hypoxia where positive pressure oxygen does not bring a prompt response.
   d. The dose of sodium bicarbonate may be repeated.
   e. Effective ventilation must be continued to prevent respiratory acidosis.

12–29. A drug that can be used to correct respiratory depression caused by meperidine or other opioids is _____ .

12–30. Which of the following causes hypovolemia in the newborn?

   a. Sepsis
   b. Fetal to maternal hemorrhage
   c. Placental trauma
   d. Pooling of blood in the placenta due to cord compression
   e. Twin-to-twin transfusion

12–31. External cardiac massage is indicated if cardiac activity was present just before birth and stops thereafter or if the heart stops after birth.

   a. True
   b. False

12–32. Which of the following statements about cardiac massage for resuscitation of the newborn is correct?

   a. Adequate ventilation must also be established.
   b. External cardiac massage is effected using two fingers to the anterior chest wall in the lower midline.
   c. The rate of massage should be about 80 per minute.
   d. Ten chest compressions should be alternated with each lung inflation.
   e. A delay in cardiac massage may have fatal consequences.

12–33. In the resuscitation of the neonate, epinephrine should first be administered intravenously to avoid trauma to the heart with intracardiac injection tried as a last resort.

   a. True
   b. False

12–34. Estimates of gestational age based on physical and neurologic examination of the neonate are frequently unacceptably inaccurate in preterm and growth-retarded infants.

   a. True
   b. False

12–35. Which of the following statements about the prevention of gonorrheal ophthalmia is correct?

   a. Use of a 1 percent silver nitrate solution eliminates the possibility of gonorrheal ophthalmia.
   b. In all cases where it is used, silver nitrate causes a transient chemical conjunctivitis.
   c. Prophylaxis with penicillin, either as an ointment or by intramuscular injection, reduces the frequency of gonorrheal ophthalmia but does not prevent chlamydial infection.
   d. Tetracycline or erythromycin ointment instilled into the newborn's eyes affords effective prophylaxis against gonorrhea and chlamydia.

12–36. Which of the following statements about proper infant identification procedures is correct?

   a. A system should be available at all hours.
   b. It is only necessary to retain identification records until the infant leaves the hospital.
   c. Fingerprints are superior to footprints because the ridges are more pronounced.
   d. Close attention must be paid to technique or the prints will be unsatisfactory.

12–37. Which of the following statements about the temperature of the newborn is correct?

   a. The infant's temperature drops rapidly after birth.
   b. Chilling increases oxygen requirements.
   c. After the first hour of life, the infant's temperature stabilizes and becomes less responsive to external stimuli.

12–38. Vitamin K should routinely be administered to the newborn infant.

a. True
b. False

12–39. Which of the following statements about the umbilical cord in the newborn is correct?

a. Loss of water from Wharton's jelly leads to mummification of the cord shortly after birth.
b. Separation of the cord usually occurs in the first 2 weeks of life.
c. A dressing for the cord is recommended.
d. Infection of the umbilical stump may present no physical signs.
e. Hygienic management of the cord serves to minimize the risk of neonatal tetanus.

12–40. Which of the following statements about skin care in the newborn is correct?

a. The infant should be dried promptly to eliminate heat loss due to evaporation.
b. All vernix caseosa must be removed.
c. Immediate bathing should be used to stabilize temperature.
d. The newborn infant should be handled as much as possible.

12–41. The components of meconium include

a. Intestinal tract epithelial cells
b. Epidermal cells
c. Lanugo
d. Bile pigments
e. Blood

12–42. Which of the following statements about stools in the newborn is correct?

a. For a few hours after birth, intestinal contents contain no bacteria.
b. Failure of the infant to pass meconium within the first 12 to 24 hours indicates a congenital defect such as imperforate anus.
c. After ingestion of milk, meconium is replaced by light yellow feces.
d. Stools should not have an odor until the infant is about 1 month of age.

12–43. Which of the following statements about jaundice in the newborn is correct?

a. Typically, there is hyperbilirubinemia at birth in the range of 1.8 to 2.8 mg/dL of serum.
b. About one in ten infants develop physiologic jaundice of the newborn.
c. Physiologic jaundice of the newborn always occurs before the third day of life.
d. Jaundice becomes noticeable when the serum concentration of bilirubin exceeds 5 mg/dL.
e. In premature infants, jaundice is more common and usually more severe than in term infants.
f. In infants who are mature but small-for-gestational age, jaundice is more common and usually more severe than in normal-sized infants.

12–44. Which of the following factors contribute to hyperbilirubinemia in the newborn?

a. Immaturity of hepatic cells
b. Reduced production and excretion of conjugated bilirubin
c. Reabsorption of free bilirubin
d. Increased erythrocyte destruction

12–45. Weight loss in the newborn may be attributed to

a. Lack of nutriment
b. Urine production
c. Sweat production
d. Feces production

12–46. Which of the following statements about weight changes in the infant is correct?

a. Premature infants lose relatively more weight than term infants.
b. Premature infants regain weight more rapidly than term infants.
c. Healthy but small-for-gestational age infants gain weight more rapidly than premature infants.
d. The normal infant regains its birth weight by about the 10th day.
e. The average healthy infant will triple its birth weight by 6 months of age.

12–47. Which of the following statements about feeding the newborn is correct?

a. Nursing should be initiated within the first 12 hours postpartum.
b. All infants thrive best when fed every 6 hours.
c. Only one breast should be used for each feeding.
d. The proper length of each feeding depends on the quantity and availability of breast milk and on the infant's appetite.

12–48. Circumcision should be performed routinely at the time of delivery.

 a. True
 b. False

12–49. Which of the following are contraindications to circumcision?

 a. Prematurity
 b. Neonatal illness
 c. Family history of penile cancer
 d. Presence of coagulation defects

13. THE PUERPERIUM

13–1. The puerperium is commonly defined as the time from the birth of an infant to the beginning of the first postpartum menstrual period.

 a. True
 b. False

Instructions for Items 13–2 to 13–7: Match the time after delivery with the appropriate events.

 a. Just after delivery
 b. 1 day after delivery
 c. 2 days after delivery
 d. 3 to 5 days after delivery
 e. 1 week after delivery
 f. 2 weeks after delivery
 g. 3 weeks after delivery
 h. 4 weeks after delivery
 i. 6 weeks after delivery

13–2. The fundus of the uterus is about midway between the umbilicus and the symphysis
13–3. The uterus has descended into the true pelvis
13–4. The uterus has regained its nonpregnant size
13–5. The uterus weighs about 1 kg
13–6. The uterus weighs about 500 g
13–7. The uterus weighs about 300 g

13–8. Which of the following statements about involution of the uterus is correct?

 a. Immediately after expulsion of the placenta, the fundus is palpable just above the pubic symphysis.
 b. The uterus reaches its nonpregnant weight within 2 weeks.
 c. Due to involution, the uterus at 1 week postpartum weighs one-half what it did just after delivery.
 d. The connective tissue framework of the uterus undergoes rapid involution after delivery.

13–9. During involution the total number of myometrial cells ____(1)____ and the size of an individual myometrial cell ____(2)____ .

 a. Increases
 b. Remains the same
 c. Decreases

13–10. How long does it take for the entire endometrium to be regenerated after delivery?

 a. 1 week
 b. 2 weeks
 c. 3 weeks
 d. 4 weeks
 e. 6 weeks

13–11. Incomplete extrusion of the placental site may result in what clinical problem?

13–12. Which of the following statements about involution of the placental site is correct?

 a. The process may take up to 6 weeks.
 b. An intermediate step in involution is thrombus formation.
 c. The final step in involution is absorption in situ.
 d. Each pregnancy leaves a fibrous scar in the endometrium.

13–13. The placental site regenerates endometrium more slowly than does the remainder of the uterus.

 a. True
 b. False

13–14. Which of the following return to their prepregnant condition (size or appearance) after delivery?

 a. Cervix
 b. Lower uterine segment
 c. Vagina
 d. Hymen
 e. Abdominal wall

13–15. Which of the following statements about the puerperal abdominal wall is correct?

 a. It takes several weeks for the abdominal wall to return to normal.
 b. Exercise does not aid the recovery of the abdominal wall.
 c. Striae may be eliminated with hormonal salves.
 d. Diastasis recti may persist.

13-16. Which of the following statements about the urinary tract during the puerperium is correct?

   a. The postpartum bladder is often hyperemic and edematous.
   b. The puerperal bladder has an increased capacity.
   c. After an uncomplicated delivery, the puerperal urinary tract is at relatively low risk for the development of infection.
   d. The effect of labor on postpartum bladder function almost always shows marked hypotonia.

13-17. Which of the following statements about breast development is correct?

   a. Mammary gland anlagen are contained in the ectodermal ridges that form on the ventral surface of the embryo.
   b. Normally only one pair of breast buds develops.
   c. The fetal mammary buds begin to grow and divide near term.
   d. Thelarche is due to progesterone stimulation.
   e. The constituents of milk are synthesized in the alveolar epithelium.

13-18. Colostrum has more _____ than mature milk.

   a. Protein
   b. Fat
   c. Sugar
   d. Minerals

13-19. Which of the following statements about colostrum is correct?

   a. Colostrum is secreted during the first 2 postpartum days.
   b. Colostrum contains immunoglobulin A which may help protect the newborn against enteric infection.
   c. Colostrum contains no vitamins.
   d. The colostrum corpuscles are large fat globules of uncertain origin.

13-20. Which of the following statements about human milk is correct?

   a. Milk is isotonic with plasma.
   b. Most proteins in milk are not found elsewhere.
   c. All vitamins except vitamin K are present in human milk.
   d. Increasing maternal iron stores increases the amount of iron in breast milk.
   e. The mammary gland concentrates iodine, which appears in breast milk.
   f. Thirty to forty hours postpartum breast milk undergoes a vast increase in lactose concentration.

13-21. Which of the following appear to help stimulate growth and development of the milk-secreting apparatus of the mammary gland?

   a. Estrogen
   b. Progesterone
   c. Cortisol
   d. Prolactin
   e. Insulin
   f. Placental lactogen

13-22. A decrease in the level of which two hormones serves to initiate lactation?

13-23. Which of the following statements concerning lactation is correct?

   a. Prolactin is essential for lactation.
   b. Suckling triggers a rise in prolactin.
   c. Suckling stimulates the neurohypophysis to release oxytocin.
   d. Expression of milk is due to contractions of myoepithelial cells in the breast alveoli.
   e. Milk letdown may be inhibited by stress.

13-24. Which statements concerning breast milk and immunology are correct?

   a. The antibodies present in human colostrum and milk are poorly absorbed from the infant's gut.
   b. The predominant immunoglobulin in milk is IgA.
   c. Breast milk contains IgA against *Escherichia coli*.
   d. Human milk has T but no B lymphocytes.
   e. There are greater amounts of protective factors in the milk of older women.

13-25. Which of the following statements about breast feeding is correct?

   a. The frequency of breast feeding among women in the United States is greater now than 25 years ago.
   b. Nursing accelerates uterine involution.
   c. If a woman's milk supply is insufficient at first, even with suckling it will not become sufficient later.
   d. Drugs are secreted in milk at higher concentration than they are present in maternal plasma.

13-26. What factors are associated with more severe afterpains?

   a. Primiparity
   b. Retained placental fragments.
   c. Breast feeding
   d. Forceps delivery
   e. Blood clots in the uterus

13-27. Which of the following are contained in lochia?

   a. Erythrocytes
   b. Microorganisms
   c. Shreds of decidua
   d. Epithelial cells

13-28. Which of the following statements about lochia is correct?

   a. Lochia rubra precedes lochia alba.
   b. Foul-smelling lochia proves that infection is present.
   c. Women who receive methylergonovine maleate are likely to lose less blood postpartum.
   d. The amount of lochia is the same in women who received methylergonovine maleate in the immediate puerperium and those who did not.
   e. Lochia rubra that lasts longer than 2 weeks is abnormal.

13-29. Which of the following statements is true?

   a. Postpartum diuresis is likely to occur even without the infusion of extra solutions.
   b. The resolution of preeclampsia is often associated with massive diuresis.
   c. Marked glycosuria in the puerperium is not uncommon.
   d. Ketones in the urine are abnormal after a long labor.

13-30. Which of the following statements about clinical aspects of the puerperium is correct?

   a. Breast fever, a commonly occurring physiologic temperature elevation beginning on the third or fourth day of lactation, often lasts 3 to 4 days.
   b. A rise in temperature in the puerperium usually implies a maternal infection, most likely somewhere in the genitourinary tract.
   c. Afterpains usually decrease in intensity by the third day after delivery.
   d. Puerperal diuresis is common in the second to fifth postpartum days.
   e. A blood leukocyte count in the puerperium of greater than 12,000 per microliter is always indicative of maternal infection.

13-31. Which are normal findings in the blood during the first postpartum week?

   a. Leukocytosis
   b. Relative lymphopenia
   c. Marked anemia
   d. Elevated sedimentation rate
   e. Decreased fibrinogen

13-32. There is significant weight loss during the puerperium that cannot be attributed to the involution of the uterus and normal blood loss.

   a. True
   b. False

13-33. Which of the following statements about the care of the mother immediately postpartum is correct?

   a. As long as the fundus is firm, there is no danger of postpartum hemorrhage.
   b. Progressive uterine enlargement may be an indication of bleeding.
   c. During the immediate postpartum period, the vulva should be cleansed after each bowel movement and before any local treatment or examination.
   d. The episiotomy should be nearly asymptomatic by the end of the third week.
   e. Perineal discomfort at the episiotomy site that is unresponsive to local analgesics may indicate that a hematoma has formed.

13-34. Which of the following statements are true regarding postpartum depression?

   a. It is usually mild and self-limited to 2 or 3 days.
   b. Symptoms of severe postpartum depression are much different than depressive symptoms in the nonpregnant patient.
   c. Those women with unwanted pregnancies or marital problems are much more susceptible to postpartum depression.
   d. Situational aspects or long-standing psychiatric problems predispose to postpartum depression.

13-35. What are the benefits of early postpartum ambulation?

   a. The patient feels better.
   b. There is less constipation.
   c. There is less chance of pulmonary emboli.
   d. There is improved lactation.

13-36. Which of the following statements about the abdominal wall during the puerperium is correct?

   a. An abdominal binder is usually unnecessary.
   b. A girdle should be worn to help in involution.
   c. Abdominal wall exercises may be started at any time after a vaginal delivery.
   d. Abdominal wall exercises after cesarean section should be started after the 6-week check-up.

13-37. Which of the following dietary considerations should apply to the postpartum woman?

   a. Nothing should be given by mouth for the first 12 hours.
   b. Only liquids should be administered for the first 2 days.
   c. Fluids should be restricted for women who do not nurse.
   d. As compared to the diet of the pregnant woman, the diet of the lactating woman should be increased in calories and protein.

13–38. Which of the following factors lead to bladder overdistention during the puerperium?

   a. Intravenous fluid administration
   b. Cessation of oxytocin administration
   c. Anesthesia
   d. Pain in the pelvic region

13–39. If the bladder becomes palpable postpartum and the patient is unable to spontaneously void, one-time catheterization should be considered.

   a. True
   b. False

13–40. Which of the following may normally be expected postpartum?

   a. Constipation
   b. Nipple irritation
   c. Nausea
   d. Urinary urgency

13–41. The postpartum hospital stay does not normally exceed _____ days.

   a. 1
   b. 2
   c. 3
   d. 4

13–42. Which statements about the return of ovulation and menstruation is correct?

   a. In the nonnursing woman, menstruation usually returns within 6 to 8 weeks.
   b. In lactating women, the first period occurs after the cessation of nursing.
   c. Ovulation may be reestablished within 2 weeks of birth.
   d. Pregnancy can occur while a woman is nursing.
   e. Amenorrhea during lactation is due to lack of pituitary gonadotropin stimulation of the ovary.

13–43. Which of the following activities should be curtailed until 6 weeks postpartum?

   a. Bathing
   b. Household work
   c. Driving
   d. Coitus
   e. Contraception

PART IV MANAGEMENT OF NORMAL PREGNANCY

14. PRENATAL CARE

14–1. Which of the following statements about prenatal care is correct?

   a. The goal is delivery of a healthy baby without impairing the health of the mother.
   b. Bad prenatal care may be worse than no care at all.
   c. Prenatal care should be a continuation of comprehensive health care prior to pregnancy.

14–2. Prenatal care is a special kind of medical treatment for the pathophysiologic changes in maternal physiology that are engendered by pregnancy.

   a. True
   b. False

Instructions for Items 14–3 to 14–9: Match the terms with their definitions.

   a. Nulligravida
   b. Gravida
   c. Nullipara
   d. Primipara
   e. Multipara
   f. Parturient
   g. Puerpera

14–3. A woman delivered once of a fetus or fetuses who reached the state of viability
14–4. A woman who is or has been pregnant
14–5. A woman who has never completed a pregnancy beyond an abortion
14–6. A woman who has just given birth
14–7. A woman in labor
14–8. A woman who has completed two or more pregnancies to the stage of viability
14–9. A woman who has never been pregnant.

14–10. A woman who was delivered of one set of twins and has had no other pregnancies would be defined as a

_____ .

14-11. A woman whose obstetrical history is described by the digits 4-0-1-3 has how many living children?

  a. 4
  b. 0
  c. 1
  d. 3

14-12. The mean duration of a normal pregnancy from the first day of the last normal menstrual period is about

  a. 250 days
  b. 260 days
  c. 270 days
  d. 280 days
  e. 290 days

14-13. According to Naegele's rule, if a pregnant woman's last menstrual period began on June 3, her expected date of delivery would be _____ .

14-14. Gestational age is synonymous with

  a. Ovulatory age
  b. Menstrual age
  c. Fertilization age

14-15. Clinically, the most useful and appropriate unit of measure for a pregnancy is the

  a. Trimester
  b. Months of gestation completed
  c. Weeks of gestation completed

14-16. The goals of the initial comprehensive obstetrical evaluation include

  a. Defining the health status of the mother
  b. Defining the health status of the fetus
  c. Determining the gestational age of the fetus
  d. Identifying women at risk for preterm labor

14-17. Which of the following contributes to difficulties in determining gestational age?

  a. Menstrual cycle significantly longer than 30 days
  b. Irregular menstrual cycles
  c. Use of steroidal contraceptives
  d. Presence of an intrauterine device

14-18. Which of the following are standard procedures at the initial prenatal obstetrical examination?

  a. Obtaining specimens for cervical cytology
  b. Obtaining urethral culture
  c. Performing colposcopy
  d. Obtaining cervical culture for gonorrhea
  e. Biopsying suspected Nabothian cysts

14-19. Which of the following types of vaginal secretions is normal in pregnancy?

  a. Foamy yellow liquid
  b. Curdlike discharge
  c. White mucoid discharge
  d. Frothy, red tinged discharge

14-20. Characterization of the bony architecture of the pelvis is the most important aspect of the internal examination in pregnancy.

  a. True
  b. False

14-21. Between 18 and 32 weeks, what is the relationship between the gestational age of the fetus and the height of the uterine fundus?

14-22. During the prenatal examination, carious teeth should be identified but dental repair should be postponed as it is dangerous during pregnancy.

  a. True
  b. False

14-23. List the ten danger signs that a pregnant woman should be warned to report immediately.

14-24. Factors which may warrant classification of a pregnancy as ''high risk'' include

  a. Preexisting medical illness
  b. Previous poor pregnancy outcome
  c. Previous placental accidents or maternal hemorrhage
  d. Evidence of maternal malnutrition

Instructions for Items 14-25 to 14-27: Match the appropriate interval of prenatal visits with the phase of pregnancy.

  a. Every week
  b. Every 2 weeks
  c. Every 4 weeks
  d. Every 6 weeks

14-25. Weeks 1 to 28
14-26. Weeks 28 to 36
14-27. Weeks 36 through delivery

14-28. Which of the following statements about findings during routine prenatal return visits is correct?

    a. Using a DeLee fetal stethoscope, fetal heart sounds are first audible in essentially all pregnancies between 16 and 19 weeks' gestation.

    b. A common cause of error in fundal height measurement is a full maternal bladder.

    c. Fundal height measurements correlate exactly with gestational age from the time the fundus is palpable until delivery.

    d. The time of first reported fetal movement can aid in the accuracy of gestational age determinations.

    e. An accurate date for the LMP and serially appropriate fundal heights may firmly establish gestational age.

14-29. Which of the following should be routinely monitored at prenatal visits?

    a. Fetal movement
    b. Presenting part
    c. Amount of amnionic fluid
    d. Fetal heart rate
    e. Size of fetus

14-30. Which maternal physical signs are monitored at every prenatal visit?

    a. Blood pressure
    b. Weight
    c. Fundal height
    d. Cervical dilation
    e. Measurement of bony pelvis

14-31. Which of the following laboratory tests should be repeated at every prenatal visit?

    a. Hematocrit
    b. Serologic test for syphilis
    c. Cervical culture for gonorrhea
    d. Urine test for protein
    e. Urine test for glucose

14-32. Which of the following is generally recommended guidelines for prenatal screening?

    a. Screening of maternal serum for alphafetoprotein concentration at 16 to 18 weeks' gestation

    b. For women at risk, diabetic screening between 24 and 28 weeks' gestation

    c. Those women with previous venereal disease should be screened for *Chlamydia trachomatis* at the first prenatal visit and again in the third trimester

    d. Serologic testing for human immunodeficiency virus in all gravidas

14-33. The neonatal mortality rate for low birth weight infants (less than 2,500 g) is approximately _____ times as high as for infants weighing more than 2,500 g.

14-34. The nutritional status of the expectant mother is more likely to be compromised in which of the following circumstances?

    a. She is less than 16 years old.
    b. She is economically deprived.
    c. She is pregnant for the third time within 2 years.
    d. She smokes, drinks, or uses hard drugs.
    e. She is underweight at the onset of pregnancy.
    f. Her weight gain for any month during the second and third trimesters is less than 2 pounds.

14-35. Which of the following statements about weight gain in pregnancy is correct?

    a. During a normal pregnancy with a single fetus, there is a physiologic basis for a weight gain of at least 9 kg.

    b. Birth weight is influenced by total maternal caloric intake.

    c. A balanced diet is the most appropriate way for a pregnant woman to obtain needed calories.

    d. Exact recommendations regarding maternal weight gain are difficult to determine.

14-36. The recommended daily caloric increase throughout pregnancy is _____ kcal.

14-37. Which of the following statements about protein requirements in pregnancy is correct?

    a. When insufficient calories are available, protein may be metabolized rather than being spared for fetal growth and development.

    b. An additional 30 g of protein above the normal nonpregnant requirement is recommended during pregnancy.

    c. Milk and milk products are the ideal sources for additional protein in all pregnant women.

    d. Protein from animal or vegetable sources is equally satisfactory as a source of protein during pregnancy.

14-38. List the minerals that should be added to the diet of a pregnant woman who consumes sufficient calories for appropriate weight gain.

14-39. Which of the following statements about iron ingestion in pregnancy is correct?

    a. Total average iron requirements during the latter part of pregnancy are 7 mg per day.

    b. The majority of women have sufficient iron stores for the increased requirements of pregnancy.

    c. Dietary iron can usually adequately supplement any deficient iron stores.

    d. Thirty mg of iron as a simple salt is the minimum daily supplement recommended.

    e. Calcium and magnesium contained in some vitamin-mineral supplements can impair the absorption of iron.

14–40. Iron supplementation during pregnancy

a. Is not necessary during the first 4 months
b. Can cause congenital malformations and impaired fetal well-being
c. Can exacerbate first trimester nausea and vomiting
d. Should be taken at night to minimize any adverse gastrointestinal reactions

14–41. Which of the following statements about calcium in pregnancy is correct?

a. Calcium supplementation in pregnancy is necessary in women over 30 to avoid the possibility of osteomalacia.
b. Maternal calcium is readily mobilized as needed for fetal growth.
c. There is increased absorption of calcium through the intestine in pregnancy.
d. The amount of calcium retained in pregnancy represents 25 percent of total maternal calcium.

14–42. Which of the following statements about zinc in pregnancy is correct?

a. Severe zinc deficiency may lead to impaired wound healing.
b. Profound zinc deficiency may lead to acrodermatitis enteropathica.
c. Zinc in plasma is mainly in the ionized, unbound form.
d. There is no strong evidence that zinc supplementation has any material or fetal benefits.
e. Low maternal zinc levels lead to babies who are small for gestational age.

14–43. Which of the following statements about dietary supplementation during pregnancy is correct?

a. Phosphorus is commonly inadequate in western diets.
b. Severe maternal iodine deficiency in expectant mothers predisposes the fetus to cretinism.
c. Fetal goiter may result from maternal ingestion of large amounts of seaweed or iodine.
d. Magnesium deficiency as a consequence of pregnancy alone occurs in about 25 percent of women.
e. Hypokalemia develops in the same ways in pregnant and in nonpregnant women.

14–44. Sodium restriction in pregnancy reduces the incidence of preeclampsia.

a. True
b. False

14–45. Which of the following statements concerning fluoride supplementation in pregnancy is correct?

a. Supplemental fluoride taken by the lactating mother increases the fluoride concentration in her milk.
b. Supplemental fluoride increases fetal bone density.
c. Offspring of mothers who ingest sodium fluoride during pregnancy have fewer caries.

14–46. There is abundant evidence that the usual vitamin supplements are of significant benefit to the fetus but of little benefit to the mother.

a. True
b. False

14–47. Which of the following statements about folic acid supplementation in pregnancy is correct?

a. Folic acid supply is more likely to be inadequate when pregnancy is complicated by prolonged vomiting or multiple fetuses.
b. Administration of folic acid during pregnancy can reduce the incidence of neural tube defects.
c. One mg of folic acid orally per day should provide sufficient supplementation when needed.

14–48. Which of the following statements about vitamin B_{12} in pregnancy is correct?

a. Vitamin B_{12} levels in maternal plasma decrease variably in normal pregnancies.
b. Strict vegetarians may give birth to infants whose vitamin B_{12} stores are low.
c. The breast milk of a vegetarian mother contains little vitamin B_{12}.
d. Excessive ingestion of vitamin C can lead to a functional deficiency of vitamin B_{12}.

14–49. Vitamin B_6

a. Deficiency induces excessive excretion of xanthurenic acid after ingestion of a trytophan load
b. Deficiency leads to a lowering of the biologic activity of endogenous insulin
c. Ingestion in large excess can lead to nervous system dysfunction
d. Requirements in pregnancy are twice those for nonpregnant women

14–50. Large doses of vitamin C, ingested by the pregnant woman for the prevention of colds, have been shown to have no deleterious effects on the fetus.

a. True
b. False

Instructions for Items 14–51 to 14–57: Match the following circumstances involving vitamins with the appropriate associated abnormal or pathologic conditions.

a. Vitamin C excess
b. Iodine deficiency
c. Iodine excess
d. Folic acid deficiency
e. Zinc deficiency
f. Vitamin D deficiency
g. Vitamin B$_{12}$ deficiency
h. Vitamin B$_6$ excess

14-51. Fetal cretinism
14-52. Hypersegmented neutrophils
14-53. Acrodermatitis enteropathica
14-54. Fetal goiter
14-55. Scurvy
14-56. Megaloblastic anemia
14-57. Progressive sensory ataxia

14-58. Which of the following nutritional recommendations should be made to pregnant women?

a. Eat certain foods regardless of food preferences.
b. Gain at least 20 pounds.
c. Take tablets of simple iron salts providing 30 to 60 mg of iron daily.
d. Do not add salt to food.

14-59. In general, it is not necessary for a pregnant woman to limit exercise, assuming she has been previously involved in a similar program of aerobic exercise.

a. True
b. False

14-60. Which of the following pregnancy complications may benefit from limitation of exercise?

a. Pregnancy-induced hypertension
b. Multiple fetuses
c. Intrauterine growth retardation
d. Breech presentation

14-61. Which of the following statements about employment during pregnancy is correct?

a. Severe physical strain should be avoided.
b. Work should not cause undue fatigue.
c. Adequate rest should be provided during the work day.
d. Women with repetitive complications of pregnancy should minimize physical work.

14-62. Which of the following statements about travel during pregnancy is correct?

a. Travel, especially in airplanes, should be avoided in pregnancy.
b. At least every 2 hours, the pregnant woman should walk about.
c. The greatest risk with international travel is the development of a pregnancy complication remote from adequate treatment facilities.

14-63. Which articles of clothing should be avoided in pregnancy?

a. Jeans
b. Constricting garters
c. Pantyhose
d. High-heeled shoes

14-64. All laxatives should be avoided by the pregnant woman.

a. True
b. False

14-65. Coitus should be avoided during pregnancy.

a. True
b. False

14-66. What limitations to douching in pregnancy should be emphasized?

a. Only hand bulb syringes should be used.
b. The douche bag should be not more than 2 feet above the level of the hips.
c. The nozzle should not be inserted more than 3 inches through the vulva.
d. The pregnant woman should only douche once a week.

14-67. Massage and ointments reduce the incidence of striae on the breast and the abdomen.

a. True
b. False

14-68. Smoking during pregnancy is associated with an increased incidence of

a. Perinatal death
b. Maternal hypertension
c. Low birth weight infants
d. Diabetes in pregnancy

14-69. Which of the following have been implicated to explain the adverse effects of smoking during pregnancy?

a. Inactivation of fetal and maternal hemoglobin by carbon monoxide.
b. A vasoconstrictor action of nicotine which causes reduced perfusion of the placenta.
c. Reduced appetite and, in turn, reduced caloric intake in women who smoke.
d. Decreased plasma volume in women who smoke.

14-70. Fetal alcohol syndrome is associated with

a. Craniofacial anomalies
b. Anomalies of the limbs
c. Cardiovascular defects
d. Growth retardation
e. Impaired gross and fine motor function
f. Impaired speech

14–71. The chronic use of which of the following drugs is associated with harmful fetal effects such as intrauterine distress and low birth weight?

    a. Marijuana
    b. Opium derivatives
    c. Barbiturates
    d. Amphetamines
    e. Caffeine

14–72. Which of the following immunizations are contraindicated during pregnancy

    a. Influenza
    b. Measles
    c. Mumps
    d. Typhoid
    e. Rubella
    f. Hepatitis A

14–73. The placenta serves as an effective barrier to most drugs, even those that exert a systemic effect in the mother.

    a. True
    b. False

14–74. Which of the following statements about the nausea and vomiting of pregnancy is correct?

    a. It only occurs in the morning.
    b. It usually disappears by the fourth month.
    c. The severity of vomiting is correlated with serum levels of chorionic gonadotropins.
    d. Therapeutic abortion is frequently the only successful therapy for severe nausea (hyperemesis gravidarum).
    e. Pregnancies with nausea and vomiting are more likely to have a favorable outcome.

14–75. Which of the following statements about backache in pregnancy is correct?

    a. A lightweight maternity girdle may afford relief in mild cases.
    b. Disc herniation is more frequent during pregnancy.
    c. Back pain may be due to general relaxation of pelvic ligaments and motion in the lumbosacral joints.

14–76. Surgical correction of varicosities of the lower extremities is often necessary to provide relief during pregnancy.

    a. True
    b. False

14–77. Which of the following statements about hemorrhoids in pregnancy is correct?

    a. Development of hemorrhoids is related to obstruction of venous return by the enlarging uterus.
    b. Bleeding from hemorrhoidal veins may result in blood loss sufficient to cause iron deficiency anemia.
    c. Hemorrhoids usually become asymptomatic after delivery.
    d. Pain and swelling are usually relieved by stool softeners, warm soaks, and topical anesthetics.

14–78. Sodium hydroxide is the antacid of choice for the treatment of heartburn in pregnancy.

    a. True
    b. False

14–79. Pica results primarily from an unconscious response to subtle physiologic needs for trace elements.

    a. True
    b. False

14–80. Which of the following is more common early in pregnancy than late in pregnancy?

    a. Backache
    b. Fatigue
    c. Heartburn
    d. Headache
    e. Hemorrhoids

14–81. Which of the following statements about vaginitis and vaginal discharge in pregnancy is correct?

    a. Increased cervical mucus production in response to hyperestrogenemia is the most common cause of increased vaginal discharge in pregnancy.
    b. *Trichomonas vaginalis* vaginitis may be treated with metronidazole.
    c. *Candida albicans* vaginitis in pregnancy may be successfully treated with miconazole nitrate cream.
    d. Candidiasis is likely to recur during pregnancy.

15. TECHNIQUES TO EVALUATE FETAL HEALTH

15–1. Which of the following factors have contributed to the relatively recent fall in the perinatal death rate?

    a. Family planning programs
    b. Legalized elective abortion
    c. Better, more available antepartum care
    d. Selective therapeutic abortion
    e. Liberal hospitalization practices
    f. Greater attention to evaluation of fetal well-being
    g. Increased cesarean birth rate
    h. Available, high quality neonatal care

15-2. Which of the following is a risk from amniocentesis?

a. Abortion
b. Rh isoimmunization
c. Placental hemorrhage
d. Trauma to the umbilical cord
e. Intrauterine fetal infection
f. Premature labor

15-3. Which of the following categories of disorders contain diseases diagnosable by amnionic fluid analysis?

a. Chromosomal anomalies
b. Skeletal disorders
c. Fetal infections
d. Central nervous system diseases
e. Hematologic disorders
f. Inborn errors of metabolism

15-4. Undesirable outcomes from amniocentesis may be minimized by

a. Performing the amniocentesis puncture suprapubically
b. Examining the newly delivered infant as soon as possible for evidence of trauma
c. Locating the placenta sonographically in any case where clinical examination is inadequate
d. Administering prophylactic anti-Rho(D) globulin to nonsensitized Rh(D) negative women

15-5. Which of the following factors increases the risk of fetal injury during amniocentesis?

a. Small volume of amnionic fluid
b. Thick amnionic fluid
c. Postterm pregnancy
d. Repeated taps
e. Use of a large (18-gauge) needle

15-6. In what circumstances should the fetal heart rate be closely monitored following amniocentesis?

15-7. The overall accuracy of prenatal diagnosis from amniocentesis performed near midpregnancy is approximately _____ percent.

a. 70
b. 80
c. 90
d. 95
e. 99

15-8. Which of the following statements about bloody taps obtained during amniocentesis is correct?

a. Erythrocytes may inhibit the replication in culture of fetal cells.
b. Small amounts of maternal blood can lead to falsely high levels of α-fetoprotein in amnionic fluid.
c. Blood in the amnionic fluid produces a lowered L/S ratio.
d. Amnionic fluid should be considered unsatisfactory for measurement of L/S ratios if the hematocrit of a spun sample exceeds 1 percent.

15-9. Surface-active phospholipids are produced in fetal lung alveoli by _____ .

15-10. In amnionic fluid, the concentration of lecithin relative to sphingomyelin begins to rise at _____ weeks of gestation?

a. 28
b. 30
c. 32
d. 34
e. 36
f. 38

15-11. Which of the following statements about the L/S ratio in amnionic fluid is correct?

a. Slight variations in technique can significantly affect the accuracy of the results.
b. When the L/S ratio is 1.5 or below, a majority of infants develop respiratory distress.
c. An L/S ratio of less than 1.0 is incompatible with fetal survival.
d. An L/S ratio of 2.0 or greater precludes the development of respiratory distress.

15-12. When the L/S ratio is below 1.5, the death rate among newborns is approximately _____ percent.

15-13. In which of the following situations is there a significant possibility that an infant may develop respiratory distress even if the L/S ratio is 2.0 or more?

a. Class A maternal diabetes
b. Class B maternal diabetes
c. Esophageal atresia
d. Erythroblastosis fetalis
e. Gestational age less than 36 weeks

15-14. The identification of which of the following in amnionic fluid suggests that respiratory distress syndrome is less likely to develop.

a. Phosphatidylglycerol
b. Lecithin
c. Sphingomyelin
d. Phosphatidylinositol

15-15. Which of the following tests is used to determine the presence of surfactant in amnionic fluid?

a. L/S ratio
b. Phosphatidylglycerol measurement
c. Foam stability test
d. Lumadex-FSI test
e. Fluorescent polarization
f. Amnionic fluid absorbence at 650 nm

15-16. In the foam stability test, a false-positive result is more common than a false-negative result.

a. True
b. False

15-17. Which of the following statements about amnionic fluid bilirubin is correct?

a. Hemolysis yields bilirubin, most of which remains unconjugated by the fetus.
b. Fetal bilirubin reaches the amnionic fluid by way of the fetal urine.
c. The amount of bilirubin in amnionic fluid normally falls during the last few weeks of pregnancy.
d. Amnionic fluid bilirubin is best measured by chemical means.

15-18. In which of the following cases is amnionic fluid bilirubin usually elevated?

a. Maternal hyperbilirubinemia
b. Maternal sickle cell anemia
c. Fetal hemolytic disease
d. Intrauterine growth retardation

15-19. Chromosomal analysis of fetal somatic cells is often of value in which of the following circumstances?

a. Pregnancy after three or more spontaneous abortions
b. Pregnancy in a woman over 35 years of age
c. A previous child or parent with a neural tube defect
d. Down syndrome in a close family member
e. A previous infant born with multiple major malformations

Instructions for Items 15-20 to 15-25: Match the clinical state or procedure with its appropriate descriptor.

a. Increased incidence of orthopedic defects
b. Associated with increased α-fetoprotein
c. Decreases risks from amniocentesis
d. Decreases risk of placental perforation
e. Presents obstacle to growth of fetal cells in culture
f. Increases risk of serious fetal bleeding

15-20. Suprapubic amniocentesis
15-21. Ultrasound guidance
15-22. Blood contamination of amnionic fluid
15-23. Low amnionic fluid volume

15-24. Anti D globulin given to the mother
15-25. Cord around the neck

15-26. Which of the following has been clinically used to evaluate fetal blood?

a. Scalp puncture
b. Cordocentesis
c. Fetoscopy
d. Blind fetal aspiration

15-27. The L/S ratio of maternal serum is approximately

a. 0.6 to 0.9
b. 1.3 to 1.5
c. 3.0 to 3.3
d. No measurable L/S is present

15-28. The problem with the foam stability test (shake test) is most commonly _____ results.

a. false-positive
b. false-negative
c. lack of true-positive
d. truly negative

Instructions for Items 15-29 to 15-31: Match the test of pulmonary lung maturity with the appropriate descriptor.

a. Nearly 100 percent accurate in predicting fetal lung maturity
b. Slight error in the test procedure or materials may greatly influence this test
c. Interpreted as a numeric value

15-29. L/S ratio
15-30. Foam stability test
15-31. Test for phosphatidylglycerol

15-32. Fetal blood carbon dioxide tension and plasma lactate concentration _____ with gestational age.

a. Increase
b. Decrease
c. Do not change
d. None of the above are correct

15-33. Indications for fetal blood sampling include which of the following?

a. Karyotyping
b. Diagnosis of certain genetic diseases
c. Evaluation of fetal hypoxia
d. Management of hemolytic disease

15-34. Real time ultrasound works by

a. Ionizing radiation
b. Detection of movement
c. Heating of tissues
d. Listening for fetal sounds

Instructions for Items 15-35 to 15-38: Match the amnionic fluid component with the appropriate procedure.

    a. Amnionic fluid supernatant
    b. Amnionic fluid cell sample

15-35. Determination of genetic sex
15-36. Determination of fetal lung maturity
15-37. Detection of hemolytic disease of the newborn
15-38. Detection of fetal neural tube defects

15-39. Fetal breathing motion is undetectable on ultrasonography.

    a. True
    b. False

15-40. Doppler waveform analysis is a routine and widely available technique to evaluate fetal health.

    a. True
    b. False

15-41. Ultrasonography may be used to determine

    a. The presence of intrauterine pregnancy
    b. The presence of multiple fetuses
    c. Gestational age
    d. Abnormal amounts of amnionic fluid
    e. Placental location
    f. Placental abnormalities

15-42. Which of the following statements about fetal motion as detected by real time ultrasonography is correct?

    a. Fetal heart beat has been demonstrated by 7 weeks of gestation.
    b. Fetal trunk movement has been demonstrated by 8 weeks of gestation.
    c. Fetal limb movement has been demonstrated by 9 weeks of gestation.
    d. Filling and emptying of the fetal bladder have been demonstrated.

15-43. For which of the following determinations is ultrasonography more precise than radiography?

    a. Fetal age
    b. Placental localization
    c. Fetal size
    d. Identification of hydatidiform mole

Instructions for Items 15-44 to 15-46: Match the procedure with its application.

    a. Amnioscopy
    b. Fetoscopy
    c. Amniography
    d. Fetography

15-44. Direct visualization of the fetus and placenta
15-45. Visualization of meconium-stained amnionic fluid
15-46. Identification of external fetal outline
15-47. Which of the following statements regarding fetal blood sampling is true?

    a. Fetal scalp blood sampling is generally limited to an intrapartum technique.
    b. Fetoscopic blood sampling is associated with a fetal loss rate of about 5 percent.
    c. Blood from the fetal umbilical cord can be obtained by venipuncture under ultrasound guidance.
    d. Cordocentesis has about the same level of fetal risk as does amniocentesis.

15-48. Which of the following contraindicate or complicate amnioscopy?

    a. Inadvertent rupture of the membranes
    b. Inaccessible cervix
    c. Possibility of infection
    d. Lack of cervical dilation

15-49. Using Doppler ultrasound, which of the following are true?

    a. Doppler ultrasound can be used to detect the movement of fetal red blood cells within fetal vessels.
    b. The shape of the systolic portion of the fetal arterial waveform has been used to identify fetal growth retardation.
    c. It has been confirmed that the Frank-Starling mechanism is operative even in the fetus.
    d. Doppler study is generally ineffectual in the evaluation of multifetal gestation.

15-50. Which of the following statements about fetal movement is correct?

    a. The number of fetal movements increases progressively until delivery.
    b. The pattern of fetal movement may be exactly correlated with gestational age.
    c. The absolute number of fetal movements per day is less important than the degree of change in the frequency of fetal movements.
    d. A marked increase in movement is an indication of fetal well-being.
    e. A sudden decrease in movement is a sign of possible loss of fetal well-being.

15–51. Which of the following does *not* describe a contraction stress test?

  a. Usually takes 1 to 2 hours
  b. Actual intrauterine pressure is measured
  c. An ultrasound transducer is utilized
  d. Maternal blood pressure is recorded
  e. Oxytocin is administered intramuscularly

15–52. Which of the following conditions may contraindicate the use of oxytocin to perform a fetal contraction stress test?

  a. Multiple fetuses
  b. An L/S ratio less than 2
  c. Previous classical cesarean section
  d. Previous multiple pregnancy
  e. Hydramnios
  f. Threatened preterm labor
  g. Placenta previa
  h. Rupture of the membranes
  i. Previous preterm labor

15–53. A contraction stress test is indicated at any time in the second or third trimester when the fetus is suspected of being in jeopardy.

  a. True
  b. False

Instructions for Items 15–54 to 15–58: Match the following interpretations for a contraction stress test with their best descriptions.

  a. Positive
  b. Negative
  c. Suspicious
  d. Hyperstimulation
  e. Unsatisfactory

15–54. At least three contractions in 10 minutes, each lasting at least 40 seconds, are identified without late decelerations of the fetal heart rate.

15–55. If uterine contractions are more frequent than every 2 minutes, or last longer than 90 seconds, or persistent uterine hypertonus is suspected.

15–56. There is inconstant late deceleration that does not persist with subsequent contractions.

15–57. The frequency of contractions is less than three per 10 minutes or the tracing is poor.

15–58. There is consistent and persistent late deceleration of the fetal heart rate.

15–59. If a contraction stress test is negative, it is usually repeated.

  a. Monthly
  b. Biweekly
  c. Weekly
  d. Weekly for 2 weeks, than monthly

15–60. A negative contraction stress test is *not* always compatible with placental function sufficient to maintain the fetus alive for at least 1 week.

  a. True
  b. False

15–61. False-negative contraction stress tests occur about _____ percent of the time.

15–62. A positive contraction stress test is sufficiently ominous to warrant interruption of pregnancy within 24 hours.

  a. True
  b. False

15–63. Fetal movement is typically accompanied by transient _____ of the fetal heart rate.

  a. Acceleration
  b. Deceleration

15–64. A nonstress test is generally considered reactive when

_____ .

15–65. No test of fetal well-being provides complete reassurance.

  a. True
  b. False

15–66. The biophysical profile entails which of the following components?

  a. A reactive nonstress test
  b. A negative contractions stress test
  c. Fetal movement with three or more discrete body or limb movements within 30 minutes
  d. A minimum of ten fetal movements per day felt by the gravida
  e. Fetal tone defined as one or more episodes of limb extension with return to flexion within 30 minutes.
  f. One or more pockets of amniotic fluid, 1 or more cm in diameters in two perpendicular planes
  g. Absence of meconium fluid on amniocentesis
  h. Apgar score of 7 or greater or a fetal scalp sampling of pH 7.2 or greater
  i. Fetal breathing movements consisting of at least one episode of at least 30 seconds

15–67. Which of the following statements about biophysical profile are true?

  a. A modified test has been performed that omits fetal breathing movements.
  b. The false-negative rate for this test is about 1 per 1,000.
  c. Scores of 4 or less are very predictive of intrapartum distress.
  d. Some examiners have added placental grading to the biophysical profile.

15-68. The internal spiral electrode should *not* be attached to the

a. Face
b. Buttocks
c. Genitalia
d. Fontanels
e. Extremities

15-69. Which method of monitoring the fetal heart rate is most accurate?

a. Ultrasound Doppler principle
b. Internal spiral electrode
c. Phonocardiography
d. Fetal electrocardiogram

15-70. Which of the following statements about intrapartum fetal monitoring is correct?

a. Dependable monitoring requires electronic detecting and recording devices.
b. Internal monitoring of heart rate requires a spiral electrode to be propelled through the fetal skin.
c. Intrauterine pressure measurement equipment presents a potential risk to the placenta.
d. External monitoring of uterine pressure and fetal heart rate is less precise than internal monitoring.

15-71. Fetal acidosis (pH < 7.2) is unlikely as long as a fetal heart rate beat-to-beat variability is present.

a. True
b. False

Instructions for Items 15-72 to 15-74: Match the baseline fetal heart rate with the appropriate description.

a. Marked bradycardia
b. Mild bradycardia
c. Normal
d. Mild tachycardia
e. Marked tachycardia

15-72. 120 to 160 beats per minute
15-73. <100 beats per minute
15-74. 161 to 180 beats per minute

15-75. Periodic fetal heart rate is defined as _____ .

Instructions for Items 15-76 to 15-78: Match the fetal heart rate deceleration pattern listed below with the clinical cause with which it is best associated.

a. Early (type I)
b. Late (type II)
c. Variable

15-76. Cord compression
15-77. Uteroplacental insufficiency
15-78. Compression of fetal head

Instructions for Items 15-79 to 15-84: Match the type of deceleration with the appropriate description.

a. Early (type I)
b. Late (type II)
c. Variable

15-79. Associated with vagus nerve stimulation
15-80. Corrected by administering atropine to the mother
15-81. A change in maternal position may be helpful
15-82. Potentially dangerous for the fetus
15-83. Slowing of heart at the beginning of a contraction
15-84. Slowing of heart as contraction peaks

15-85. Which of the following may result in the absence of beat-to-beat variability in fetal heart rate?

a. Prematurity
b. Fetal sleep state
c. Morphine
d. Magnesium sulfate
e. Meperidine

15-86. Which of the following statements about fetal heart rate patterns is correct?

a. A sinusoidal pattern may be due to maternal medication.
b. Mild bradycardia without acceleration or deceleration is usually associated with fetal distress.
c. Persistent tachycardia without deceleration may be due to hypoxia.
d. Fetal bradycardia may be associated with maternal hypothermia.
e. Distinguishing fetal from maternal heart rate is often difficult.
f. Fetal arrhythmias must be corrected to a normal rate and rhythm to assure fetal well-being.

Instructions for Items 15-87 to 15-89: Match the fetal heart rate pattern with the appropriate statement.

a. Sinusoidal
b. Persistent fetal tachycardia
c. Mild persistent fetal bradycardia
d. Severe persistent fetal bradycardia

15-87. Identified in severely anemic fetuses
15-88. Present with congenital fetal heart block
15-89. Response to maternal febrile illness

15–90. Which of the following is an integral part of fetal blood sampling?

  a. Ruptured membranes
  b. Ethyl chloride spray
  c. Skin incision
  d. Heparinized capillary tube

Instructions for Items 15–91 to 15–93: Match the confirmed fetal blood pH with the appropriate management.

  a. Observation of labor
  b. Repeat pH determination in less than 30 minutes
  c. Immediate delivery (abdominal or vaginal)

15–91. pH 7.10
15–92. pH 7.20
15–93. pH 7.30

15–94. Which of the following statements about fetal blood pH is correct?

  a. A fall in pH is an early indication of hypoxia.
  b. Fetal blood pH is appreciably influenced by maternal pH.
  c. Fetal blood pH is a better indication of hypoxia than P_{O_2}.
  d. Continuous transcutaneous monitoring of fetal oxygen is a better predictor of fetal distress than pH.

15–95. What are potential direct dangers of amniotomy?

  a. Fetal trauma
  b. Infection
  c. Cord prolapse
  d. Precipitous loss of amnionic fluid
  e. Hemorrhage

15–96. Which of the following is a potential danger from internal fetal monitoring?

  a. Early amniotomy
  b. Fetal trauma
  c. Placental trauma
  d. Fetal infection

15–97. External monitoring techniques are without known direct or indirect risk to mother and fetus.

  a. True
  b. False

15–98. In which conditions can bleeding from the site of fetal blood sampling be particularly troublesome?

  a. Diabetes
  b. Hypertension
  c. Delivery by vacuum extractor
  d. Deficiency of vitamin K-dependent coagulation factors
  e. Hemophilia

15–99. Systematic clinical monitoring has in no case been shown to be as effective as electronic monitoring for ensuring fetal well-being.

  a. True
  b. False

16. CONDUCT OF NORMAL LABOR AND DELIVERY

16–1. Which of the following are elements of natural childbirth?

  a. Elimination of fear
  b. Elimination of pain
  c. Antepartum education
  d. Exercises to promote relaxation
  e. Elimination of anesthetics

Instructions for Items 16–2 to 16–6: Select the characteristics of the contractions of true or false labor.

  a. True labor
  b. False labor

16–2. Occur at irregular intervals
16–3. Cervix dilates
16–4. Not stopped by sedation
16–5. Intensity remains the same
16–6. Discomfort mostly in the lower abdomen

16–7. A woman should be told to be sure she is in true labor before reporting to her health care provider.

  a. True
  b. False

16–8. Questions that should be a routine part of the basic admission procedures for a woman in labor include

  a. Frequency of uterine contractions
  b. Intensity of uterine contractions
  c. Time when uterine contractions became uncomfortable
  d. Degree and quality of uterine contraction discomfort
  e. Whether fluid has leaked from the vagina
  f. Whether there has been bleeding from the vagina

16–9. The best way to ascertain the significance of vaginal bleeding in late pregnancy is a pelvic examination at the time of admission to the labor area.

  a. True
  b. False

16–10. Which statements about the initial vaginal examination during labor are correct?

 a. If bleeding greater than a bloody show is present, the examination must be done with a sterile speculum.
 b. A sterile speculum examination always precedes the digital examination.
 c. The cervix is examined for softness, position, dilation, and effacement.
 d. The presenting part and station should be ascertained.
 e. X-ray pelvimetry to evaluate pelvic architecture should be obtained as early in labor as possible.
 f. Distensibility of the vagina and firmness of the perineum should be assessed.

16–11. If the cervix is one-fourth of its original length, it is _____ effaced.

 a. 25 percent
 b. 50 percent
 c. 75 percent
 d. 100 percent

16–12. The cervix is fully dilated when it has opened about _____ cm.

 a. 8
 b. 9
 c. 10
 d. 11

16–13. Which of the possible positions of the cervix is suggestive of premature labor?

 a. Anterior
 b. Midposition
 c. Posterior

16–14. Which of the following statements about the evaluation of station is correct?

 a. It identifies the level of the presenting part in the birth canal.
 b. If the presenting part is at the level of the ischial spines, it is at 0 station.
 c. Progressive dilation of the cervix without a change of station implies fetopelvic disproportion.
 d. If the vertex is at 0 station, it is certain that engagement of the fetal head has occurred.

16–15. If the presenting part is located two-thirds of the distance from the plane of the pelvic inlet to the midplane of the pelvis, its station is said to be

 a. −3
 b. −2
 c. −1
 d. 0
 e. +1
 f. +2
 g. +3

16–16. Which of the following make rupture of the membranes a significant occurrence?

 a. Risk of infection
 b. Imminent onset of labor
 c. Risk of cord prolapse
 d. Risk of maternal hypovolemia

16–17. The normal pH of vaginal fluid is about _____ $_{(1)}$, whereas that of amnionic fluid is usually _____ $_{(2)}$.

16–18. Which of the following statements about rupture of the membranes is correct?

 a. No test for detection of rupture of the membranes is completely reliable.
 b. Amnionic fluid is more acidic than vaginal secretions.
 c. Nitrazine paper turns blue if in contact with amnionic fluid.
 d. The nitrazine test may provide a falsely positive reading if there is excessive bloody show.

16–19. Which of the following statements about the care of a woman in labor is correct?

 a. Shaving of the perineum is necessary for hygiene.
 b. For the fetus, rectal examinations are considerably safer than vaginal examinations.
 c. Enemas are recommended to stimulate labor.
 d. The hematocrit or hemoglobin concentration should be rechecked on admission.

16–20. Since the average duration of the first stage of labor is 8 hours in the nullipara and 5 hours in the multipara, a woman in the first stage of labor may be given reasonably accurate assurances as to the time of delivery.

 a. True
 b. False

16–21. Which of the following statements about monitoring fetal heart rate during labor is correct?

 a. All women must be electronically monitored during labor.
 b. The best interval for monitoring of fetal heart tones in the first stage of labor is undetermined.
 c. Fetal distress is suspected if the fetal heart rate is less than 120 beats per minute.
 d. Maternal tachycardia may be misinterpreted as a normal fetal heart rate.

16–22. Which statements about the management of labor are correct?

  a. Intensity of uterine contractions may be gauged manually.
  b. Trained labor room personnel can provide care that may lead to outcomes as good as with electronic monitoring.
  c. The patient must not be allowed to lie in the supine position.
  d. There is some evidence that routine electronic monitoring of ''low risk'' pregnancy may increase the chance of cesarean section with improving perinatal morbidity or mortality.
  e. Maternal vital signs may vary relative to a contraction.

16–23. Which of the following contribute to the decision to administer analgesia in labor?

  a. Degree of discomfort
  b. Amount of cervical dilation
  c. Pattern of labor
  d. Estimated interval of time until delivery

16–24. Which of the following statements about amniotomy is correct?

  a. Amniotomy will significantly shorten the first stage of labor.
  b. Amniotomy is beneficial to the fetus.
  c. Aseptic technique is required.
  d. Care must be taken not to dislodge the fetal head from the pelvis.
  e. Amniotomy is hazardous to maternal health.

16–25. Which of the following statements about nutrition in labor is correct?

  a. Gastric emptying time is reduced during labor.
  b. Intravenous fluids should be initiated upon admission to the hospital.
  c. Fluids should be minimized in order to reduce urine production.
  d. Food and oral fluids should be withheld during active labor.

16–26. Which of the following statements about urinary bladder function in labor is correct?

  a. Bladder distention can obstruct labor.
  b. A woman in labor is unable to void without catheterization.
  c. All women should have an indwelling bladder catheter.
  d. Bladder hypotonia and infection may be sequelae of overdistention.

16–27. Active management of labor

  a. Refers to attempts to speed delivery by augmentation
  b. Has been shown in at least one randomized trial not to reduce rates of cesarean section
  c. Dramatically lowers cesarean section rates
  d. Results in lowered perinatal mortality and morbidity

16–28. For all term singleton pregnancies, the second stage of labor lasts between 20 and 50 minutes.

  a. True
  b. False

16–29. Which of the following statements about fetal heart rate in the second stage of labor is correct?

  a. The fetal heart rate should be identified more frequently than during the first stage.
  b. Slowing of the fetal heart rate is due solely to fetal head compression.
  c. Reduction of uterine volume due to fetal descent may trigger premature placental separation.
  d. Blood flow through the umbilical cord may be compromised as loops of cord tighten around the fetus.
  e. Failure of the fetal heart rate to recover between uterine contractions is abnormal.

16–30. During the second stage of labor,

  a. The desire to bear down is reflex and spontaneous
  b. The woman should be coached to ''push'' as much as possible regardless of the duration of the contraction
  c. Expulsion of feces indicates imminent delivery
  d. The mother should be informed of the progress of labor

16–31. The most common position used for vaginal delivery is the _____ .

16–32. Leg cramping during delivery may occur as a result of pressure on pelvic nerves, and requires no action beyond reassurance to the mother.

  a. True
  b. False

16–33. Which of the following measures assures a noninfected outcome after vaginal delivery?

  a. Use of scrub suit, mask, and hat
  b. Perineal scrubbing
  c. Sterile drapes
  d. Sterile gloves
  e. Careful hand washing

16–34. The encirclement of the largest diameter of the fetal head by the vulvar ring is known as _____ .

16-35. Which statements about the delivery of the fetal head are correct?

   a. The vulvovaginal opening may become smaller between contractions.
   b. As the perineum thins, the anterior wall of the rectum may become visible through the anus.
   c. A properly timed episiotomy can prevent the long-term sequelae of pelvic relaxation.

16-36. The obstetric maneuver by which the physician facilitates delivery of the head is called the _____ .

16-37. What should always be done before delivery of the fetal shoulders?

   a. Wipe face
   b. Aspirate nares
   c. Aspirate mouth
   d. Check for nuchal cord

16-38. Which of the following statements about the delivery of the fetal shoulders is correct?

   a. In most cases the shoulders are born spontaneously.
   b. Any traction should be directed in the long axis of the fetus.
   c. Delivery of the shoulders occurs when they are in the transverse diameter of the pelvis.
   d. Hooking a finger in the axillae should be done to deliver the anterior shoulder only.
   e. Gushing of amnionic fluid tinged with blood after delivery of the infant is an ominous sign.

16-39. Direct causes of fetal nerve injury during delivery include

   a. Traction in the axillae
   b. Oblique traction to the fetal head
   c. Pressure on the uterine fundus
   d. Poorly timed episiotomy

16-40. Which of the following statements about the management of the placenta and umbilical cord at delivery is correct?

   a. Nuchal cord occurs in about 55 percent of cases.
   b. If a nuchal cord cannot be slipped over the baby's head, it may be clamped and cut provided the infant is delivered promptly thereafter.
   c. After delivery of the baby, the cord should usually be clamped within about 1 cm of the baby's abdomen.
   d. If the infant is placed at the level of the vaginal introitus or below before the cord is clamped, blood will be shifted from the placenta to the infant (infant transfusion).
   e. Infant transfusion should be avoided as the circulatory overload is always dangerous to the infant.
   f. Neonatal hyperbilirubinemia may result from infant transfusion.

16-41. Which of the following is a sign of placental separation?

   a. The uterus becomes globular and usually firmer.
   b. A sudden gush of blood occurs in many cases.
   c. A sudden transient drop in maternal blood pressure and rise in pulse rate occurs.
   d. The uterus rises in the abdomen.
   e. The umbilical cord protrudes farther out of the vaginal opening.
   f. A significant decrease in uterine pain occurs.

16-42. Which of the following is a correct statement about the management of the third stage of labor?

   a. Signs of placental separation usually appear within 1 to 5 minutes after delivery of the baby.
   b. As long as the uterus remains firm and there is no unusual bleeding, watchful waiting for spontaneous placental separation is usually acceptable practice.
   c. During placental separation and delivery, abdominal palpation of the uterus is indicated to be sure that the uterus is contracting and remaining firm.
   d. Placental expulsion should be hastened by traction on the umbilical cord.
   e. The placenta and membranes should be examined immediately after their delivery to ascertain their completeness.

16-43. Attempts to express the placenta before placental separation may result in _____ .

16-44. If there is brisk bleeding and the placenta cannot be expressed, manual removal is indicated.

   a. True
   b. False

16-45. Routine manual removal of the placenta has proven safe only under which of the following circumstances?

   a. A minimal number of vaginal examinations during labor
   b. A multiparous patient
   c. A properly prepared and draped perineum
   d. A delivery uncomplicated by bacterial contamination of the genital tract
   e. Satisfactory anesthesia

16-46. Following delivery of the placenta, which of the following should occur?

   a. Inspection of the placenta, membranes, and cord
   b. Administration of oxytocics
   c. Frequent monitoring for uterine atony
   d. Frequent inspection of the perineum for excessive bleeding

16-47. The primary mechanism by which hemostasis is achieved at the placental site is _____ .

16-48. Which of the following is an oxytocic commonly used in the third or fourth stage of labor?

a. Oxytocin
b. Ergonovine maleate
c. Epinephrine
d. Methylergonovine maleate

16-49. Which of the following statements about oxytocin is correct?

a. It is a naturally occurring decapeptide.
b. The half-life for intravenously infused oxytocin is about 3 minutes.
c. Oxytocin may cause postpartum uterine rupture.
d. It is effective if given by mouth, intravenously, or intramuscularly.
e. If given as a large intravenous bolus, it may cause maternal hypotension.
f. It may cause water intoxication if administered in a large volume of electrolyte-free IV solution.

16-50. Which of the following are characteristics of ergonovine and methylergonovine?

a. They stimulate myometrial contractions.
b. They can be administered intravenously, intramuscularly, or orally.
c. Parenteral administration can initiate transient hypertension.
d. They are dangerous to the fetus if administered before delivery.
e. The effects of these drugs may persist for hours.

16-51. What is a potential danger of oxytocin administration before delivery of the placenta?

Instructions for Items 16-52 to 16-55: Match the degree of laceration with the affected anatomy.

a. First degree
b. Second degree
c. Third degree
d. Fourth degree

16-52. Fascia and muscles of the perineal body
16-53. Anal sphincter
16-54. Vaginal mucous membrane and perineal skin
16-55. Rectal mucosa

16-56. Episiotomy

a. Substitutes a neat, straight surgical incision for a ragged laceration of the perineum and vagina
b. Is easier to repair, heals better, and is less painful than a birth canal laceration
c. Provides additional room for difficult deliveries (large babies, forceps deliveries, the breech)
d. Is commonly performed when the head is visible to a diameter of 3 to 4 cm during a contraction
e. Is commonly repaired after delivery of the placenta
f. Helps prevent the development of cystocele, rectocele, and urinary stress incontinence

Instructions for Items 16-57 to 16-63: Match the statement to the type of episiotomy with which it is best associated.

a. Median (midline)
b. Mediolateral

16-57. Less painful in puerperium
16-58. Blood loss greater
16-59. Extension through the anal sphincter is uncommon
16-60. Faulty healing is rare
16-61. Possibility of a fourth degree extension greater with forceps delivery
16-62. More difficult to repair
16-63. Type most frequently performed

16-64. What are the two essentials for success in episiotomy repair?

16-65. Which of the following are helpful measures in caring for the routine adjunctive second degree episiotomy?

a. Prophylactic antibiotics
b. Enemas
c. Stool softeners
d. Ice packs
e. Heat lamp
f. Local anesthetics

16-66. What are the conditions that may cause persistent severe pain after episiotomy?

17. ANALGESIA AND ANESTHESIA

17-1. Which of the following distinguishes obstetrical from surgical anesthesia?

a. Number of patients to consider
b. Absolute necessity of using anesthesia
c. Duration of anesthesia
d. Preoperative time to prepare the patient

17-2. Which of the following statements about the general principles of obstetrical analgesia and anesthesia is correct?

    a. The proper psychological management of the mother throughout the antepartum period and labor is of great importance in successful analgesia.

    b. Maintenance of satisfactory fetal oxygenation is essential for safe obstetric pain relief.

    c. Obstetrical pain relief requires close supervision of the laboring woman.

    d. Whatever agents are used must have little or no deleterious effect upon uterine contractions or maternal voluntary expulsive forces.

    e. Constant attention to the status of both mother and unborn child are basic to safe obstetric analgesia and anesthesia.

17-3. Regarding nonpharmacologic methods of pain control, which of the following statements are true?

    a. Proper management psychologically is a valuable aid in pain control in labor.

    b. Preparatory classes for childbirth may aid significantly in pain control.

    c. Breathing techniques may provide analgesic effect.

    d. Psychoprophylaxis training only sets the patient up to fail.

17-4. Which of the narcotics and tranquilizers used for analgesia during labor do not reach the fetus?

17-5. What is the drug of choice for treating narcotic depression in the newborn?

    a. Naloxone hydrochloride (Narcan)

    b. Levallorphan (Lorfan)

    c. Nalorphine (Nalline)

    d. Phenergan

17-6. Which of the following statements about Narcan (naloxone hydrochloride) is correct?

    a. It displaces the narcotic from receptors in the central nervous system.

    b. It does not inhibit the analgesic effects of narcotics.

    c. It does not inhibit narcotic-related euphoria.

    d. It may precipitate withdrawal symptoms in the physically dependent.

    e. An intravenous dose acts within 2 minutes.

    f. A single dose is sufficient to treat either mother or newborn.

17-7. Which of the following statements about general anesthesia is correct?

    a. The placenta is a selective barrier for some anesthetic agents.

    b. Fasting before anesthesia is an effective safeguard against aspiration.

    c. Endotracheal intubation minimizes the risk of aspiration.

    d. The concentration of inhalation anesthetic increases more rapidly in the lungs of pregnant women than in nonpregnant women.

17-8. Nitrous oxide

    a. May be used during both labor and delivery

    b. Provides true anesthesia

    c. Does not interfere with uterine contractions

    d. Should not be used in concentrations higher than 70 percent

    e. Use requires the close supervision of qualified personnel

17-9. Which of the following volatile anesthetics does not cross the placenta and potentially cause fetal narcosis?

    a. Isoflurane

    b. Halothane (Fluothane)

    c. Methoxyflurane (Penthrane)

    d. Enflurane (Ethrane)

Instructions for Items 17-10 to 17-12: Match the volatile anesthetic with the appropriate description.

    a. Isoflurane

    b. Halothane

    c. Methoxyflurane

    d. Enflurane

17-10. Causes uterine relaxation

17-11. Nephrotoxic

17-12. Hypotensive effect

17-13. Which of the following is an advantage of intravenous thiopental?

    a. Rapid induction

    b. Allows for ample oxygenation

    c. Controllability

    d. Minimal association with postpartum bleeding

    e. Prompt recovery without vomiting

17-14. Thiopental

    a. Is an excellent analgesic agent

    b. Is best used as the sole anesthetic agent

    c. Is commonly used to induce general anesthesia

    d. Is commonly used in conjunction with succinylcholine and nitrous oxide

17-15. General anesthesia always causes appreciable respiratory depression in the newborn infant.

  a. True
  b. False

17-16. Ketamine

  a. Produces appreciable anesthesia when administered intravenously
  b. May accentuate maternal hypertension
  c. May cause unpleasant delirium and hallucinations
  d. May cause respiratory depression in the newborn

17-17. The *most* common cause of anesthetic death in obstetrics is _____ .

17-18. Which of the following statements about the prevention of aspiration during general anesthesia is correct?

  a. Fasting for 12 hours will rid the stomach of acidic liquid.
  b. Ingestion of antacids before induction of anesthesia can reduce the acidity of gastric juice.
  c. Emptying the stomach by use of a nasogastric tube is totally effective.
  d. Intubation should be performed in the supine position.
  e. Extubation should be performed with the patient awake and in the lateral recumbent position.

17-19. Aspiration of strongly acidic gastric juice is probably more common than aspiration of gastric contents containing particulate matter.

  a. True
  b. False

17-20. Which of the following statements about aspiration pneumonitis is correct?

  a. If the pH of aspirated fluid is below 2.5, severe chemical pneumonitis is more likely to ensue.
  b. The right lower lobe of the lung is most often involved.
  c. The woman who aspirates always develops respiratory distress immediately.
  d. Roentgenographic changes occur early in aspiration pneumonitis.
  e. Chest x-ray alone should not be used to exclude aspiration pneumonitis.

17-21. Which of the following is of *proven* benefit in the treatment of aspiration pneumonitis?

  a. Suction of the pharynx and trachea
  b. Saline lavage
  c. Steroids
  d. Oxygen
  e. Antibiotics

17-22. Which of the following statements about anesthetic gas exposure and pregnancy outcome is correct?

  a. The embryo and fetus may be exposed to some danger if the pregnant woman works in an operating room.
  b. The congenital malformation rate is markedly higher in children of women who work in operating rooms.
  c. The midtrimester abortion rate is markedly higher for women who work in an operating room.
  d. Women chronically exposed to anesthetic gases should be advised to stop working as soon as pregnancy is confirmed.

17-23. Which of the following statements about the innervation of the uterus is correct?

  a. Visceral sensory fibers from the uterus, cervix, and upper vagina travel to the pelvic plexus via Frankenhaüser's ganglion.
  b. Sensory fibers enter the spinal cord in association with the 10th, 11th, and 12th thoracic and 1st lumbar nerves.
  c. Motor pathways to the uterus leave the spinal cord at the level of the seventh and eighth thoracic vertebrae.
  d. Only sensory blocks that do not block motor pathways should be used for analgesia during labor.

17-24. The pudendal nerve provides sensory innervation for the

  a. Perineum
  b. Anus
  c. Medial and inferior parts of the vulva and clitoris
  d. Superior parts of the vulva and clitoris
  e. Upper vagina

17-25. The sensory nerve fibers of the pudendal nerve are derived from the ventral branches of the _____ nerves.

17-26. Which of the following statements about central nervous system toxicity induced by agents used to produce local or regional anesthesia and analgesia is correct?

  a. Symptoms are limited to convulsions and loss of consciousness.
  b. Immediate management includes airway control (with intubation if needed) and oxygenation.
  c. Succinylcholine may be used to abolish peripheral neural manifestations.
  d. Thiopental may be used as a central inhibitor of convulsions.
  e. Diazepam may be used as a central inhibitor of convulsions.
  f. Rapid fluid administration, intravenous ephedrine, and placement on the left side are useful to treat hypotension associated with CNS toxicity reactions.
  g. In cases of convulsions, the fetus should be delivered immediately by cesarean section.

17-27. Local infiltration of the genital tract with anesthetics is useful

  a. For analgesia during labor
  b. Before episiotomy and delivery
  c. After delivery for episiotomy repair
  d. For inspection of the genital tract after delivery
  e. For its relative safety
  f. For its immediate effectiveness

17-28. Which of the following statements about pudendal block is correct?

  a. After needle placement, aspiration is always attempted to avoid intravenous injection of local anesthetic.
  b. Injection is made at the site where the pudendal nerve passes adjacent to the sacrospinous ligament.
  c. Pudendal block is usually effective within 3 to 4 minutes.
  d. An anesthetic with high tissue penetration and rapid action should be used.
  e. Before pudendal block, it is useful to infiltrate the site where episiotomy will be made.
  f. Cardiovascular toxicity may also occur, generally requiring higher blood levels than CNS toxicity.

17-29. For which types of delivery is pudendal block likely to provide adequate anesthesia?

  a. Cesarean section
  b. Midforceps delivery
  c. Low forceps delivery
  d. Spontaneous delivery

17-30. Which of the following are possible complications of pudendal block?

  a. Infection
  b. Hematoma formation
  c. Convulsions
  d. Fetal distress
  e. Protracted labor

17-31. Paracervical block

  a. Is useful to relieve the pain of uterine contractions
  b. May need to be repeated during labor
  c. Is useful for delivery
  d. May cause fetal bradycardia

17-32. Which of the following statements about the use of spinal block is correct?

  a. Spinal block involves the injection of local anesthetic into the subarachnoid space.
  b. For vaginal and cesarean deliveries, block at the level of tenth thoracic dermatome (T10) is appropriate.
  c. For vaginal deliveries, the anesthetic should not be administered until the cervix is fully dilated and all other requirements for delivery are completed.
  d. A somewhat larger dose of anesthetic is used for cesarean deliveries than for vaginal deliveries.
  e. Spinal block may be utilized for pain relief during labor.

17-33. Which of the following are possible complications of spinal anesthesia?

  a. Hypotension
  b. Respiratory paralysis
  c. Anxiety
  d. Headache
  e. Bladder dysfunction
  f. Meningitis

17-34. Which of the following is effective in the prophylaxis and treatment of maternal hypotension following spinal anesthesia?

  a. Uterine displacement
  b. Hydration with balanced salt solution
  c. Intravenous injection of ephedrine
  d. Use of a small-gauge needle to administer the anesthetic

17-35. The most common cause of complete spinal blockade with respiratory paralysis is _____ .

17-36. Which of the following is useful in supplementing a spinal anesthetic that is providing inadequate analgesia?

  a. Nitrous oxide
  b. Morphine
  c. Meperidine
  d. Fentanyl

17-37. Spinal headaches are caused by _____ .

17-38. Which of the following is a *proven* preventive or treatment measure for spinal headaches?

  a. Use of a small-gauge needle
  b. A single puncture to administer the anesthetic
  c. Supine position
  d. Hyperhydration
  e. Blood patch
  f. Saline patch
  g. Abdominal binder

17–39. Hypertension from ergot medication is most common in women who have received spinal or epidural block.

  a. True
  b. False

17–40. List the *major* maternal contraindications to spinal anesthesia.

17–41. Which of the following statements about epidural (peridural) block is correct?

  a. Epidural block may be used to provide both analgesia and anesthesia for labor and anesthesia for delivery.
  b. Block from T10 to S5 is indicated for analgesia and anesthesia in vaginal delivery.
  c. Block from T8 to S1 is indicated for anesthesia in abdominal delivery.
  d. The spread of epidural anesthesia depends only on the location of the injection site.
  e. Epidural block is usually made through a thoracic level injection.

17–42. Which of the following is a potential complication of epidural anesthesia?

  a. Inadvertent spinal anesthesia
  b. Ineffective anesthesia
  c. Hypotension
  d. Central nervous system stimulation
  e. Depression of uterine activity

17–43. There is likely to be an increased incidence of midforceps deliveries in patients given epidural anesthesia.

  a. True
  b. False

17–44. List the *major* maternal contraindications to the use of epidural block.

17–45. Epidural opiate analgesia

  a. Refers to direct injection of opiates into the epidural space
  b. Provides no motor paresis
  c. Is commonly complicated by pruritus
  d. Is likely to replace local anesthetic injection into the epidural space for cesarean section

PART V ABNORMALITIES OF LABOR AND DELIVERY

18. DYSTOCIA DUE TO ABNORMALITIES OF THE EXPULSIVE FORCES AND PRECIPITATE LABOR

18–1. List the four distinct abnormalities that, alone or in combination, cause dystocia.

18–2. The most common cause of dystocia is _____ .

18–3. As a generalization, uterine dysfunction is common whenever there is disproportion between the presenting part of the fetus and the birth canal.

  a. True
  b. False

Instructions for Items 18–4 and 18–5: Match the stage of labor with the appropriate cervical changes.

  a. Latent phase
  b. Active phase

18–4. Cervix undergoes softening and effacement
18–5. Rapid cervical dilation occurs

18–6. Complete the following table characterizing contractions during labor using the following descriptors: strong, mild, irregular, regular, long or short.

	LATENT PHASE	ACTIVE PHASE
Strength	(1)	(2)
Duration	(3)	(4)
Frequency	(5)	(6)

18–7. Which of the following statements about lack of progress in labor is correct?

    a. Lack of progress in the first stage of labor presents no real danger to the mother or fetus.
    b. Prolongation of the latent phase of labor is defined as 20 hours in both nulliparas and multiparas.
    c. A protracted active phase is defined as cervical dilation of less than 1.2 cm per hour in nulliparas.
    d. A protracted active phase is defined as cervical dilation of less than 1.5 cm per hour in multiparas.

Instructions for Items 18–8 to 18–14: Match the type of uterine dysfunction with the appropriate description.

    a. Hypotonic uterine dysfunction
    b. Hypertonic (incoordinate) uterine dysfunction

18–8. Basal hypertonous may be present

18–9. No basal hypertonus

18–10. There is a normal uterine pressure gradient during a contraction

18–11. The uterine pressure gradient during a contraction may be distorted

18–12. Occurs during the active phase of labor after the cervix has dilated to more than 4 cm

18–13. Contractions are especially painful but ineffective

18–14. Contractions become less frequent and intense during labor

18–15. Complete the following table that describes the diagnostic criteria for abnormal labor patterns (according to Friedman)

LABOR PATTERN	DIAGNOSTIC CRITERIA	
	NULLIGRAVIDA	MULTIGRAVIDA
Prolongation disorder:		
Prolonged latent phase	>20 hr	_____ (1)
Protraction disorder:		
Protracted active phase dilation	_____ (2)	<1.5 cm/hr
Protracted descent	<1 cm/hr	_____ (3)
Arrest disorder:		
Prolonged deceleration phase	_____ (4)	>1 hr
Secondary arrest of dialation	_____ (5)	>2 hr
Arrest of descent	>1 hr	_____ (6)
Failure of descent	_____ (7)	No descent in the deceleration phase or in the second stage

18–16. According to Cohen and Friedman, in a prolonged latent phase the preferred treatment is _____ (1) and the exceptional treatment is _____ (2) . In cases of protracted active phase or protracted descent, the preferred treatment is _____ (3) and the exceptional treatment is _____ (4) .

18–17. The most common cause of dystocia associated with uterine dysfunction is the presence of a cervix too rigid to dilate.

    a. True
    b. False

18–18. Which of the following is a potential complication of prolonged dysfunctional labor?

    a. Intrauterine infection
    b. Maternal exhaustion
    c. Psychological effects on mother
    d. Fetal or neonatal death

18–19. What two general conditions must be met before treatment of hypotonic uterine dysfunction with intravenous oxytocin may be initiated?

18–20. Why is uterine rupture not a common outcome in cases of cephalopelvic disproportion?

18–21. Which of the following factors contribute to the decision to augment labor in cases of hypotonic uterine dysfunction?

    a. Fetal size
    b. Presentation
    c. Position
    d. Parity
    e. Pelvic size

18–22. According to Bottoms and co-workers, arrest disorders in labor are treated just as effectively with amniotomy or ambulation as with the use of intravenous oxytocin.

    a. True
    b. False

18–23. If the criteria for a noncontracted pelvis are not met, oxytocin stimulation should not be used.

    a. True
    b. False

18–24. What potential problem is associated with the infusion of dextrose in water during oxytocin stimulation?

18–25. In which of the following situations at Parkland Hospital is the use of oxytocin to stimulate labor generally be avoided?

    a. High parity
    b. Oligohydramnios
    c. Uterine overdistention
    d. Presence of a dead fetus
    e. Presence of a uterine scar

18-26. Which of the following statements about the use of oxytocin to stimulate labor is correct?

   a. A dilute solution of 10 units of oxytocin in 1 liter of balanced salt solution should be utilized.
   b. The infusion rate of oxytocin may be increased every 10 minutes until a clinically adequate labor pattern is established.
   c. Infusion rates of more than 10 mU/min for augmentation or 30 to 40 mU/min for induction are rarely needed.
   d. The mean half-life of oxytocin is about 30 minutes.
   e. Continuous clinical monitoring of the patient during oxytocin stimulation is necessary.
   f. The hypotonic uterus often requires 4 to 5 hours to respond to oxytocin.

18-27. If oxytocin fails to stimulate labor within a few hours, cesarean delivery should be performed.

   a. True
   b. False

18-28. Prolonged latent phase is always due to either injudicious use of analgesics or anesthetics, false labor or hypertonic uterine dysfunction.

   a. True
   b. False

18-29. Which of the following statements about the use of prostaglandins in the stimulation of labor is correct?

   a. Prostaglandins $F_{2\alpha}$ and E_2 have been approved by the FDA for use in the United States.
   b. Prostaglandins are capable of augmenting but not inducing labor.
   c. Prostaglandins have been shown to be effective in ripening the cervix preparatory to the induction of labor.
   d. Use of prostaglandins has been associated with a higher rate of cesarean deliveries.

18-30. Hypertonic uterine dysfunction

   a. Is characterized by pain that is more severe than expected for the intensity of the contractions
   b. Characteristically appears after the cervix is dilated 4 cm or more
   c. Is relatively infrequent compared to hypotonic uterine dysfunction
   d. Is best treated by dilute oxytocin infusion to create a more rhythmic uterine contraction pattern

18-31. Which of the following statements about inadequate voluntary expulsive force is correct?

   a. Conduction anesthesia may reduce the reflex to "push."
   b. Conduction anesthesia may impair a woman's ability to contract her abdominal muscles sufficiently to generate the needed force.
   c. Insufficient expulsive forces may be the consequence of longstanding paralysis of the abdominal muscles.
   d. Nitrous oxide may be used with women who cannot bear down with each contraction due to great discomfort.

18-32. Precipitate labor

   a. May result from low resistance of the cervix and birth canal
   b. May result from abnormally strong contractions
   c. May cause amnionic fluid embolism, especially if there is resistance from the cervix and birth canal
   d. Does not affect perinatal mortality or morbidity rates because of the shortened time the fetus is exposed to the stresses of labor
   e. May be effectively treated by β-mimetic tocolytics
   f. Is associated with an increased incidence of postpartum hemorrhage

18-33. Which of the following statements about localized abnormalities of the uterus is correct?

   a. Prolonged labor may result in localized rings or contractions of the uterus.
   b. The pathologic retraction ring of Bandl is the most common type of retraction ring.
   c. In modern obstetrics, pathologic contraction rings are rarely seen because prolonged labor is relatively uncommon.
   d. The most likely time for the occurrence of a contraction ring is after the delivery of the first of twins.

18-34. Describe the circumstances surrounding missed labor.

19.   DYSTOCIA DUE TO ABNORMALITIES IN PRESENTATION, POSITION, OR DEVELOPMENT OF THE FETUS

19-1. About _____ percent of singleton pregnancies are breech at the (1) start of the second half of pregnancy, whereas at term the incidence of breech presentations is _____ .
(2)

19-2. Which of the following conditions is associated with an increased incidence of breech presentation?

    a. Grand multiparity
    b. Multifetal pregnancy
    c. Hydramnios
    d. Contracted pelvis
    e. Hydrocephalus
    f. Protracted labor
    g. Anencephalus
    h. Oligohydramnios
    i. Previous breech delivery
    j. Uterine anomalies
    k. Uterine tumors
    l. Cornual-fundal placental implantation
    m. Placenta previa
    n. Abruptio placentae

19-3. List the complications that occur with increased frequency in association with a breech delivery.

Instructions for Items 19-4 to 19-6: Match the type of breech presentation with the appropriate description.

    a. Frank breech
    b. Complete breech
    c. Incomplete breech

19-4. Lower extremities flexed at the hips; one or both knees are flexed

19-5. Lower extremities flexed at the hips and extended at the knees; the feet lie in close proximity to the head

19-6. One or both hips are not flexed and one or both feet or knees lie below the breech

19-7. The most common breech presentation near term is the

    a. Frank breech
    b. Complete breech
    c. Incomplete breech

19-8. In cases of breech presentation, the maneuvers of Leopold are ineffective for determining fetal presentation and position.

    a. True
    b. False

19-9. In a breech presentation, the location where fetal heart sounds are usually best heard is _____, whereas with a cephalic presentation the fetal [1] heart sounds are loudest _____ [2] .

19-10. Which of the following statements about the vaginal examination in cases of breech presentation is correct?

    a. The ischial tuberosities, the sacrum, and the anus are usually palpable.
    b. The diagnosis of position and variety are based on the location of the sacrum and its spinous processes.
    c. In footling presentations, the feet may be felt alongside the buttocks.
    d. Due to swelling caused by prolonged labor, it may be hard to differentiate the fetal buttocks and face.

19-11. Sonography is better than x-ray for identifying the relationship of the lower extremities to the fetal pelvis.

    a. True
    b. False

19-12. Which of the following contributes to the increased maternal morbidity and mortality for pregnancies complicated by persistent breech presentation?

    a. Greater frequency of operative delivery
    b. Greatly prolonged labor
    c. Increased incidence of preeclampsia–eclampsia

19-13. List the main contributing factors to the increased perinatal morbidity and mortality in breech presentation.

19-14. Which organ is most frequently found to be injured during traumatic vaginal deliveries of breech presentations?

    a. Liver
    b. Adrenal glands
    c. Spleen
    d. Spinal cord
    e. Brain

19-15. Use of cesarean delivery in all breech presentations reduces the risk of neonatal mortality to approximately that of the overall population.

    a. True
    b. False

19-16. Which of the following statements about breech presentation in mature fetuses ($>$2,500 g) is correct?

    a. The overall perinatal mortality rate for breech presentation is about equal to that for cephalic presentations.
    b. Major congenital anomalies are more frequent in breech than in vertex presentations.
    c. The incidence of fetal distress of undetermined cause is greater in breech than in vertex presentations.
    d. The incidence of overt prolapse of the umbilical cord is approximately equal in frank breech and in vertex presentations.

19–17. In cases of breech presentation in mature fetuses (>2,500 g), the mortality and morbidity rates from delivery trauma are _____ to fetal weight.

   a. Directly proportional
   b. Inversely proportional
   c. Unrelated

19–18. Perinatal mortality associated with vaginal delivery as a breech in premature infants is _____ in term breech infants.

   a. Greater than
   b. The same as
   c. Less than

19–19. Which of the following statements about external version in a breech presentation is correct?

   a. External version is more readily accomplished in multiparous women.
   b. Conduction, or occasionally general, anesthesia should be used to relax the abdominal walls.
   c. External version is more likely to be successful early in the third trimester than later.
   d. Attempts at external version may be complicated by antepartum hemorrhage, premature labor, fetal death, and fetomaternal hemorrhage.

19–20. Which of the following problems is associated with the vaginal delivery of breech presentations?

   a. Delivery of the breech draws the cord into the pelvis, which can lead to cord compression.
   b. Once the breech has passed the vaginal introitus, the parts still to be delivered are readily compressible.
   c. The time required for accommodation of the fetal head may lead to fetal acidosis and hypoxia.
   d. With a premature fetus, the disparity between the size of the head and the buttocks is less than with a larger fetus.

19–21. List the clinical circumstances where cesarean delivery of breech presentations is recommended.

19–22. Which of the following pelvic shapes is unfavorable for vaginal delivery of breech presentations.

   a. Gynecoid
   b. Android
   c. Anthropoid
   d. Platypelloid

19–23. Vaginal delivery in cases of hyperextension of the fetal head may lead to what injury?

19–24. Vaginal delivery should be relatively safe for a frank breech presentation if

   a. A previous cephalic delivery was successful
   b. The fetus is judged to weigh less than 8 pounds
   c. Orderly effacement and dilation of the cervix and descent of the breech occurs
   d. Individuals skilled in breech delivery are available

19–25. In face presentations, the fetal head is

   a. Hyperflexed
   b. Hyperextended

19–26. Which of the following factors is associated with face presentations?

   a. Contracted pelvis
   b. Small fetus
   c. Pendulous maternal abdomen
   d. Anencephalic fetus

19–27. Face presentation

   a. Has a reported incidence of <1 percent
   b. Generally starts as a brow presentation with extension of the head as descent occurs during labor
   c. Cannot be easily confirmed by roentgenogram because of interference from the maternal pelvic bones
   d. Is usually best managed by cesarean delivery because of its association with pelvic contraction

19–28. Which of the following statements about brow presentation is correct?

   a. The fetal head occupies a position midway between full flexion and full extension.
   b. Except where the head is small or the pelvis is large, vaginal delivery is difficult.
   c. Brow presentation is usually unstable and in a majority of cases converts to occiput or face presentations.
   d. Caput succedaneum may be so extensive over the forehead that identification of the brow by palpation is difficult.

Instructions for Items 19–29 and 19–30: Match the type of presentation with the features that can be felt on vaginal examination.

   a. Face presentation
   b. Brow presentation

19–29. Frontal sutures, large anterior fontanel, orbital ridges, and eyes can be felt but the mouth and chin cannot

19–30. Mouth and nose, malar bones, and orbital ridges can be felt

Instructions for Items 19-31 and 19-32: Match the type of shoulder presentation with the appropriate description.

    a. Transverse lie
    b. Oblique lie

19-31. Fetal long axis forms an acute angle with the maternal long axis

19-32. Fetal long axis is approximately perpendicular to the maternal long axis

19-33. Transverse lie

    a. Is designated as right or left depending on the orientation of the fetal acromion to the maternal pelvis
    b. Occurs in <1 percent of singleton pregnancies
    c. Is suspected when the abdomen is wide from side to side and the uterine fundus does not extend much above the umbilicus
    d. Is associated with an increased incidence of prolapse of the hand and arm, especially as labor progresses

19-34. Transverse lie is more common in

    a. Nulliparous patients
    b. Grand multiparity
    c. Postmature gestations
    d. Premature gestations
    e. Placental abruption
    f. Placenta previa
    g. Women with a large pelvis
    h. Women with a contracted pelvis

19-35. Most maternal deaths associated with transverse lie occur in neglected cases from _____ .

19-36. Even with appropriate care, the reasons for increased maternal morbidity and mortality in transverse lie include

    a. Association with placenta previa
    b. Increased incidence of cord accidents
    c. Necessity for major operative procedures
    d. Likelihood of sepsis associated with extrusion of the arm into the vagina

19-37. Transverse lie

    a. Does not allow vaginal delivery except in the case of conduplicato corpore
    b. Is usually managed by external version although this is difficult after 8 cm dilation
    c. Is usually managed by lower segment transverse cesarean section
    d. Is best treated by including antibiotic therapy after delivery, whether or not there are signs of infection

19-38. In cases of transverse lie a vertical incision may be preferable to a transverse uterine incision for cesarean section.

    a. True
    b. False

19-39. Compound presentation

    a. Occurs when an extremity prolapses alongside the presenting part
    b. Is more common in premature pregnancies
    c. Is associated with a reported 25 percent perinatal loss rate
    d. Is best managed by cesarean section

19-40. The persistent occiput posterior position

    a. Undergoes spontaneous anterior rotation in about 65 percent of cases
    b. Rarely results in spontaneous vaginal delivery
    c. May in most instances be managed by forceps delivery under local anesthesia with a midline episiotomy
    d. May be managed by forceps rotation (Scanzoni maneuver)

19-41. In persistent occiput posterior position as compared with occiput anterior position

    a. Labor is usually prolonged
    b. The perinatal mortality rate is increased threefold
    c. Significantly lower Apgar scores are common
    d. Extended episiotomies are required

19-42. The persistent occiput transverse position

    a. Usually converts spontaneously to occiput anterior position when pelvic anatomy is normal
    b. May remain persistent in cases of hypotonic uterine dysfunction
    c. May remain persistent because of pelvic contraction
    d. May take the form of deep transverse arrest, requiring cesarean delivery in most cases

19-43. Describe deep transverse arrest as it occurs in persistent occiput transverse presentations.

19-44. Fetal macrosomia is defined as an infant weighing

_____ .

19-45. Fetal macrosomia is associated with

    a. A large mother
    b. A large father
    c. Multiparity
    d. Primaparity
    e. Maternal diabetes
    f. Maternal obesity
    g. Prolonged gestation
    h. Previous delivery of a large infant

19-46. Which of the following statements about fetal macrosomia is correct?

   a. It occurs in about 5 percent of newborns.
   b. It cannot be diagnosed clinically.
   c. Sonographic evaluation of the dimensions of the head, thorax, and abdomen provides a fairly accurate estimate of fetal size.
   d. Fetal macrosomia is associated with increased perinatal morbidity and mortality.

19-47. The incidence of shoulder dystocia is _____ to fetal weight.

   a. Directly proportional
   b. Inversely proportional

19-48. Describe the danger to the fetus associated with shoulder dystocia.

19-49. Which of the following statements about the prevention and management of shoulder dystocia is correct?

   a. There is an increased likelihood of shoulder dystocia following a prolonged second stage of labor managed by instrumental vaginal delivery of the head from the midpelvis.
   b. Comparison of chest and head circumference measurements reveal situations where there is a high likelihood of shoulder dystocia.
   c. Cesarean delivery is required in cases of shoulder dystocia.

19-50. Describe five of the sequences of maneuvers used in the management of shoulder dystocia.

19-51. Which of the following is true regarding ultrasound and the diagnosis of shoulder dystocia?

   a. A chest measurement of 1.6 cm greater than the head has a good predictive value for shoulder dystocia.
   b. The head to abdominal ratio is the best predictor of shoulder dystocia.
   c. Estimated fetal weights by ultrasound are so inaccurate that they have no predictive value regarding shoulder dystocia.
   d. Total intrauterine volume is the best predictor of shoulder dystocia.

19-52. Which of the following statements about internal hydrocephalus is correct?

   a. Internal hydrocephalus is best diagnosed radiographically by the appearance of an enlarged fetal head of a fetus in the breech position.
   b. Diagnosis is confirmed by ultrasonographic demonstration of enlarged fetal ventricles and decreased brain cortex.
   c. Internal hydrocephalus is associated with an increased danger of uterine rupture.
   d. Aspiration of excess cerebrospinal fluid can be accomplished by transvaginal or transabdominal puncture.
   e. The intrapartum use of a ventricular ''shunt'' is now widely possible.

19-53. Which of the following criteria aid the radiographic identification of hydrocephalus?

   a. The face is small in relation to the head.
   b. The hydrocephalic cranium tends to be ovoid rather than globular.
   c. The shadow of the hydrocephalic cranium is often thin or scarcely visible.

19-54. Which of the following can enlarge the fetal abdomen enough to potentially cause dystocia?

   a. Greatly distended bladder
   b. Ascites
   c. Enlarged kidneys
   d. Enlarged liver

19-55. In general, after excess fluid is removed from the abdomen the prognosis for the fetus is good regardless of the route of delivery.

   a. True
   b. False

20.   DYSTOCIA DUE TO PELVIC CONTRACTION

20-1. Contraction of which of the following pelvic diameters may cause dystocia?

   a. The pelvic inlet
   b. The midpelvis
   c. The pelvic outlet

20-2. The pelvic inlet is considered to be contracted when the

   a. Shortest anteroposterior diameter is less than 10 cm
   b. Greatest transverse diameter is less than 12 cm
   c. Diagonal conjugate is less than 11.5 cm

20-3. The incidence of obstetric difficulty when either the anteroposterior or the transverse diameters of the pelvic inlet is contracted is _____ when both diameters are contracted.

a. Greater than
b. The same as
c. Less than

20-4. Maternal size is _____ related to pelvic size and _____ related to fetal size.
(1)   (2)

a. Directly
b. Inversely

20-5. Which of the following methods is most reliable in determining whether the fetal head will navigate the pelvis successfully?

a. Clinical pelvimetry
b. Radiographic pictures
c. Ultrasound
d. Trial of labor

20-6. Elongation in the occipitofrontal diameter of the fetal head is referred to as

a. Brachycephaly
b. Kinesiocephaly
c. Dolichocephaly
d. Platycephaly

20-7. Which of the following statements about fetal presentations associated with a contracted pelvic inlet is correct?

a. When the pelvic inlet is contracted, descent into the pelvic cavity does not usually begin until after the onset of labor.
b. Vertex presentations occur in about one-third of cases.
c. Face and shoulder presentations are three times more frequent in women with contracted pelves.
d. Prolapse of the umbilical cord and of the extremities occurs four to six times more frequently in women with contracted pelves.

20-8. Contraction of the pelvic inlet is associated with

a. Precipitate labor and delivery
b. Early spontaneous rupture of the membranes
c. Slow or absent dilation of the cervix during labor
d. An increased incidence of vesicovaginal, vesicocervical, or rectovaginal fistulas
e. An increased incidence of intrapartum infection
f. The possibility of uterine rupture

20-9. The appearance of a pathologic retraction ring in a laboring patient with a clinically contracted pelvic inlet is indication for immediate cesarean delivery.

a. True
b. False

20-10. Which of the following statements about the fetal head in labors associated with a contracted pelvis is correct?

a. A large caput succedaneum may develop, causing diagnostic error from overestimation of the degree of fetal descent.
b. Pressure from uterine contractions may cause overlapping of the fetal skull bones at their sutures (molding).
c. Fetal tentorial tears and intracranial hemorrhage may result from molding that reduces the biparietal diameter more than 0.2 cm.
d. Accommodation of the fetal head to a contracted pelvis is easier when the bones of the head are completely ossified.

Instructions for Items 20-11 to 20-18: Determine the effects of the following situations on the prognosis for vaginal delivery in a patient with a borderline contracted pelvic inlet (anteroposterior diameter only slightly below 10 cm).

a. Favorable prognosis for vaginal delivery
b. Unfavorable prognosis for vaginal delivery

20-11. Occiput presentation
20-12. Breech presentation
20-13. Large fetus
20-14. Android pelvis
20-15. Orderly progression of cervical dilation
20-16. Uterine dysfunction
20-17. Previous difficult labor
20-18. Asynclitism

20-19. In the management of a contracted pelvic inlet,

a. A trial of labor is always indicated
b. Conduction anesthesia is preferred because of the anticipated protracted extent of labor
c. Close monitoring of the mother and fetus for signs of impending uterine rupture is essential
d. The infusion of dilute oxytocin solution may facilitate molding and engagement of the fetal head

20-20. Describe the anatomic constituents that make up the plane of the obstetric midpelvis.

20-21. A transverse line connecting the _____ divides the midpelvis into fore and hind portions.

20-22. Supply the following average measurements of the diameters of the midpelvis.

Transverse (interspinous) diameter: _____ cm
(1)
Anteroposterior diameter: _____ cm
(2)
Posterior sagittal diameter: _____ cm
(3)

20–23. The midpelvis should be considered contracted when the sum of the interischial spinous and the posterior sagittal diameters falls at or below _____ .

a. 10.5 cm
b. 11.5 cm
c. 12.5 cm
d. 13.5 cm
e. 14.5 cm

20–24. There is reason to suspect the existence of midpelvic contraction whenever the interischial spinous diameter is less than

a. 8 cm
b. 9 cm
c. 10 cm
d. 11 cm
e. 12 cm

20–25. Midpelvic contraction may be precisely diagnosed by a combination of x-ray and ultrasonographic evaluations.

a. True
b. False

20–26. Midpelvic contraction is probably _____ inlet contraction.

a. More common than
b. As common as
c. Less common than

20–27. Which of the following statements about the treatment of labor complicated by midpelvic contraction is correct?

a. Use of forceps before the head has passed the contracted midpelvis facilitates flexion.
b. Early use of forceps reduces the space available for the fetal head.
c. Midforceps delivery is contraindicated in cases where the biparietal diameter of the fetal head has not passed beyond the level of contraction.
d. Vacuum extraction may be useful after complete cervical dilation.
e. Oxytocin should not be used in the treatment of dystocia caused by pelvic contraction.

20–28. Contraction of the pelvic outlet is defined as _____ .

20–29. Supply the anatomic constituents of the two triangles that comprise the pelvic outlet.

TRIANGLES

	Anterior	Posterior
Base	(1)	(2)
Sides	(3)	(4)
Apex	(5)	(6)

20–30. Outlet contraction without simultaneous contraction of the midpelvis never occurs.

a. True
b. False

20–31. What is a possible complication of a contracted pelvic outlet when disproportion with the fetal head is not sufficiently great to cause serious dystocia?

20–32. Previous history of pelvic fracture is an automatic indication for cesarean delivery.

a. True
b. False

20–33. Complete the following table by listing the complications of labor associated with the kyphotic patient.

GIBBUS LOCATION	COMMON COMPLICATION
Thoracic	(1)
Lumbar	(2)
Thoracolumbar	(3)

20–34. Which of the following statements concerning the effects of an anatomically deformed bony pelvis is correct?

a. Mechanisms of labor in the kyphotic pelvis favor abnormal positions of the fetus.
b. Kyphosis generally causes no problems in labor.
c. All dwarf pelves are characterized by incomplete ossification and the presence of varying amounts of cartilage.
d. All patients with bony abnormalities of the pelvis should be delivered by cesarean section.

21. DYSTOCIA DUE TO SOFT TISSUE ABNORMALITIES OF THE REPRODUCTIVE TRACT

21–1. Which of the following statements about dystocia associated with abnormalities of the vulva is correct?

a. Complete vulvar atresia is usually incompatible with conception unless it is surgically corrected.
b. Incomplete vulvar atresia resulting from adhesions or scars may allow vaginal delivery at the cost of deep perineal tears.
c. When the vulvovaginal outlet is small, rigid, and inelastic, adequate episiotomy will usually prevent dystocia and lacerations.
d. An extremely edematous vulva commonly results in dystocia.
e. Presence of *Condylomata acuminata* is an absolute indication for cesarean delivery.

21-2. Which of the following statements about dystocia associated with abnormalities of the vagina is correct?

   a. Both complete and incomplete vaginal septa usually do not cause dystocia.
   b. Annular stricture of the vagina usually causes significant dystocia that requires cesarean delivery.
   c. Transverse vaginal septa do not allow a normal course of labor.
   d. The softening of tissues in pregnancy usually overcomes the obstruction caused by vaginal scarring.
   e. Gartner duct cysts seldom cause dystocia, but may have to be asceptically aspirated during vaginal delivery.
   f. Tetanic contraction of the levator ani muscle usually responds to anesthesia, thus allowing vaginal delivery.

21-3. Which of the following can cause cervical stenosis?

   a. Conization
   b. Cauterization
   c. Corrosives used to induce abortion
   d. Cervical amputation
   e. Infection and tissue destruction

21-4. Which of the following statements about atresia or stenosis of the cervix is correct?

   a. Complete cervical atresia prevents the possibility of future conception.
   b. Normal tissue softening during pregnancy usually reduces stenosis sufficiently to allow cervical dilation during labor.
   c. Conglutination of the cervical os usually causes dystocia severe enough to require cesarean delivery.
   d. Congenital abnormalities of the cervix that cause dystocia are frequently associated with other abnormalities of the genital and urinary tracts.

21-5. Extensive invasion of the cervix by carcinoma will usually impede dilation.

   a. True
   b. False

Instructions for Items 21-6 to 21-9: Match the type of extreme uterine displacement with the circumstances with which it is associated.

   a. Anteflexion
   b. Retroflexion

21-6. Associated with diastasis recti and a pendulous abdomen
21-7. Associated with spontaneous abortion in the first half of pregnancy
21-8. Associated with sacculation and a risk of uterine rupture
21-9. Associated with impeded cervical dilation

21-10. Which of the following statements about the management of uterine displacement is correct?

   a. Marked anteflexion of the uterus may be corrected by use of a properly fitting abdominal binder.
   b. Persistent retroflexion of the uterus requires cesarean delivery.
   c. Operative shortening of the round ligaments to affect uterine suspension does not adversely influence labor in a subsequent pregnancy.
   d. Pregnancy after fixation of the uterine fundus to the anterior abdominal wall may be complicated by considerable discomfort.

Instructions for Items 21-11 to 21-14: Match the type of uterine myoma with the appropriate description.

   a. Submucous myoma
   b. Subserous myoma
   c. Intramural myoma
   d. Pedunculated myoma

21-11. Confined to the myometrium
21-12. Located immediately beneath the uterine serosa
21-13. Located immediately beneath the endometrial or decidual surface
21-14. Attached to the uterus by a stalk

21-15. Which of the following statements about uterine myomas is correct?

   a. Uterine myomas increase greatly in size during pregnancy and remain large thereafter.
   b. Implantation over the site of a submucous myoma is either unsuccessful or leads to faulty placentation and abortion.
   c. Hemorrhagic infarction of myomas ("red" degeneration) is usually life threatening for the mother.
   d. With a submucous myoma, pregnancy occasionally progresses to term, with the myoma then prolapsing through the cervix at delivery.

21-16. The signs and symptoms of hemorrhagic infarction may make it difficult to distinguish from

   a. Appendicitis
   b. Placental abruption
   c. Placenta previa
   d. Ureteral stone
   e. Pyelonephritis

21-17. Which of the following statements about the treatment of uterine myomas in pregnancy is correct?

a. Complications of the antepartum or intrapartum periods are common in women with uterine myomas.
b. While dystocia from fundal myomas is uncommon, postpartum hemorrhage is a frequent and serious complication.
c. Uterine myomas shown by ultrasonography to be in the lower uterine segment require cesarean delivery because of the dystocia that they will cause.
d. Myomectomy during pregnancy should be limited to tumors with discrete pedicles.

21-18. Which of the following statements about ovarian tumors in pregnancy is correct?

a. The two most common ovarian tumors in pregnancy are cystic teratoma and mucinous cystadenoma.
b. About one-quarter of ovarian tumors in pregnancy are malignant.
c. The most common complication of ovarian tumors in pregnancy is rupture of a cystic ovarian mass.
d. Torsion of an ovarian tumor is most common in the first trimester.
e. Most ovarian tumors during pregnancy are symptomatic.
f. It is almost always possible to make the diagnosis of an ovarian tumor clinically.

21-19. Which of the following statements about treatment of ovarian tumors in pregnancy is correct?

a. The safest time to perform laparotomy is the fourth month of gestation.
b. When the diagnosis of a benign ovarian tumor is made late in pregnancy, it is best to delay laparotomy until the fetus is mature.
c. With all ovarian tumors, cesarean delivery is usually preferable to vaginal delivery.

21-20. Which of the following statements about pelvic masses causing dystocia is correct?

a. A distended bladder, with or without cystocele, will not delay the normal course of labor.
b. Pelvic kidneys, either natural or transplanted, usually necessitate cesarean delivery.
c. Enteroceles frequently cause dystocia.
d. Bladder tumors rarely cause dystocia severe enough to require cesarean delivery.
e. Tumors or inflammation in the lower part of the rectum or the pelvic connective tissue may cause dystocia.

22. TECHNIQUES FOR BREECH DELIVERY

22-1. Which of the following statements about the mechanism of labor in the breech presentation is correct?

a. Descent usually takes place with the bitrochanteric diameter of the breech in one of the oblique diameters of the pelvis.
b. Internal rotation occurs as a response to resistance from the pelvic floor.
c. The anterior hip is born before the posterior hip.
d. The posterior portion of the neck is normally brought to a position just under the pubic symphysis.
e. The head is born in extension.

22-2. Concerning the evaluation of a breech presentation in labor, which of the following statements are true?

a. Mother and fetus are at increased risk compared with a cephalic presentation.
b. Assessment of cervical dilatation and effacement and station of the fetal presenting part are essential in planning the route of delivery.
c. Sonography or x-ray should be used to best determine the presence or absence of fetal anomalies.
d. Continuous electronic fetal monitoring or heart rate and uterine contraction strength should be begun immediately.
e. Route of delivery is based on the type of breech, flexion of the head, fetal size, maternal pelvic size, and a normal progress in labor.

Instructions for Items 22-3 to 22-5: Match the type of breech delivery with the correct description.

a. Spontaneous breech delivery
b. Partial breech extraction
c. Total breech extraction

22-3. The infant is delivered spontaneously as far as the umbilicus
22-4. No traction or manipulation is required except support of the infant
22-5. The entire body of the fetus is extracted by the obstetrician

22-6. List the members of the delivery team (and their functions) that must be present at a vaginal breech delivery.

22-7. Delivery is easier and perinatal mortality and morbidity are lower when the breech is allowed to deliver spontaneously.

a. True
b. False

22-8. What options are available if fetal distress develops during labor in a breech presentation?

22-9. Which of the following statements about extraction of the complete or incomplete breech is correct?

a. The obstetrician's hand is introduced through the vagina and the infant's ankles are grasped.
b. The anterior foot should be brought through the introitus first.
c. Episiotomy is required only in a preterm birth.
d. As the buttocks emerge, the operator's thumbs should be placed over the sacrum with the fingers over the hips and downward traction should be continued.
e. The legs are wrapped in a towel to allow a better grip as downward traction is exerted.
f. No attempt should be made to deliver the shoulders and arms until one axilla becomes visible.

22-10. In a successful breech extraction, gentle steady downward traction is applied until the lower halves of the scapulas are delivered outside the vulva.

a. True
b. False

22-11. What two methods are available to deliver the shoulders in a breech extraction?

22-12. In extraction of the complete or incomplete breech, attempts to deliver the arms immediately after the costal margins emerge should be avoided.

a. True
b. False

22-13. Which of the following statements apply when it is necessary to first free and deliver the arms in a breech extraction?

a. Free the posterior arm first.
b. Apply downward traction at all times.
c. Splint the infant's arm with two fingers.
d. Never manipulate the scapulas.

22-14. Which of the following statements about a nuchal arm is correct?

a. One or both fetal arms may be draped around the back of the neck.
b. The presence of a nuchal arm usually requires cesarean delivery.
c. In cases where the arm cannot be delivered, rotation of the fetus so as to force the elbow toward the face may be effective.
d. To free the nuchal arm, the fetus should be pulled downward.
e. Forcible extraction of a nuchal arm by hooking a finger over it often leads to fracture of the humerus or clavicle.
f. Fracture of a humerus or clavicle usually leads to permanent deformity.

22-15. The Mauriceau maneuver is used to help _____ the fetal head.

a. Flex
b. Extend

22-16. What are important aspects of the Mauriceau maneuver?

a. Index and middle finger placed over infant's maxilla
b. Infant's body resting on operator's palm and forearm
c. Two fingers of operator's other hand hooked over fetal neck, grasping shoulders
d. Downward traction until suboccipital region appears under symphysis
e. Moderate suprapubic pressure by assistant
f. Body of fetus elevated toward maternal abdomen

22-17. Which of the following statements about the extraction of a frank breech is correct?

a. Moderate traction exerted by a finger in each groin may be adequate.
b. A generous episiotomy can facilitate delivery.
c. Breech decomposition converts the frank breech into a footling breech.
d. Breech decomposition can be more readily accomplished if there has been prolonged rupture of the membranes.
e. The Pinard maneuver should be used to aid in the delivery of the anterior shoulder.

22-18. Forceps should not be applied to the aftercoming head until it has been brought into the pelvis and is engaged.

a. True
b. False

22-19. Why is the fetal body suspended in a towel while forceps are applied to the aftercoming head?

22-20. "Abdominal rescue" refers to the delivery of an infant

a. By cesarean section after delivery of the body vaginally but with entrapment of the fetal head
b. From the breech presentation by employing strong fundal pressure to overcome dystocia
c. By cesarean section when the breech presentation is first noted
d. The performance of a transabdominal and uterine incision during breech delivery to allow an assistant to push the fetal head out the vagina

22-21. Which of the following statements about anesthesia for breech delivery is correct?

   a. Pudendal block and local infiltration are usually adequate.
   b. Nitrous oxide should never be used in a breech delivery.
   c. Halothane can be used to relax the uterus for decomposition and extraction.
   d. Conduction anesthesia (spinal, epidural, caudal) may prolong the second stage of labor.

22-22. List the increased maternal risks due to manipulation and anesthesia in cases of complicated breech delivery.

22-23. In general, the prognosis for the mother whose fetus is delivered by breech extraction is probably _____ as compared to cesarean delivery and the prognosis for the fetus is _____.

   a. More favorable
   b. Less favorable

22-24. Which of the following are potential risks to the fetus in breech extraction?

   a. Intracranial hemorrhage
   b. Tentorial tears
   c. Umbilical cord prolapse
   d. Fractures
   e. Epiphyseal separations
   f. Paralysis

22-25. What is a version operation?

Instructions for Items 22-26 to 22-29: Match the type of version with the appropriate description.

   a. Cephalic version
   b. Podalic version
   c. External version
   d. Internal version

22-26. Breech is made the presenting part
22-27. Head is made the presenting part
22-28. Manipulations are performed through the abdominal wall
22-29. Manipulations are performed by a hand introduced into the uterine cavity

22-30. Which of the following conditions is necessary before attempting external version?

   a. Presenting part must be engaged
   b. Abdominal wall must not be flaccid
   c. Uterine wall must not be irritable
   d. Uterus must contain enough amnionic fluid to permit easy movement of the fetus

22-31. Which of the following statements about external cephalic version is correct?

   a. It should be attempted in the last few weeks of pregnancy in all cases of breech or shoulder presentation.
   b. It should not be attempted in the presence of marked disproportion between the fetus and the pelvis.
   c. General anesthesia is preferable to conduction anesthesia for the version procedure.
   d. Version can be attempted early in labor.
   e. Version can usually be accomplished most easily after the membranes have ruptured and the cervix has fully dilated.

22-32. Which of the following is necessary whenever an external cephalic version is attempted?

   a. Fetal presentation and position must be determined.
   b. Fetal heart rate should be continuously monitored.
   c. Version should be performed in a labor and delivery unit.
   d. Use of tocolytic agents is required.

22-33. Which of the following may be an indication for an internal podalic version?

   a. Delivery of a first twin
   b. Delivery of a second twin
   c. Delivery of a dead fetus
   d. Transverse lie
   e. Lack of descent after full cervical dilation

23. INJURIES TO THE BIRTH CANAL

23-1. In cases of deep perineal laceration, suturing of the external integuments without repair of underlying fascia and muscle may contribute to

   a. Relaxation of the vaginal outlet
   b. Rectocele
   c. Cystocele
   d. Uterine prolapse

23-2. Which of the following statements about obstetrical injuries to the vagina is correct?

   a. Isolated lacerations unassociated with lacerations of the perineum or cervix are equally likely in the lower, middle, and upper thirds of the vagina.
   b. Lacerations of the anterior vaginal wall in close proximity to the urethra are relatively common.
   c. Laceration in the periurethral area may cause difficulty in voiding, a complication that should be treated by intermittent catheterization.
   d. Injuries to the levator ani as a result of birth canal overdistention may interfere with the function of the pelvic diaphragm.
   e. The likelihood of urinary incontinence resulting from injury to the pubococcygeus muscle is minimized by appropriate use of episiotomy.

23-3. Bleeding while the uterus is firmly contracted is evidence of

   a. A genital tract laceration
   b. Retained placental fragments
   c. The presence of a uterine tear

23-4. Which of the following statements about obstetrical injury to the cervix is correct?

   a. Extensive lacerations of the cervix and/or the upper vagina are usually associated with difficult forceps deliveries.
   b. Any cervical laceration greater than 1 cm should be considered to be the result of improper obstetrical management.
   c. Operative forceps deliveries should be followed by extensive inspection of the cervix only when there is profuse bleeding immediately after delivery.
   d. Annular cervical detachment is associated with difficult midforceps deliveries.
   e. Persistent leukorrhea sometimes results from cervical laceration.

23-5. Which of the following statements about the management of cervical lacerations is correct?

   a. Postpartum digital examination of the cervix is usually sufficient.
   b. To ensure correct anatomical approximation of cervical lacerations, suturing is best started from the distal end.
   c. Packing as a treatment for cervical lacerations generally results in a poorer outcome than surgical repair.
   d. Treatment of extensive cervical lacerations includes evaluation of extension superiorly and laterally, by laparotomy if needed.
   e. An assistant using right angle retractors and the operator grasping the cervix with a ring forceps will usually provide the best surgical exposure.

23-6. The nontraumatized, normally laboring uterus rarely undergoes spontaneous rupture.

   a. True
   b. False

23-7. List the causes of uterine rupture associated with injury before the current pregnancy that are related to: (1) surgery involving the myometrium and (2) coincidental trauma to the uterus.

23-8. List the causes of uterine rupture associated with injury during the current pregnancy that can occur: (1) before delivery and (2) during delivery.

23-9. Which of the following uterine defects is least likely to lead to uterine rupture?

   a. Pregnancy in an incompletely developed uterus or uterine horn
   b. Placenta increta
   c. Placenta percreta
   d. Placenta accreta
   e. Choriocarcinoma
   f. Sacculation of an adherent retroverted uterus

Instructions for Items 23-10 and 23-11: Match the type of uterine rupture with the correct definition.

   a. Incomplete
   b. Complete

23-10. Laceration communicates directly with the peritoneal cavity

23-11. Laceration is separated from the peritoneal cavity by the uterine or broad ligament peritoneum

23-12. Incomplete uterine ruptures rarely become complete.

   a. True
   b. False

23-13. Which of the following statements about scars from a previous cesarean section is correct?

   a. Rupture of a cesarean section scar is defined as the separation of the old incision throughout most of its length without accompanying rupture of the fetal membranes.
   b. In the dehiscence of a cesarean section scar, the fetal membranes are usually ruptured and all or part of the fetus is extruded into the peritoneal cavity.
   c. The degree of obstetric hemorrhage in rupture or dehiscence is approximately equal.
   d. Dehiscence usually occurs gradually, while rupture of a previous scar is a more rapid process.

23-14. A classical cesarean section scar is derived from an incision made in what location?

23-15. Which of the following statements about cesarean section scars is correct?

   a. In the rupture of a classical cesarean section scar, the maternal mortality rate is about 25 percent and the perinatal mortality rate is about 50 percent.
   b. The probability of rupture of a classical cesarean section scar is several times greater than the probability of rupture of a lower segment scar.
   c. About two-thirds of classical cesarean section scars that will rupture do so before labor begins.
   d. Early repeat cesarean section of patients with classical cesarean section scars will prevent most ruptures.
   e. In patients with lower segment uterine scars, dehiscence is much more frequent than rupture.

23–16. Cesarean section scars show evidence of healing by scar tissue formation.

    a. True
    b. False

23–17. Which of the following statements about the rupture of the unscarred uterus is correct?

    a. During pregnancy, uterine rupture is more commonly caused by blunt trauma to the abdomen than by placental abruption.
    b. Oxytocin should probably not be administered antepartum to women of high parity because of their increased risk of spontaneous uterine rupture.
    c. Excessive stretching of the lower uterine segment with the formation of a pathologic contraction ring is highly associated with spontaneous uterine rupture.
    d. Formation of a retroperitoneal hematoma is equally likely with complete and incomplete uterine rupture.
    e. Development of a uteroabdominal pregnancy is a rare outcome of uterine rupture.

23–18. Spontaneous uterine rupture during labor may be associated with

    a. Cessation of most labor pain
    b. Abrupt shock
    c. Severe immediate vaginal hemorrhage
    d. Massive hemoperitoneum formation

23–19. Which of the following statements about the detection of a uterine rupture during labor is correct?

    a. When the fetus is totally extrauterine, abdominal palpation or vaginal examination are helpful in identifying fetal parts.
    b. A contracted uterus may be felt alongside the fetus.
    c. Failure to detect a tear on vaginal examination means that uterine rupture has not occurred.
    d. Abdominal paracentesis or culdocentesis may be employed to detect hemoperitoneum.

23–20. The perinatal mortality rate associated with uterine rupture is between _____ .

23–21. Which of the following statements about the management of a uterine rupture is correct?

    a. Surgical control of bleeding and treatment of hypovolemia and shock are the critical components of immediate management.
    b. Hysterectomy is usually required, although uterine repair may be possible in selected cases.
    c. Oxytocin administration should be avoided in all cases because it extends the uterine laceration.
    d. Antibiotic therapy is only indicated in cases where there is antecedent chorioamnionitis.
    e. Ligation of the hypogastric arteries to control bleeding interferes with subsequent reproductive function.

23–22. A _____ fistula is the most frequent type formed as a result of obstructed labor.

24. ABNORMALITIES OF THE THIRD STAGE OF LABOR

24–1. Postpartum hemorrhage has most often been defined as the loss of more than _____ mL of blood during the first 24 hours after delivery.

24–2. Late postpartum hemorrhage is defined as _____ .

24–3. The most common cause of serious blood loss in obstetrics is

    a. A low implanted placenta
    b. Postpartum hemorrhage
    c. Placental abruption
    d. Ectopic pregnancy
    e. Uterine rupture
    f. Hemorrhage from abortion

24–4. Which of the following may contribute to the development of uterine atony?

    a. Prolonged labor
    b. Very rapid labor
    c. High parity
    d. An overdistended uterus
    e. Use of general anesthesia
    f. Use of vigorous oxytocin stimulation
    g. Uterine infection

24–5. Which of the following are the two most common causes of immediate postpartum hemorrhage?

    a. Coagulation defects
    b. A large episiotomy
    c. Lacerations of the vagina and cervix
    d. A hypotonic myometrium
    e. Retained placental tissue

24–6. Retention of part or all of the placenta may cause

    a. Immediate postpartum hemorrhage
    b. Delayed postpartum hemorrhage

24-7. Which of the following is characteristic of postpartum hemorrhage?

a. It is usually difficult to predict in advance of delivery which women will hemorrhage.
b. May be exacerbated in preeclampsia by the already contracted intravascular volume.
c. The effects of the hemorrhage depend on the nonpregnant blood volume, the degree of pregnancy-induced hypervolemia, and the presence of anemia at the time of delivery.
d. Pulse and blood pressure may only undergo moderate alterations until a large amount of blood has been lost.

24-8. Kneading and squeezing of a contracted uterus aids the mechanism of placental separation and shortens the third stage of labor.

a. True
b. False

24-9. The determination of whether postpartum hemorrhage is the result of uterine atony or genital tract lacerations begins with an examination of _____ .

Instructions for Items 24-10 to 24-13: Match the clinical situation with the appropriate postpartum management to prevent hemorrhage.

a. Inspection of the cervix
b. Inspection of the vagina
c. Examination of the uterine cavity

24-10. After a breech extraction
24-11. After every delivery
24-12. After internal podalic version
24-13. After a vaginal delivery in a woman with a previous cesarean delivery

24-14. Describe the clinical picture of complete Sheehan syndrome that follows severe intrapartum or early postpartum hemorrhage.

24-15. The risk of acquiring human immunodeficiency virus infection from transfusion with screened donor blood after postpartum hemorrhage has been estimated to be about

a. 1 in 250
b. 1 in 2,500
c. 1 in 25,000
d. 1 in 250,000

Instructions for Items 24-16 and 24-17: Match the type of third stage bleeding with the mechanism of placental separation.

a. Mechanism of Duncan
b. Mechanism of Schultze

24-16. Immediate escape of blood into the vagina
24-17. Blood concealed behind the placenta and fetal membranes until the placenta is delivered

24-18. Which of the following statements about the management of the placenta in the third stage of labor is correct?

a. Uterine massage is indicated when external hemorrhage precedes the expulsion of the placenta.
b. Uterine massage and gentle traction will often result in placental separation and expulsion.
c. Placental separation is usually first recognized by a slackening of the umbilical cord or a gush of blood.
d. Manual removal of the placenta is mandatory in the case of continued third stage bleeding.
e. Manual placental removal is accomplished by inserting a gloved hand into the uterine cavity and gently peeling the placenta from its attachment, then grasping it with the hand, which is gradually withdrawn.
f. The membranes should not be removed during the process of manual placental removal.

24-19. Which of the following statements about management after the delivery of the placenta is correct?

a. Palpation of the uterine fundus is only necessary when hemorrhage persists after the delivery of the placenta.
b. Ergonovine (Ergotrate) or methylergonovine (Methergine) should be administered only if vigorous fundal massage and the intravenous infusion of dilute oxytocin solution do not result in a firm, contracted uterus.
c. Bimanual compression of the uterus is often effective in the management of postpartum bleeding after the removal of all placental remnants.
d. Uterine packing is often effective in the management of postpartum bleeding after the removal of all placental remnants.
e. The 15-methyl derivative of prostaglandin $F_{2\alpha}$ has proven to be effective in the management of postpartum bleeding after the removal of all placental remnants.

24-20. Describe the technique of bimanual compression.

24-21. Describe the essential steps in the management of postpartum hemorrhage that is not controlled by uterine massage or oxytocics.

24–22. Lacerations of the vagina and the cervix are repaired by interrupted single or figure-of-eight sutures starting _____ the apex of the laceration.

a. Just above
b. At
c. Just below

24–23. What should be done to stabilize the patient prior to performing a therapeutic hysterectomy for the treatment of postpartum hemorrhage?

Instructions for Items 24–24 to 24–26: Match the type of abnormally adherent placenta with the appropriate description.

a. Placenta increta
b. Placenta percreta
c. Focal placenta accreta
d. Partial placenta accreta
e. Total placenta accreta

24–24. Placental villi penetrate through the myometrium
24–25. Placental villi invade the myometrium
24–26. Several cotyledons are firmly attached to the myometrium

24–27. The direct attachment of placental villi to the myometrium occurs because of what abnormal events in placental development?

24–28. The incidence of abnormally adherent placenta is about 1 in every 55 deliveries.

a. True
b. False

24–29. Which of the following is associated with placenta accreta in approximately one-quarter or more of cases?

a. Placenta previa
b. Previous cesarean delivery
c. Previous uterine curretage
d. Grand multiparity
e. Maternal age greater than 35 years

24–30. The clinical characteristics of placenta accreta include

a. Frequent antepartum bleeding, usually due to associated placenta previa
b. An increased incidence of uterine rupture, especially over a uterine scar
c. A high incidence of dysfunctional labor
d. An inverse relationship between the extent of the placenta accreta and the extent of obstetrical hemorrhage, before manual placental removal is attempted

24–31. Which of the following statements about the management of an abnormally adherent placenta is correct?

a. Placenta increta may be identified ultrasonographically by the absence of a subplacental sonolucent area.
b. Hysterectomy is usually necessary in all types of placenta accreta.
c. Manual removal is often possible in both partial and total placenta accreta.
d. Conservative management of abnormally adherent placentas (by packing) is as effective as hysterectomy in preventing maternal mortality.

24–32. Uterine inversion is

a. Almost always the consequence of strong traction on the umbilical cord of a fundally implanted placenta
b. Almost always associated with some degree of placenta accreta
c. Associated with massive blood loss, the extent of which is often underestimated
d. Associated with shock disproportionate to the degree of blood loss
e. Can at times be more easily accomplished with the use of tocolysis

24–33. Outline in sequential order the major steps in the management of uterine inversion.

24–34. If transvaginal reposition of the uterus is not possible, laparotomy should be performed so that the fundus can both be pushed upward from below and pulled from above.

a. True
b. False

25. FORCEPS DELIVERY AND RELATED TECHNIQUES

25-1. Obstetrical forceps are designed for what basic purpose?

25-2. List the parts of each forceps branch.

25-3. The cephalic curve of the forceps blade conforms to the shape of the _____ , while the pelvic curve conforms to the shape of the _____ .
₍₁₎
₍₂₎

a. Birth canal
b. Fetal head

25-4. Fenestrated forceps blades permit a firmer hold on the fetal head.

a. True
b. False

Instructions for Items 25-5 to 25-9: Match the type of forceps with the correct lock.

a. English lock
b. Sliding lock
c. French lock

25-5. Kielland forceps
25-6. Simpson forceps
25-7. Barton forceps
25-8. Tucker-McLane forceps
25-9. Vacuum extractor

25-10. In an outlet forceps operation, the instrument is applied after the fetal head has reached the _____ , the sagittal suture is in the _____ , and the scalp is visible at _____ .
₍₁₎
₍₂₎
₍₃₎

25-11. Which of the following statements about midforceps operations is correct?

a. Forceps are applied before the criteria for low forceps are met but after the fetal head is engaged.
b. The fetal head is usually engaged when the lowermost part of the skull has descended to the level of the ischial spines.
c. All midforceps operations are of approximately equal difficulty.
d. A midforceps delivery requires that the biparietal diameter be at or below the level of the ischial spines and the leading part be above +2 station (in centimeters).
e. In a midforceps delivery, the head does not contact the hollow of the sacrum.

25-12. Which of the following types of midforceps deliveries has the greater potential for fetal and maternal trauma?

a. The fetal head has never reached the perineum and the sagittal suture has never achieved the anteroposterior diameter.
b. Due to uterine contraction and maternal expulsive efforts the fetal head lay firmly on the perineum, but receded slightly after anesthesia.

25-13. Under what circumstances is a high forceps delivery indicated?

25-14. Increased perinatal morbidity and mortality and maternal morbidity result from midforceps delivery as compared to spontaneous delivery.

a. True
b. False

25-15. Which of the following influences the decision to use low forceps delivery as opposed to spontaneous delivery?

a. Parity of the mother
b. Type of analgesia used in labor
c. Type of anesthesia used in labor
d. Attitudes of staff

25-16. What two physical forces can forceps apply?

25-17. Which of the following are possible treatments for deep transverse arrest?

a. Cesarean delivery
b. Forceps delivery
c. Oxytocin stimulation

25-18. Which of the following maternal or fetal conditions may be an indication for forceps delivery?

a. Maternal heart disease
b. Maternal pulmonary edema
c. Maternal intrapartum infection
d. Maternal exhaustion
e. Prolapse of the umbilical cord
f. Fetal distress
g. Placental abruption

25-19. Which of the following statements about the elective outlet forceps operation is correct?

a. It constitutes the vast majority of forceps operations in the United States.
b. It is commonly the most reasonable procedure when anesthesia interferes with the patient's voluntary expulsive efforts.
c. If enough time is allowed, the strict criteria for outlet forceps can usually be met despite the effects of analgesia and anesthesia.
d. Forceps should not be used electively until the criteria for outlet forceps are fulfilled.

25-20. When is ''prophylactic'' forceps delivery used?

25-21. Prophylactic outlet forceps delivery improves neonatal outcome in low birth weight infants.

a. True
b. False

25-22. List the prerequisites for the successful application of forceps.

25-23. Which of the following forms part of an outlet forceps delivery?

a. The bladder should be catheterized
b. The patient's buttocks should rest on the edge of the delivery table
c. The patient's legs should rest in stirrups
d. The patient should be scrubbed and draped
e. General anesthesia should be administered

25-24. Which of the following statements about the technique of forceps application is correct?

a. The biparietal diameter of the fetal head corresponds to the greatest distance between appropriately applied blades.
b. The long axis of appropriately applied blades corresponds to the occipitomental diameter.
c. The tips of the blades should be over the cheeks, while the concave blade margins should be directed toward either the sagittal suture or the face.
d. If one blade is applied over the brow and the other over the occiput, most forceps cannot be locked.
e. The position of the head can be determined by examination of the sagittal suture and fontanels.
f. The posterior ear of the fetus can be helpful in determining the exact position of the head.

25-25. The term pelvic application means that the left blade is applied to the _____ side and the right blade to the _____ side of the woman's pelvis, irrespective of the position of the fetal head (does not apply to the breech fetus).

a. Left
b. Right

25-26. Pelvic application of forceps should not be practiced because the procedure can potentially cause injury to the fetus.

a. True
b. False

25-27. What are the major obstacles to delivery with a outlet forceps operation?

25-28. Which of the following statements about outlet forceps application is correct?

a. The left blade of the forceps is inserted with the left hand.
b. The palmar surface of the fingers of the right hand serve as a guide for the left blade.
c. The handle and blade are inserted directly horizontally.
d. An assistant must be utilized to stabilize one blade while the other is being applied.
e. Application should be checked prior to applying traction.

25-29. Describe the locations of appropriately applied blades for the occiput anterior and occiput posterior positions.

25-30. If cervical tissue has been grasped in an outlet forceps application, it is appropriate to apply gentle traction for three to five contractions to free the fetal head from the incompletely dilated cervix.

a. True
b. False

25-31. Which of the following statements about traction during an outlet forceps delivery is correct?

a. Gentle intermittent horizontal traction is applied until the perineum bulges.
b. After vulvar distention, the handles are gradually elevated.
c. Episiotomy usually precedes the application of forceps.
d. During the birth of the head, traction should be intermittent.
e. The modified Ritgen maneuver, when used in conjunction with forceps, predisposes to maternal lacerations.

25-32. Which of the following statements about midforceps operations is correct?

a. The first blade should always be applied over the posterior ear.
b. In the occiput transverse position, one blade lies in front of the sacrum and the other lies behind the symphysis.
c. If the occiput is obliquely anterior, it rotates spontaneously to the symphysis as traction is exerted.
d. In exerting traction and rotation, the operator's body weight must often be used.

25–33. The fetal head is often improperly flexed when it is in the right occiput posterior or left occiput posterior positions.

    a. True
    b. False

25–34. A vital part of manual rotation of the fetal head in posterior positions is the disengagement of the head from the pelvis.

    a. True
    b. False

25–35. If manual rotation of the head to the occiput anterior position is accomplished, the need for forceps delivery is eliminated.

    a. True
    b. False

25–36. Which of the following statements about forceps delivery from the occiput posterior position is correct?

    a. If manual rotation cannot be accomplished easily, delivery from the persistent occiput posterior position may be the safest procedure.
    b. Extraction is easier from the posterior position than from the anterior position.
    c. Perineal laceration is less common in the posterior position than in the anterior position.
    d. Forceps rotation should only be done with Kielland forceps.
    e. Forceps rotation is less traumatic to the mother and the fetus than delivery of the head in the occiput posterior position.

25–37. Which of the following is characteristic of the Scanzoni-Smellie maneuver?

    a. It is used for the obliquely posterior occipital position.
    b. There is a double application of forceps.
    c. The head must be disengaged from the pelvis.
    d. An exaggerated arc is described by the forceps handles.

25–38. Which of the following statements about Kielland midforceps rotation operations is correct?

    a. The Kielland forceps have virtually no cephalic curve.
    b. The safer approach for applying the anterior blade is the ''wandering'' method.
    c. Rotation is performed at the station at which it can be most easily accomplished.
    d. The procedure should only be utilized for occiput transverse positions.
    e. The same forceps may be used for both rotation and extraction.

25–39. The following description best identifies which of the forceps listed? A narrow bayonet-shaped blade, often applied to the sides of the fetal head for the purpose of rotation in the transverse position.

    a. Kielland
    b. Tucker-McLane
    c. Simpson
    d. Barton

25–40. In which of the following situations could midforceps delivery be a substitute for cesarean section?

    a. Fetal distress
    b. Prolapse of the umbilical cord
    c. Maternal exhaustion
    d. Secondary arrest of labor due to conduction anesthesia

25–41. As compared with cesarean delivery, midforceps procedures generally carry _____ risk of maternal morbidity and _____ risk of short-term fetal morbidity.
<small>(1)</small> <small>(2)</small>

    a. Decreased
    b. Increased

25–42. It has been well documented that midforceps rotation operations are associated with a higher incidence of cerebral palsy and lower intelligence that persists over time.

    a. True
    b. False

25–43. Forceps should not be applied in a face presentation when the chin is directed to the _____ .

Instructions for Items 25–44 to 25–46: Match the procedure with the appropriate description.

    a. Trial forceps
    b. Failed forceps

25–44. Performed in an operating room ready for cesarean delivery
25–45. Vigorous but unsuccessful attempt to deliver with forceps
25–46. The possibility of fetopelvic disproportion is known to the operator in advance

25–47. What are the fundamental factors responsible for failed forceps?

25–48. Which of the following is a theoretic advantage associated with vacuum extraction?

    a. It is a simpler operation than forceps delivery.
    b. Rotation can be accomplished with less trauma to the mother.
    c. Less intracranial pressure is applied during traction.

25–49. What are the reported complications of vacuum extraction?

25-50. Which of the following is a commonly used obstetrical procedure in the United States?

    a. Craniotomy
    b. Pubiotomy
    c. Symphysiotomy
    d. Hysterostomatomy (Dührssen incision)
    e. Manual dilation of the cervix

26. CESAREAN SECTION AND CESAREAN HYSTERECTOMY

26-1. Cesarean section is defined as the delivery of the fetus through _____ .

26-2. Removal of the fetus from the abdominal cavity in the case of uterine rupture or abdominal pregnancy is a special case of cesarean delivery.

    a. True
    b. False

26-3. In general, what temporal factors affect the decision to use cesarean delivery?

26-4. Specific indications for cesarean delivery may include

    a. Previous cesarean delivery
    b. Breech presentation
    c. Fetal distress
    d. Dystocia

26-5. Increased use of cesarean delivery is the major reason for the absolute decrease in perinatal mortality.

    a. True
    b. False

26-6. Based on data from other countries, neonatal morbidity and mortality would be minimized if the cesarean delivery rate was below 10 percent.

    a. True
    b. False

26-7. The lower the birth weight, the _____ the risk for a vaginal breech delivery.

    a. Lower
    b. Higher

26-8. Which of the following statements about the morbidity and mortality associated with cesarean delivery is correct?

    a. Maternal mortality is due primarily to blood loss.
    b. The most frequent cause of maternal morbidity is associated with the use of anesthesia.
    c. The incidence and severity of maternal morbidity is similar to that seen with vaginal delivery.
    d. Cesarean delivery provides a guarantee against fetal injury.
    e. Fetal morbidity is decreased if cesarean delivery is utilized in breech presentations and transverse lie.
    f. Respiratory distress is more common following cesarean delivery.

26-9. Which of the following statements about the timing of repeat cesarean delivery is correct?

    a. A preset delivery date allows better arrangements to be made by hospital personnel and by the family.
    b. Uterine rupture is more likely if labor occurs in a woman with a previous vertical uterine incision than with a previous horizontal uterine incision.
    c. All repeat cesarean sections should first undergo amniocentesis to determine fetal lung maturity.
    d. Sonography can be used in place of amniocentesis to determine fetal lung maturity.

26-10. At Parkland Hospital, what information is used to determine fetal maturity so as to correctly time repeat cesarean section?

26-11. Which of the following is an absolute contraindication to cesarean delivery?

    a. Presence of a dead fetus
    b. Prematurity
    c. Placenta previa
    d. Neglected transverse lie
    e. Maternal coagulation defect

26-12. Which of the following statements about the use of vaginal delivery in a woman with a previous cesarean delivery is correct?

    a. Vaginal delivery should only be considered in a young patient.
    b. The cesarean delivery must have utilized a low transverse uterine incision.
    c. The cesarean delivery cannot have been performed because of cephalopelvic disproportion.
    d. When attempting a trial of labor, an operating room and all relevant personnel and equipment must be available.

26-13. Describe a classical cesarean incision.

Instructions for Items 26–14 to 26–21: Match the description with the appropriate indication

- a. Contraindication to a trial of labor
- b. Not a contraindication to a trial of labor
- c. Undetermined as to whether contraindicated or not

26–14. Less likely to inadvertently extend

26–15. More likely to result in decreased tensile strength

26–16. Premature breech infant

26–17. Two prior cesarean sections

26–18. Twin gestation

26–19. Desire for epidural analgesia in labor

26–20. Oxytocin augmentation needed

26–21. Estimated fetal weight greater than 4,000 g

26–22. For a cephalic presentation, a transverse incision through the lower uterine segment is usually the procedure of choice.

- a. True
- b. False

26–23. Which of the following steps in preparation for cesarean delivery should be completed before the induction of general anesthesia?

- a. Abdomen shaved
- b. Bladder emptied through an indwelling catheter
- c. Operative field scrubbed
- d. Operating team fully prepared

26–24. Which of the following types of anesthesia used in cesarean delivery is administered before the abdomen is scrubbed and draped?

- a. Epidural
- b. General
- c. Spinal

26–25. Which of the following statements about the abdominal infraumbilical midline vertical incision for cesarean delivery is correct?

- a. It is the quickest to make.
- b. For all deliveries, the length of the incision should be 10 cm.
- c. There is greater risk of incising underlying structures if the fascia is opened with scissors.
- d. The peritoneum should be opened at the inferior end of the incision.
- e. Bleeding sites anywhere in the abdominal incision should be ligated as soon as encountered.

26–26. Which of the following is characteristic of the Pfannenstiel incision?

- a. Transverse skin incision
- b. Incision just below the umbilicus
- c. Transverse muscle incision
- d. Longitudinal muscle incision

26–27. Which of the following statements about abdominal incisions used for cesarean delivery is correct?

- a. The transverse incision has a cosmetic advantage.
- b. There is less likelihood of dehiscence with a transverse incision.
- c. With a vertical incision, there is superior exposure of the uterus and its appendages.
- d. The horizontal incision should be used with obese women.
- e. The horizontal incision should be used by a less skilled operator.
- f. At repeat cesarean section, reentry through the transverse incision is more time consuming.

26–28. The uterus is palpated upon entry into the abdominal cavity to identify _____ .

26–29. During cesarean section, placement of laparotomy packs in the lateral peritoneal gutters minimizes the chance of uterine artery laceration.

- a. True
- b. False

26–30. Describe the process by which the upper margin of the bladder is pushed off the lower uterine segment during cesarean section.

26–31. Which of the following constitutes correct technique when incising the uterus for cesarean delivery?

- a. The uterine incision is made 2 cm above the detached bladder.
- b. The incision is begun transversely and made with a scalpel.
- c. The incision is extended laterally and upward with a scalpel.
- d. The incision should never exceed 8 cm in length.

26–32. What steps should be taken if the placenta is encountered in the line of the uterine incision?

26–33. Describe the method for delivery of the infant through the uterine incision.

26–34. In cesarean section, what can be done to aid the delivery of an infant whose head is tightly wedged into the pelvis?

26–35. After the body of the fetus is delivered,

- a. 20 Units of oxytocin should be administered as an IV bolus
- b. The nares and mouth should be aspirated with a bulb syringe.
- c. The cord should be clamped
- d. The newborn should be given to a member of the resuscitation team
- e. A sample of cord blood should be obtained
- f. Fundal massage should be initiated

26-36. At the time of cesarean section, manual removal of the placenta should never be attempted.

   a. True
   b. False

26-37. A longitudinal incision through the lower uterine segment might be advantageous when

   a. The fetus is not in a vertex presentation
   b. The fetus is macrosomic
   c. There are multiple fetuses
   d. A placental abnormality is present

26-38. What are the advantages and disadvantages of extra-abdominal exteriorization for repair of the uterus after cesarean delivery?

26-39. The principal reason that the uterus should not be exteriorized for repair is that the procedure markedly increases the risk of infection.

   a. True
   b. False

26-40. Which of the following steps is involved in repairing the uterus after cesarean delivery?

   a. Inspect and wipe uterine cavity.
   b. Probe endocervical canal to ensure patency.
   c. Ligate large vessels individually with a suture ligature.
   d. Incorporate posterior uterine wall into closure.

26-41. Describe the suturing technique that should be used for uterine repair after cesarean section.

26-42. After the uterine incision is closed, the peritoneal edge should be sutured above the bladder to strengthen the incision.

   a. True
   b. False

26-43. If tubal sterilization is to be performed along with cesarean section, it should be done after the repair of the uterus.

   a. True
   b. False

26-44. Outline the preferred method of tubal sterilization that is used at the time of cesarean section at Parkland Hospital.

26-45. Which of the following statements about closure of the abdomen after cesarean section is correct?

   a. Blood and amnionic fluid are left in the abdomen to decrease the formation of adhesions.
   b. If possible, the abdominal contents should be palpated.
   c. The uterus is compressed to express blood.
   d. As each layer is closed, identified bleeding sites are clamped and ligated.
   e. A tight pressure dressing should always be applied.

Instructions for Items 26-46 to 26-49: Match the layer of the abdominal wall with the correct suture that is used to close it after cesarean delivery.

   a. Interrupted 0 nonabsorbable sutures
   b. Continuous 00 chromic catgut
   c. Vertical 000 silk mattress sutures
   d. Interrupted 000 plain catgut

26-46. Peritoneum
26-47. Rectus fascia
26-48. Subcutaneous adipose tissue
26-49. Skin

26-50. Which of the following is an indication for classical cesarean section?

   a. Inability to expose the lower uterine segment
   b. Presence of a myoma in the lower uterine segment
   c. Invasive cervical carcinoma
   d. Transverse lie of a large fetus
   e. Placenta previa

26-51. Which of the following statements about classical cesarean section is correct?

   a. The abdominal incision is the same as that used in a lower segment cesarean.
   b. The uterine incision is begun in the fundus and carried caudad as far as necessary.
   c. Bleeders in the uterine wall should be clamped and tied as soon as they are encountered.
   d. One layer is usually sufficient for closure.
   e. An assistant should compress the myometrium medially to aid in closure of the uterus.

26-52. Extraperitoneal cesarean section is particularly useful in patients with a bleeding disorder.

   a. True
   b. False

26-53. Fetal outcome from a postmortem cesarean section is dependent upon which of the following factors?

a. Anticipation of maternal death
b. Fetal gestational age
c. Adequate personnel and equipment
d. Postmortem support of the mother
e. Prompt delivery
f. Effective infant resuscitation

26-54. Which of the following may be indications for cesarean hysterectomy?

a. Intrauterine infection
b. Defective uterine scar
c. Uterine atony
d. Uterine vessel laceration
e. Invasive cervical carcinoma
f. History of abnormal menses
g. Placenta increta

26-55. What are the two major dangers/complications of cesarean hysterectomy?

Instuctions for Items 26-56 and 26-57: Match the average blood loss with the procedure.

a. 500 mL
b. 1000 mL
c. 1500 mL
d. 2000 mL

26-56. Cesarean section
26-57. Cesarean hysterectomy

26-58. Which of the following statements about cesarean hysterectomy is correct?

a. The adnexa usually must be removed.
b. The tissue planes are usually easy to develop.
c. Administration of oxytocin is unnecessary.
d. The bladder and its peritoneal flap should be fully developed before ligating the round ligaments.
e. All pedicles should be doubly ligated.

26-59. In a cesarean hysterectomy, the ureters are most likely to be injured when the round ligament is incised.

a. True
b. False

26-60. In a supracervical hysterectomy, the body of the uterus is amputated after doubly clamping and ligating what structures?

26-61. Which of the following is an important step in performing a total cesarean hysterectomy?

a. Extensive mobilization of the bladder
b. Identification of the cervix
c. Ligation of the pedicles to include only a small volume of tissue in each clamp
d. Excision of the entire cervix

26-62. In a total cesarean hysterectomy, what is the advantage of using a running-lock stitch around the vaginal mucosal edge rather than a series of figure-of-eight sutures?

26-63. Which of the following should be routinely performed as part of a cesarean hysterectomy?

a. Appendectomy
b. Oophorectomy
c. Reperitonealization
d. The peritoneum and fascia closed as a single layer with permanent nonreactive sutures
e. The skin and subcutaneous tissue left open

26-64. Which of the following is a recommended preoperative step when elective repeat cesarean section is contemplated?

a. Type and cross-match so as to have at least 1000 mL of blood available.
b. Administer a sedative 1 hour before surgery.
c. Administer nothing by mouth for 8 hours before surgery.
d. Administer an antacid shortly before the induction of anesthesia.

26-65. Which of the following statements about the management of fluids at the time of cesarean section is correct?

a. Each milliliter of blood lost at surgery should be replaced by a milliliter of transfused blood.
b. The only intravenous fluid that should be used is 5 percent dextrose in water.
c. Oxytocin should be added to the IV infusion when the shoulders of the infant are delivered.
d. Throughout the procedure, blood pressure and urine flow should be monitored.
e. Urine flow need not be monitored in the recovery area.

26-66. What might contribute to the underestimation of blood loss from cesarean delivery?

26-67. Which of the following statements about recovery room care after cesarean delivery is correct?

a. The best method to assure that the uterus is well contracted is to watch for excessive vaginal bleeding.
b. Withholding analgesia in the recovery room allows for better monitoring of clinical signs.
c. A thick abdominal dressing should be applied if only a small one was applied in the operating room.
d. Deep breathing and coughing should be encouraged.

26-68. A woman may be returned to her room when she

    a. Is fully awake
    b. Has minimal bleeding
    c. Has a satisfactory blood pressure
    d. Has a urine output of at least 30 mL per hour

26-69. What type of dosage of analgesia is recommended for the postoperative cesarean section patient?

26-70. At what intervals should the vital signs of the patient be monitored during the first 24 hours after cesarean section?

26-71. Which of the following should routinely be monitored at the prescribed intervals during the first day after cesarean delivery?

    a. Blood pressure
    b. Pulse rate
    c. Urine flow
    d. Hematocrit
    e. Temperature
    f. Amount of bleeding
    g. Status of the fundus
    h. Degree of dilation of pupils

26-72. Due to the sequestration of large amounts of extracellular fluid, patients undergoing an uncomplicated cesarean section usually require approximately 6 liters of IV fluids in the first 24 hours.

    a. True
    b. False

26-73. After cesarean section, a urine output of less than 30 ml per hour should be evaluated only if it persists for at least 12 consecutive hours.

    a. True
    b. False

Instructions for Items 26-74 to 26-81: Match the time after cesarean section with the events that should normally occur.

    a. Postoperative day 1
    b. Postoperative day 2
    c. Postoperative day 3
    d. Postoperative day 4

26-74. Oral fluids tolerated
26-75. General diet tolerated
26-76. Bladder catheter removed
26-77. Active bowel sounds
26-78. Gas pains from incoordinate bowel action
26-79. Ambulation with assistance
26-80. Bathing by shower or tub
26-81. Skin sutures removed

26-82. Which of the following statements about the routine management of a patient after cesarean delivery is correct?

    a. A complete blood count is preferred over a hematocrit.
    b. Initial blood testing is performed 2 days after surgery.
    c. Blood transfusion should be immediately instituted if the initial hematocrit is low.
    d. If the patient is stable and no further blood loss is anticipated, iron therapy is preferable to transfusion.

26-83. Which of the following statements about postcesarean section breast feeding is correct?

    a. Breast feeding should begin on the third postoperative day.
    b. A breast binder may suppress lactation in a woman not wishing to breast feed.
    c. Bromocriptine is effective for suppressing lactation.
    d. Suppression of lactation removes a possible source of postpartum fever.

26-84. In the absence of complications, the mother can be safely released from the hospital after cesarean delivery on the _____ postpartum day.

26-85. What instructions for home care and follow-up visits are advisable at the time of discharge after cesarean delivery?

26-86. Which of the following statements about the use of prophylactic antibiotics in cesarean delivery is correct?

    a. Prophylactic antibiotics should be administered to all women having a cesarean delivery.
    b. Febrile morbidity appears to be more common among indigent women.
    c. Women undergoing cesarean delivery whose membranes have been ruptured for more than 6 hours are at greater risk of infection.
    d. Antibiotics should be administered before clamping the cord.

PART VII ABNORMALITIES OF THE PUERPERIUM

27. PUERPERAL INFECTION

27-1. Puerperal infection is defined as _____ .

27-2. Puerperal morbidity

  a. Is defined as a temperature of at least 38.0°C, occurring on any 2 of the first 10 postpartum days (exclusive of the first 24 hours), when measured by a standard technique at least four times daily
  b. Is used as an estimate of the incidence of puerperal infection
  c. Only includes infectious causes of temperature elevation

27-3. What causes other than infection of the reproductive tract may result in a temperature elevation during the puerperium?

  a. Pyelonephritis
  b. Thrombophlebitis
  c. Upper respiratory infection
  d. Breast engorgement
  e. Postpartum hemorrhage

27-4. The general factors that are associated with a likelihood of serious postpartum infection include

  a. Preterm ruptured membranes and preterm labor
  b. The length of labor
  c. The number of vaginal examinations that were performed
  d. The extent of intrauterine manipulations that were required during delivery
  e. The number and size of obstetric incisions and lacerations

27-5. Which of the following statements about antepartum factors that may predispose to puerperal infection is correct?

  a. Maternal anemia of any cause is associated with a twofold increase in the incidence of serious puerperal infection.
  b. Transferrin may decrease maternal resistance to infection.
  c. Poor nutrition decreases cell-mediated immunity, causing a significant increase in the incidence of infection.
  d. Sexual intercourse in the 6 weeks before the onset of labor causes a significantly increased incidence of infection.

27-6. Which of the following statements about intrapartum factors that may predispose to puerperal infection is correct?

  a. Iatrogenic introduction of bacteria into the upper genital tract through intrapartum vaginal examination is a major factor causing infection.
  b. Significant sources of infection are the bacteria already present on the pudenda or vagina and nasopharyngeal droplet contamination from obstetrical personnel.
  c. Trauma that destroys and devitalizes tissue predisposes to puerperal infection.
  d. Obstetrical hemorrhage of greater than 1,200 mL is a predisposing factor.

27-7. Explain the statement that puerperal infection is basically a wound infection.

27-8. Which of the following statements about puerperal infection associated with lesions of the perineum, vulva, vagina, and cervix is correct?

  a. In the localized infection of a repaired laceration or episiotomy, the wound edges become necrotic and pus may exude from the opening created.
  b. Infection in lacerations of the vagina is more likely to remain localized than infection in deep lacerations of the cervix.
  c. Dysuria, with or without urinary retention, is an indication of severe infection.
  d. The first treatment for puerperal infections of the lower genital tract is antibiotic therapy, followed after 48 hours by surgical drainage if no improvement has occurred.

27-9. Which of the following statements about puerperal metritis (endometritis) is correct?

  a. Metritis refers to infection of the decidua and adjacent myometrium.
  b. True metritis involves a uniform infection of the entire decidual surface.
  c. Metritis is characterized by a profuse, foul, bloody, and sometimes frothy discharge.
  d. β-Hemolytic streptococci are most often associated with the foul, profuse discharge of metritis.
  e. Metritis is always characterized by a spiking high fever associated with chills, tachycardia, and uterine tenderness.
  f. In severe cases, breast feeding should be discontinued.
  g. All patients with metritis should be treated with intravenously administered broad-spectrum antibiotics.

Instructions for Items 27-10 to 27-12: Match the vessels initially involved in thrombophlebitis with the sites to which infection may spread.

    a. Right ovarian vein
    b. Left ovarian vein
    c. Uterine veins

27-10. Involvement of the renal vein and kidneys
27-11. Extension to the inferior vena cava
27-12. Extension to the common iliac veins

27-13. Which of the following statements about puerperal thrombophlebitis is correct?

    a. Anaerobic bacteria can exist and grow in venous thrombi.
    b. In almost all cases, the sole method for the spread of puerperal infection is along the veins.
    c. The uterine veins are usually involved bilaterally, whereas the right ovarian vein is more commonly involved than the left ovarian vein.
    d. The most frequent occurrence is the development of large emboli which reach the pulmonary artery.

27-14. Multiple small septic thromboemboli are more often associated with cor pulmonale and sepsis, whereas large emboli are more frequently associated with sudden death.

    a. True
    b. False

27-15. Venous thrombi associated with metritis may

    a. Block the spread of infection along venous routes
    b. Suppurate, causing the vascular wall to become edematous and necrotic
    c. Reach the terminal branches of pulmonary vessels, resulting in pleurisy, pneumonia, pulmonary infarcts, and abscesses
    d. Lead to septic shock through the release of bacterial products into the circulation

27-16. Which of the following statements about the bacteriology of puerperal infections is correct?

    a. Most puerperal infections result from contamination with organisms that normally exist in the bowel and lower genital tract.
    b. Iatrogenic infection with organisms carried to the patient by obstetric staff is relatively uncommon, although β-hemolytic streptococcal infections sometimes occur.
    c. Anaerobic and aerobic cultures of the infection site are more likely to be of diagnostic benefit than blood cultures.
    d. Only anaerobic bacteria are involved in puerperal infections.
    e. Usually only one species of bacteria is involved in a given case of puerperal infection.

27-17. It is usually possible to precisely identify the bacterial species responsible for any given puerperal infection.

    a. True
    b. False

Instructions for Items 27-18 to 27-20: Select the appropriate description for the following conditions.

    a. Chlamydia trachomatis
    b. Gardnerella vaginalis
    c. Genital mycoplasma

27-18. Questionable role in the etiology of puerperal metritis
27-19. Indolent late onset metritis
27-20. Not a proven pathogen in puerperal infections

27-21. Which of the following statements about antibiotic therapy used for puerperal infections is correct?

    a. First line treatment with either clindamycin or penicillin in combination with gentamicin has been shown to be an effective therapy.
    b. When coverage for a pelvic abscess must be provided, metronidazole and an aminoglycoside are a good combination.
    c. Chloramphenicol may be substituted for clindamycin and gentamicin in patients with impaired renal function.
    d. Ileus may be an indication for the use of chloramphenicol rather than clindamycin and gentamicin.
    e. Pseudomembranous colitis is associated with *Clostridium difficile,* which is best treated by the addition of vancomycin to the regimen.
    f. Metronidazole is the agent of choice for all anaerobic infections of the upper genital tract.

27-22. Pelvic cellulitis (parametritis) must be treated by antibiotic therapy and may require surgical drainage of abscesses.

    a. True
    b. False

27-23. Necrotizing fascitis is

    a. A rare but frequently fatal complication of perineal and vaginal wound infections
    b. More common in the diabetic patient
    c. Known for extending from the perineum to the abdominal wall
    d. Cured with low-dose penicillin in most cases

27-24. Which of the following statements about the clinical course of pelvic cellulitis (parametritis) is correct?

    a. The condition should be suspected when persistent, steady elevations of temperature occur in the puerperium.
    b. Unilateral or bilateral abdominal tenderness and tenderness on vaginal examination are common.
    c. The uterus may become fixed due to the parametrial exudate.
    d. Rectovaginal examination may help to identify a posterior extension of the exudate into the broad ligament along the sacrouterine folds.
    e. Suppuration of the parametrial mass occurs in the majority of patients.
    f. Adhesion and abscess formation are common and serious complications.

27-25. Which of the following statements about pelvic cellulitis (parametritis) is correct?

    a. Pelvic cellulitis is more often unilateral.
    b. Direct extension of pelvic cellulitis may ultimately cause a pointing abscess along the upper border of Poupart's ligament.
    c. Retrocervical extension of pelvic cellulitis may result in localized abscess formation in the cul-de-sac of Douglas.
    d. After cesarean section, infection of the tissue anterior to the cervix results in cellulitis in the space of Retzius.

27-26. Toxic shock syndrome is

    a. An acute febrile illness confined to the lower reproductive tract
    b. Characterized by fever, headache, mental confusion, scarlatiniform rash, subcutaneous edema, nausea, vomiting, watery diarrhea, marked hemoconcentration, oliguria, and renal failure
    c. Associated with *Staphylococcus* species and their endotoxin
    d. Best treated with broad-spectrum antibiotics

27-27. Regarding puerperal infection, which of the following statements is true?

    a. The term phlegmon refers to induration that is a complication of infection.
    b. Cellulitis extends along natural lines of the pelvic cleavage.
    c. Puerperal metritis with pelvic cellulitis is typically a retroperitoneal infection.
    d. The primary treatment for pelvic phlegmon remains surgical excision.

27-28. Persistent fever postpartum should alert one to the possibility of

    a. Parametrial phlegmon
    b. Sheehan's syndrome
    c. Occult episiotomy infection
    d. Milk fever

27-29. Which of the following statements are true regarding septic pelvic thrombophlebitis?

    a. The etiology is probably secondary to extension of infection along venous channels.
    b. Ovarian vein involvement is seen.
    c. It is characterized by hectic fever spikes.
    d. Diagnosis relies on the finding of a palpable posterior pelvic mass.

27-30. Septic shock is

    a. Most common in pregnancy secondary to abortion, pyelonephritis, and puerperal infection
    b. Most common bacteria-causing septic shock are of the family Enterobacteriaceae
    c. Exotoxin release is the most common etiologic mechanism
    d. Is actually a form of high output cardiac failure
    e. Failure to correct hypotension with fluid administration is a poor prognostic sign
    f. Classical clinical signs would include hypotension and oliguria
    g. Treatment involves immediate surgery

27-31. Differential diagnosis of postpartum fever

    a. Should consider foremost genital tract infection
    b. Can include extrapelvic sites of infection, most commonly respiratory atelectasis
    c. Should include breast engorgement, especially if the fever persists for days despite therapy
    d. In a woman with a painful, swollen leg should include treatment with diuretics

28. OTHER DISORDERS OF THE PUERPERIUM

28-1. Deep venous thrombosis and thromboembolism are limited to the puerperium.

    a. True
    b. False

28-2. The strongest single predisposing factor to deep vein thrombosis is _____ .

28-3. The increasing incidence of venous thromboembolic disease during the puerperium is due to increases in the use of oral contraceptives before conception and in the number of women who work at sedentary jobs.

   a. True
   b. False

28-4. Puerperal thromboembolic disease can be decreased by

   a. Early ambulation
   b. Prohibition of ambulation

Instructions for Items 28-5 to 28-6: Match the type of venous thrombosis with the appropriate description.

   a. Thrombophlebitis
   b. Phlebothrombosis

28-5. Venous thrombosis associated with an inflammatory response

28-6. Venous thrombosis without evidence of inflammation

28-7. Deep and superficial venous thrombosis of the legs have an equal potential for generating pulmonary emboli.

   a. True
   b. False

28-8. The standard used for diagnostic confirmation of deep venous thrombosis in pregnancy is

   a. Impedance plethysmography
   b. Intravenous pyelogram
   c. Doppler flow measurement
   d. Phlebography or venography

28-9. Which of the following statements about deep venous thrombosis of the legs is correct?

   a. Puerperal pelvic thrombosis is commonly associated with uterine infection.
   b. It is characterized by an abrupt onset of swelling and pain in one or both extremities, usually with the demonstration of a positive Homan sign.
   c. It may be definitively identified by doppler and impedance plethysmography.
   d. Puerperal deep vein thrombosis is treated with antibiotics (if there is associated fever), anticoagulation, bed rest, and analgesia.
   e. Antepartum deep venous thrombosis is treated by prolonged anticoagulation.

Instructions for Items 28-10 to 28-14: Match the drug utilized for anticoagulation therapy with the appropriate statement.

   a. Heparin
   b. Warfarin (coumadin)

28-10. Inhibits the synthesis of vitamin K-dependent coagulation factors

28-11. May result in congenital malformations if administered early in pregnancy

28-12. May produce maternal thrombocytopenia

28-13. Crosses the placenta

28-14. Does not cross the placenta

28-15. Which of the following statements about the anticoagulant therapy of deep venous thrombosis is correct?

   a. In pregnancy, warfarin (coumadin) is as effective as heparin in the long-term treatment of deep venous thrombosis.
   b. Thrombosis with embolization is less likely to recur after heparin therapy than after warfarin therapy.
   c. Warfarin is the drug of choice for long-term prophylaxis in the absence of pregnancy.
   d. Aspirin and other drugs that impair platelet function are useful adjuvants to low dose heparinization.

28-16. Which of the following statements about pelvic venous thrombosis is correct?

   a. Pelvic vein thrombosis, which occurs very infrequently, is characterized by the acute onset of deep pelvic pain.
   b. Ovarian vein thrombophlebitis rarely occurs in the left vein.
   c. Ovarian vein thrombophlebitis is characterized by the acute onset of pain, with or without fever, in the second or third postpartum day.
   d. Optimal therapy for ovarian vein thrombophlebitis is operative removal of the firm tumefaction of the ovarian vein and the overlying inflamed peritoneum, ligation of the inferior vena cava, followed in 48 hours by heparinization.

28-17. Which of the following statements about delivery in the presence of anticoagulation therapy is correct?

   a. Treatment with warfarin continued until just before delivery may result in fetal hemorrhage.
   b. Slow intravenous administration of 10 mg of vitamin K, increases the levels of vitamin K-dependent coagulation factors to safe levels in both the mother and fetus in about 8 hours.
   c. Infusion of plasma or plasma fractions rich in Factors II, VII, IX, and X results in immediate reversal of low levels in both mother and fetus.
   d. In most cases, heparin therapy may be continued during labor and delivery.
   e. Protamine sulfate will promptly neutralize the effect of heparin.
   f. Given in excess, protamine has an anticoagulant effect.

28–18. List the variables that influence the risk of excessive blood loss/hematoma formation during labor and delivery for a patient undergoing therapy with heparin.

28–19. If a woman who has recently suffered a pulmonary embolism must be delivered by cesarean, ligation of the inferior vena cava above the insertion of the right renal vein and of the left ovarian vein near its insertion into the renal vein will yield the most favorable outcome.

a. True
b. False

28–20. The incidence of pulmonary embolism associated with pregnancy has been reported to be about

a. 1 in 100
b. 1 in 5,000
c. 1 in 100,000
d. 1 in 1,000,000

28–21. Which of the following signs and symptoms are characteristic of puerperal pulmonary embolism?

a. Chest discomfort
b. Shortness of breath
c. Respiratory rate <16 per minute
d. Air hunger
e. Obvious apprehension

28–22. Which of the following statements about the diagnosis of pulmonary embolism is correct?

a. Physical examination of the chest characteristically identifies an accentuated pulmonic valve second sound, rales, and friction rub.
b. Right axis deviation may or may not be observed in an electrocardiogram.
c. The classic triad of hemoptysis, pleuritic chest pain, and dyspnea are present in over 80 percent of patients.
d. A combination of ventilation–perfusion scintigraphy and pulmonary angiography is required for an accurate diagnosis to be made.

28–23. Which of the following statements about heparin therapy for pulmonary embolism during pregnancy is correct?

a. Treatment with heparin, either 5,000 to 7,500 units intravenously every 4 hours or by a constant infusion pump at a rate of approximately 1 IU/mL of estimated blood volume every 4 hours, is effective.
b. Measurement of the whole blood clotting time and the plasma partial thromboplastin time are useful for monitoring the effectiveness of heparin therapy.
c. Frequent measurement of the hematocrit is useful to detect hemorrhage during heparin therapy.
d. Heparin therapy may be discontinued in 10 days to 2 weeks if the disease process has abated and factors predisposing to recurrence are absent.
e. If anticoagulation with warfarin is desired, therapy with it should overlap the therapy with heparin for about 6 days until the prothrombin time has reached therapeutic levels.

28–24. What is the treatment of choice when heparin therapy fails to prevent recurrent pulmonary embolism from the pelvis or legs?

28–25. Which of the following statements about problems of the puerperium involving the uterus is correct?

a. Unless therapy is instituted, subinvolution of the uterus is always associated with leukorrhea followed by hemorrhage.
b. The diagnosis of subinvolution is made by bimanual examination.
c. Subinvolution is associated with retained placental fragments and pelvic infection (metritis).
d. Subinvolution is treated with ergonovine or methylergonovine in addition to antibiotics if there is associated metritis.

28–26. Cervical erosions or eversions, a complication of the early puerperium, can best be treated by cone biopsy.

a. True
b. False

28–27. What are the possible causes of hemorrhage that occurs late in the puerperium?

28–28. Hemorrhage late in the puerperium is best treated by

a. Prompt curettage
b. Oxytocics
c. Hysterectomy

28–29. Which of the following statements about puerperal hematomas is correct?

   a. Hematomas of the vulva are characterized by the acute onset of a painful, swollen mass in the vulva or vagina.

   b. Hematomas may infrequently be located above the pelvic fascia and may progress by a retroperitoneal route all the way to the diaphragm.

   c. Vulvar hematomas, even those that are subperitoneal, ultimately cause external bleeding, which may take the form of hemorrhage or the discharge of large clots.

   d. Vulvar hematomas should be incised, the bleeding points ligated, and the remaining cavity obliterated with mattress sutures.

   e. Broad-spectrum antibiotics are of value in the treatment of vulvar hematomas.

   f. The blood loss in vulvar hematomas is usually slight.

28–30. Which of the following statements about urinary tract disease in the puerperium is correct?

   a. The puerperal bladder is less sensitive to intravesical pressure than the bladder in a nonpregnant woman.

   b. In most patients, there is postpartum bladder distention and overflow incontinence of small amounts of urine.

   c. The distended bladder and/or residual urine may serve as a site for bacterial infection, requiring antibiotic therapy.

   d. If there is continued overdistention of the bladder, 24 hours of continuous catheter drainage is the appropriate initial therapy.

   e. Catheterization should be reinitiated if a woman cannot void within 4 hours after removal of the catheter or if there is more than 200 mL of urine in her bladder.

28–31. Which of the following statements about breast engorgement in the puerperium is correct?

   a. For the first 24 to 48 hours after the development of lacteal secretion, it is not uncommon for the breasts to become distended, firm, and nodular.

   b. Engorged or ''caked breasts'' are the result of overdistention of the lacteal system with milk.

   c. Fever is uncommon with simple breast engorgement.

   d. The treatment of breast engorgement is support with a binder or brassiere, ice packs, and analgesics as needed.

28–32. Which of the following statements about the suppression of lactation is correct?

   a. Suppression may be accomplished by support with a comfortable binder, application of cold, and administration of mild analgesics.

   b. If the breasts are not stimulated by pumping, signs and symptoms disappear after several weeks.

   c. Some estrogens used to suppress lactation may predispose to venous thrombosis and thromboembolism.

   d. Bromocriptine is an effective but expensive method to suppress lactation.

28–33. Mastitis

   a. Is as common antepartum as in the puerperium

   b. Usually becomes symptomatic in the puerperium during the third or fourth weeks

   c. Is characterized by breast engorgement followed by inflammation, fever, tachycardia, and discomfort

   d. Always pursues an acute course

   e. Is most commonly caused by *Staphylococcus aureus*

28–34. The immediate cause of mastitis is usually the introduction of bacteria from the nursing infant's nose and throat through a fissure or abrasion in the nipple.

   a. True

   b. False

28–35. Which of the following statements about the prevention of mastitis is correct?

   a. Careful screening of infants in the newborn nursery for bacterial infection and frequent handwashing by personnel will reduce the risk of iatrogenic infection.

   b. Bacterial interference techniques have not proven effective for control of staphylococcal epidemics in the newborn nursery.

   c. Nasopharyngeal cultures with phage typing of nursery personnel to identify asymptomatic carriers is useful in a suspected outbreak of staphylococcal infection.

   d. Suppurative mastitis outbreaks in the postpartum ward are often associated with staphylococcal infections in the nursery.

28–36. If an examination of breast milk would show a leucocyte count of 106 per mL in conjunction with more than 103 bacteria per mL on culture, it indicates

   a. No evidence of infection

   b. A probable infection of the breast

   c. No prognostic value

28-37. Which of the following statements about the treatment of mastitis is correct?

a. Culture of milk expressed from the breast will usually identify the responsible organism and its sensitivities.
b. Prompt antibiotic therapy (with either penicillin G or a penicillinase-resistant compound) will usually prevent a suppurative infection.
c. Nursing should be discontinued when the diagnosis of suppurative mastitis is confirmed.
d. Antibiotic therapy may be discontinued as soon as the patient has been asymptomatic for 24 hours.
e. An abscess should be treated by a radial incision and drainage followed by packs in decreasing sizes.

28-38. Galactocele results from _____ .

28-39. Which of the following statements about puerperal breast disorders is correct?

a. Supernumary breasts (polymastia) occur in about 1 in 10,000 women.
b. Supernumary breasts have little obstetrical significance apart from sometimes becoming enlarged and mildly painful at the start of nursing.
c. Some nipples are depressed, not allowing suckling.
d. Fissures of the nipple cause pain and harbor infection.

28-40. Galactorrhea, amenorrhea, and evidence of estrogen deficiency (formerly referred to as Chiari-Frommel syndrome) is most often associated with a pituitary adenoma.

a. True
b. False

28-41. Which of the following statements about obstetrical paralysis is correct?

a. Obstetrical paralysis is characterized by intense neuralgia or cramplike pain extending into one or both legs.
b. Obstetrical paralysis is caused by pressure on the sacral plexus branches by the fetal head during descent in labor.
c. Obstetrical paralysis/pain rarely continues into the puerperium.
d. Footdrop usually results from improper positioning of the patient in stirrups or leg holders.

28-42. Labor-associated separation of the symphysis pubis or one of the sacroiliac synchondroses is usually not associated with difficulties in the puerperium.

a. True
b. False

PART VIII COMPLICATIONS OF PREGNANCY

29. ABORTION

29-1. An abortion is defined as the elective termination of pregnancy by artificial means.

a. True
b. False

Instructions for Items 29-2 to 29-3: Match the category of abortion with the appropriate definition.

a. Elective (voluntary)
b. Therapeutic
c. Criminal

29-2. The interruption of pregnancy before viability at the request of the woman but not for reasons of impaired maternal health or fetal disease
29-3. The interruption of pregnancy before the time of fetal viability for the purpose of safeguarding the health of the mother

29-4. Which of the following is now the most common category of abortion?

a. Therapeutic
b. Criminal
c. Elective (voluntary)

29-5. According to a United States Supreme Court decision, during what period of gestation is the decision to perform an abortion left solely to the judgment of the woman's physician?

a. During the first trimester
b. After the first trimester but before the fetus is viable
c. After the fetus is viable

29-6. Define viability as it is commonly used with respect to abortion.

29-7. Describe what is meant by the preterm delivery of a premature infant.

29-8. In many states, abortion is defined as occuring at less than _____ weeks of completed gestation or less than _____ grams of fetal weight.

29-9. The determination of the degree of prematurity or immaturity should be based on

a. Fetal length
b. Fetal weight
c. Fetal gestational age
d. Reported date of the LMP

29-10. Why is the commonly quoted incidence of spontaneous abortion (10 percent of all pregnancies) believed to be unreliable?

29-11. Which of the following is a possible cause of embryonic or fetal death?

a. Abnormalities of the ovum
b. Abnormalities of the generative tract
c. Maternal systemic disease
d. Paternal disease

29-12. Which of the following statements about abnormalities of embryonic development associated with spontaneous abortion is correct?

a. In the very early months of pregnancy, spontaneous abortion is most often preceded by the death of the embryo or fetus.
b. The most common morphologic findings in early spontaneous abortions are developmental abnormalities of the embryo (fetus) or the placenta.
c. Eighty percent of abortions occur in the first 12 weeks of pregnancy, half are associated with chromosomal abnormalities.
d. Most chromosomal abnormalities involve some abnormality of chromosome structure.
e. Trisomies are the most frequent abnormalities of chromosome number.
f. Cases of abnormal chromosome number in the fetus usually reflect an abnormal chromosome number in one or both parents.

29-13. The missing chromosome in monosomic zygotes is usually a(n) _____ , and in trisomic zygotes the extra chromosome is usually a(n) _____ .
(1)   (2)

a. Autosome
b. Sex chromosome

29-14. Maternal diseases are usually associated with euploid abortion.

a. True
b. False

29-15. Which of the following factors may affect the normal intrauterine environment and, consequently, lead to a defective conceptus?

a. Hormonal control of tubal and uterine peristalsis
b. Endocrine control of the maturation of the endometrium
c. Blastocyst response to implantation
d. Trophoblast ability to obtain nutrition

29-16. Which of the following maternal infections has been clearly implicated as a cause of spontaneous abortion?

a. *Brucella abortus*
b. *Toxoplasma*
c. *Listeria monocytogenes*
d. Syphilis
e. *Ureaplasma urealyticum*

29-17. Severe hypertension is a common cause of spontaneous abortion.

a. True
b. False

29-18. Deficiency of which of the following hormones is associated with an increased incidence of abortion?

a. Progesterone
b. Human placental lactogen
c. Estrogen
d. Thyroid hormone

29-19. Which of the following situations predisposes to a greater frequency of spontaneous abortion?

a. Moderate to heavy alcohol consumption
b. Smoking
c. Severe general malnutrition
d. Micronutrient deficiency
e. Maternal–fetal Rh incompatibility

29-20. Women who share a large number of major antigens of the histocompatibility complex with their sex partners abort more often than the general population.

a. True
b. False

29-21. Which of the following statements about spontaneous abortion after laparotomy is correct?

a. Use of postoperative progesterone minimizes the risk of spontaneous abortion.
b. Abortion is more likely if surgery involves the pelvic organs.
c. Ovarian cystectomy may be performed without usually compromising pregnancy.
d. Pedunculated myomas may be removed without usually compromising pregnancy.
e. Postoperative peritonitis appears to have no adverse effect on pregnancy outcome.

29-22. Which of the following statements about spontaneous abortion is correct?

   a. Some authorities feel repetitive abortion may occur because of too many shared HLA antigens between mother and offspring.
   b. Paternal to maternal leucocyte transfusions are currently being used in the treatment of infertility.
   c. Massive doses of immunosuppressive drugs are commonly used for the treatment of habitual abortion.
   d. Formation of blocking antibodies leads to chronic recurrent abortion.

29-23. Which of the following statements regarding uterine defects and spontaneous abortion are true?

   a. Even large myomas are not usually associated with abortion.
   b. Asherman's syndrome is associated with no increased incidence of abortion.
   c. Diethylstilbestrol (DES) is associated with increased rates of pregnancy loss and late abortion.
   d. Prophylactic cervical cerclage has been reported to improve reproductive outcome in DES-exposed patients.

29-24. Which of the following statements about the pathology of abortion is correct?

   a. Hemorrhage into the decidua basalis and necrotic changes in adjacent tissues usually occur.
   b. After fetal death, the ovum or gestational sac acts as a foreign body, usually resulting in uterine contractions and expulsion of the products of conception.
   c. Fetus compressus and fetus papyraceus are progressive stages in the decomposition of a retained dead fetus.
   d. Fetus papyraceus is relatively common in twin pregnancies when one of the fetuses has died and the pregnancy continues to viability.

Instructions for Items 29-25 to 29-29: Match the type of abortion with the appropriate description.

   a. Threatened
   b. Inevitable
   c. Incomplete
   d. Missed
   e. Habitual

29-25. Vaginal bleeding with or without cramping in the first half of pregnancy
29-26. Partial expulsion of the placenta or fetus
29-27. Rupture of the membranes and cervical dilation
29-28. Repeated spontaneous abortion
29-29. Prolonged retention (>8 weeks) of a fetus who died during the first half of pregnancy

29-30. Which of the following statements about threatened abortion is correct?

   a. Signs of threatened abortion occur in about 25 percent of pregnancies.
   b. About 75 percent of women with threatened abortion will eventually abort.
   c. Bleeding at the time of the first expected menses may be physiologic.
   d. Bleeding early in pregnancy may result from cervical lesions or polyps rather than from the endometrium.

29-31. What outcomes are associated with threatened abortion?

   a. Congenital malformations
   b. Prematurity
   c. Low birth weight
   d. Perinatal death

29-32. A gush of fluid from the uterus during the first half of pregnancy always signals an inevitable abortion.

   a. True
   b. False

29-33. Which of the following statements about incomplete abortion is correct?

   a. The fetus and placenta are more likely to be expelled together before the tenth week of gestation.
   b. The main sign of incomplete abortion is bleeding.
   c. Whatever the duration of gestation, serious hemorrhage is very rare.

29-34. Which of the following statements about missed abortion is correct?

   a. Signs of a threatened abortion always occur at the time of fetal death.
   b. The uterus begins to regress in size at the time of fetal death.
   c. Most missed abortions terminate spontaneously.
   d. Maternal coagulopathy secondary to missed abortion usually occurs when the fetus has died early in gestation.

29-35. A woman should be instructed to notify her physician whenever vaginal bleeding, however slight, occurs during pregnancy.

   a. True
   b. False

29-36. In threatened abortion, usually _____ begins first, followed a few hours later by _____ .
                                    (1)   (2)

   a. Bleeding
   b. Cramping

29-37. Which of the following types of pain are commonly associated with threatened abortion?

a. Anterior pelvic pain that is clearly rhythmic
b. Persistent low back pain associated with a feeling of pelvic pressure
c. Dull, midline, suprasymphyseal discomfort, with tenderness over the uterus
d. Sharp, intermittent pain in the epigastric region

29-38. Which of the following statements about the management of threatened abortion is correct?

a. If pain and/or bleeding is minimal, physical examination is not necessary.
b. If bleeding continues after an interval of bed rest, the patient should be examined and her hematocrit determined.
c. Termination of the pregnancy is generally indicated when bleeding is sufficient to cause anemia or hypovolemic symptoms.
d. Progesterone given in regular oral doses is effective in reducing the risk of pregnancy loss.
e. Daily quantitative measurements of hCG that do not show an increase in concentration are usually indicative of eventual pregnancy loss.
f. If the uterus does not increase in size or becomes smaller over time, the fetus is almost certainly dead.

29-39. Which of the following statements about the use of ultrasonography in threatened abortion is correct?

a. A distinct, well-formed gestational ring with central echoes implies that the embryo/fetus is reasonably healthy.
b. A gestational sac with no central echoes proves the conceptus is dead.
c. Heart action in a living fetus is observable at 5 to 6 weeks of gestation.
d. A single examination is usually sufficient to determine the likelihood of abortion.

29-40. If bleeding and pain persist unabated for at least _____ , an abortion is probably inevitable.

a. 1 hour
b. 6 hours
c. 1 day
d. 3 days

29-41. Which finding accompanying or following a gush of amnionic fluid warrants uterine evacuation?

a. Fever
b. Severe pain
c. Foamy vaginal discharge
d. Bleeding

29-42. Which of the following statements about incomplete abortion is correct?

a. Dilation is often unnecessary prior to curettage.
b. Suction curettage should only be used for intact pregnancies.
c. Curettage should not be performed if the patient is febrile.
d. Hemorrhage from incomplete abortion is rarely fatal.

29-43. Optimal therapy for a missed abortion is to await the spontaneous expulsion of the uterine contents.

a. True
b. False

29-44. What is the most generally accepted definition of habitual spontaneous abortion?

Instructions for Items 29-45 and 29-46. Match the time during gestation when spontaneous abortion occurs with the most probable cause.

a. Cytogenetic abnormalities in the conceptus
b. Maternal abnormalities

29-45. Early abortions
29-46. Late abortions

29-47. Which of the following statements about recurrent spontaneous abortion is correct?

a. Following the first spontaneous abortion, the likelihood of future spontaneous abortions is about 25 percent for each subsequent pregnancy.
b. After the first spontaneous abortion, the parents should be karyotyped.
c. Chromosomal banding techniques should be used when karyotyping is done.
d. After two or more spontaneous abortions, a pregnancy carried to term is at greatly increased risk of congenital anomalies.

29-48. Which of the following is characteristic of an incompetent cervix?

a. Painless cervical dilation in the second or early third trimester
b. Rupture of the membranes
c. Expulsion of the immature fetus
d. Extremely difficult to diagnose before pregnancy

29-49. Unless treated, the events characteristic of an incompetent cervix will tend to repeat in subsequent pregnancies.

a. True
b. False

29-50. Which of the following is a potential cause of an incompetent cervix?

a. In utero exposure to stilbesterol
b. Previous trauma to the cervix
c. Early menarche
d. Heavy, irregular menstrual flows

29-51. Cervical dilation with an incompetent cervix seldom occurs before _____ weeks of gestation.

a. 12
b. 16
c. 20
d. 24

29-52. What are the contraindications to surgical treatment of an incompetent cervix?

29-53. Which of the following statements about the management of incompetent cervix is correct?

a. A surgical "purse-string" suture (cerclage) is the best treatment for incompetent cervix.
b. Cerclage is best performed in the second trimester, before the cervix has dilated 4 cm.
c. Both the McDonald and the Shirodkar cerclage techniques have an overall success rate of 85 to 90 percent.
d. The McDonald cerclage procedure is usually accompanied by greater blood loss and longer operative time than the Shirodkar procedure.
e. With the development of clinical infection, the cerclage suture should be cut and the uterus emptied.
f. Beta-mimetic tocolytics and prophylactic antibiotics will decrease the risks of premature labor and infection.

29-54. What grave consequence can occur if vigorous uterine contractions begin while the ligature used to repair an incompetent cervix is still in place?

29-55. Following the _____ procedure, the suture can be left in place for future pregnancies.

a. McDonald
b. Shirodkar

29-56. List the medical indications for therapeutic abortion proposed by the American College of Obstetricians and Gynecologists.

29-57. Elective abortion is strictly a medical issue.
a. True
b. False

29-58. Which of the following is a potential complication of transcervical abortion?

a. Infection
b. Uterine perforation
c. Cervical laceration
d. Incomplete removal of the fetus or placenta
e. Hemorrhage

29-59. The likelihood of complication is increased if suction curettage or dilation and curettage are preformed after _____ weeks of gestation.

a. 16
b. 17
c. 18
d. 19
e. 20

29-60. Dilation and curettage or suction curettage should be performed on an inpatient basis.

a. True
b. False

29-61. Which of the following statements about transcervical abortion is correct?

a. Trauma can be minimized by using laminaria tents to slowly dilate the cervix.
b. The laminaria may cause cramping pain.
c. Prostaglandins have been shown to be effective in softening the cervix.
d. Paracervical or local block anesthesia is mandatory before uterine evacuation.
e. Suction aspiration is used to remove any tissue remaining after initial vigorous curettage with a dull curet.

29-62. Which instrument, when used in the uterine cavity, is not associated with the possibility of uterine wall perforation?

29-63. What procedural elements can minimize short- and long-term morbidity from transcervical abortion?

29-64. Perforation of the uterus is associated with which step in abortion?

a. Dilation
b. Curettage
c. Sounding of the uterus

29-65. Which of the following statements about uterine performation during abortion is correct?

a. Perforation is more likely if the operator is inexperienced.
b. Uterine position does not affect the frequency of perforation.
c. All perforations require laparotomy to evaluate the potential intraabdominal damage.
d. Vacuum aspiration has a lower perforation rate than mechanical curettage.

29-66. Which of the following is a rare complication of transcervical abortion?

a. Uterine synechiae
b. Cervical incompetence
c. Consumptive coagulopathy

29-67. Which of the following terms refers to the aspiration of the endometrial cavity using a flexible 5- or 6-millimeter Karman cannula and syringe?

a. Menstrual extraction
b. Menstrual induction
c. Instant period
d. Atraumatic abortion
e. Miniabortion

29-68. List the problems that may be associated with the technique of menstrual aspiration.

29-69. Postabortion treatment of Rh negative women with anti-Rho (anti-D) immunoglobulin is recommended.

a. True
b. False

29-70. In an abortion by menstrual aspiration, the identification of placenta can only be made using standard fixation and staining techniques.

a. True
b. False

29-71. Which of the following statements about surgical methods of abortion is correct?

a. Hysterotomy or hysterectomy may be indicated after failed medical induction of abortion in the second trimester.
b. Hysterectomy is the best treatment if significant uterine disease is also present.
c. Uterine rupture in subsequent pregnancies is more likely following hysterotomy.
d. Hysterotomy is now outdated as a routine method for pregnancy termination.

29-72. Which of the following statements about the use of oxytocin in pregnancy termination is correct?

a. Intravenous oxytocin is an effective drug for terminating an intact second trimester pregnancy in a healthy woman.
b. Oxytocin is more effective after the cervix has already undergone some dilation and effacement such as with the use of laminaria tents.
c. Water intoxication may develop if a large volume of electrolyte-free solution is administered along with the oxytocin.
d. Oxytocin has no cardiovascular effects.
e. Uterine rupture is unlikely in women who are not of high parity.

29-73. Which of the following statements about the use of prostaglandins in abortion is correct?

a. Prostaglandin $F_{2\alpha}$ is the only safe prostaglandin for pregnancy termination.
b. Vaginal, transcervical, and intraamnionic administration of prostaglandins have proven effective in the induction of abortion.
c. Vaginal or intra-amnionic modes of delivery eliminate any gastrointestinal side effects.
d. A fetus with signs of life may be the result of a prostaglandin-induced abortion.
e. Consumptive coagulopathy is a rare complication of the use of prostaglandins.

29-74. Which of the following statements about the use of hyperosmotic solutions to induce abortion is correct?

a. Hyperosmotic dextrose is more effective than either urea or saline.
b. The fetus is most often killed after the administration of hyperosmotic solutions.
c. The mechanism of action may be related to damage of the fetal membranes resulting in the formation of phospholipases.
d. Hyperosmotic solutions have been largely replaced by dilatation and evaluation as a method of midtrimester abortion.

29-75. Which of the following complications has been associated with the use of hyperosmotic saline for pregnancy termination?

a. Hyperosmolar crisis
b. Septic shock
c. Cardiac failure
d. Peritonitis
e. Hemorrhage
f. Consumptive coagulopathy
g. Water intoxication
h. Myometrial necrosis
i. Uterine rupture
j. Fistula formation
k. Lacerations

29-76. Which of the following statements about the consequences of abortion is correct?

   a. The risk of death from legal abortion is about one-fourth the risk from childbirth.

   b. Abortion has not been shown to be associated with adverse late outcomes in subsequent pregnancies.

   c. Forceful dilation of the cervix may predispose to cervical incompetence.

   d. Asherman's syndrome predisposes to both infertility and obstetrical complications.

29-77. Regarding elective termination of pregnancy, which of the following statements are true?

   a. Fertility is not altered by elective abortion.

   b. Vacuum aspiration results in no increased rate of preterm delivery or low-birthweight infants.

   c. Subsequent ectopic pregnancy rate is not increased by vacuum aspiration termination of pregnancy.

   d. Multiple elective terminations of pregnancy clearly presents a risk to future obstetrical outcome.

29-78. What are the main therapeutic steps in managing a patient with septic abortion?

29-79. What pathophysiologic changes are associated with septic shock?

   a. Damage to the vascular endothelium

   b. Inappropriate vasomotor tone

   c. Impaired myocardial function

   d. Decreased cardiac output

   e. Decreased effective blood volume

29-80. Which of the following statements about the diagnosis and treatment of septic shock is correct?

   a. Hypotension or oliguria in an infected patient should arouse suspicion of septic shock.

   b. In the absence of hemorrhage, hypotension and oliguria that are unresponsive to fluid therapy are likely due to sepsis.

   c. Antibiotics should be initiated after culture results are obtained.

   d. Hysterectomy is seldom indicated.

29-81. The primary goal in treatment of septic shock is to reestablish effective _____ .

29-82. Which of the following statements about renal failure in septic shock is correct?

   a. Renal failure usually arises solely as a result of the infection.

   b. Mild bacterial shock rarely leads to renal failure.

   c. Renal failure may be especially intense when sepsis is due to the exotoxin from *Clostridium perfringens*.

   d. Intense hemoglobinemia associated with clostridial infection should be aggressively managed by dialysis.

30. ECTOPIC PREGNANCY

30-1. Ectopic pregnancy is defined as the implantation of the embryo in the fallopian tube.

   a. True

   b. False

30-2. Which of the following conditions has been implicated as a factor associated with ectopic pregnancy?

   a. Salpingitis

   b. Peritubal adhesions

   c. Developmental abnormalities of the fallopian tube

   d. Tumors that distort the fallopian tube

   e. Previous tubal surgery

   f. External migration of the ovum

   g. Menstrual reflux

   h. Ectopic endometrial elements

30-3. Ectopic pregnancy can occur after hysterectomy.

   a. True

   b. False

30-4. The incidence of ectopic pregnancies in recent years has increased by a factor of

   a. 2

   b. 3

   c. 4

   d. 5

30-5. List the causes for the increased incidence of ectopic pregnancy.

30-6. All ectopic pregnancies require surgical intervention.

   a. True

   b. False

30-7. Order the anatomical portions of the oviduct from the least frequent to the most frequent site for implantation of a tubal pregnancy.

   a. Interstitium

   b. Fimbria

   c. Ampulla

   d. Isthmus

30-8. Which of the following statements about implantation in cases of tubal ectopic pregnancy is correct?

   a. The fertilized ovum remains on the epithelial surface.

   b. The proliferating trophoblast invades the muscularis layer of the tube.

   c. Maternal vessels are eroded by the proliferating trophoblast.

   d. The fallopian tube does not form an extensive decidua.

   e. The embryo is always identifiable.

30-9. Which of the following statements about uterine changes in ectopic pregnancy is correct?

  a. The uterus enlarges.
  b. The cervix and isthmus soften.
  c. External bleeding may be associated with sloughing of the uterine decidua.
  d. The absence of decidua excludes the possibility of ectopic pregnancy.

30-10. Which of the following cellular changes are characteristic of the Arias-Stella reaction?

  a. Enlarged epithelial cells with hypertrophic nuclei
  b. Loss of mitotic capacity
  c. Loss of cellular polarity
  d. Vacuolated cytoplasm

30-11. The Arias-Stella reaction is not specific for ectopic pregnancy, but is associated with the blighting of the conceptus.

  a. True
  b. False

30-12. Which type of endometrium has been identified in cases of ectopic pregnancy?

  a. Decidua
  b. Secretory
  c. Proliferative
  d. Menstrual

30-13. Tubal abortion is defined as _____ .

30-14. Which of the following statements about tubal abortion is correct?

  a. It is more common in ampullary pregnancies than in isthmic pregnancies.
  b. Bleeding usually persists as long as the products of conception remain in the oviduct.
  c. Immediate laparotomy is required to control hemorrhage.
  d. Hematosalpinx may occur if the distal tube is occluded.
  e. Incomplete tubal abortion may result in a tubal polyp.

30-15. Which of the following statements about rupture of a tubal pregnancy is correct?

  a. Rupture will occur sooner if the pregnancy is located in the isthmus than if it is located in the interstitium.
  b. The most usual cause of tubal rupture is coital trauma.
  c. If tubal rupture is suspected, the woman should not undergo surgery.
  d. Formation of a lithopedion is the most likely outcome after tubal rupture in an early pregnancy.
  e. If the placenta is damaged extensively during the process of tubal rupture, consequent abdominal pregnancy is unlikely.

30-16. Rupture of a tubal pregnancy into the broad ligament may result in

  a. Abdominal pregnancy
  b. Broad ligament hematoma
  c. Death of the fetus

30-17. Interstitial pregnancy occurs when the fertilized ovum _____ .

30-18. Which of the following statements about interstitial pregnancy is correct?

  a. The term is synonomous with cornual pregnancy.
  b. Twenty-five percent of all tubal pregnancies are interstitial.
  c. No adnexal mass is palpable.
  d. Rupture is likely to occur later than in other types of tubal pregnancy.
  e. There is the possibility of severe hemorrhage following rupture.

30-19. Ruptured interstitial pregnancies must commonly be treated by hysterectomy.

  a. True
  b. False

30-20. A tubal pregnancy in the presence of a coexisting intrauterine pregnancy is refered to as _____ .

30-21. Which of the following statements about combined or multifetal ectopic pregnancy is correct?

  a. Combined pregnancy is difficult to diagnose clinically.
  b. A congested and enlarged uterus observed upon laparotomy confirms the presence of an intrauterine pregnancy.
  c. Combined pregnancy is relatively common following clomiphene therapy.
  d. Twin tubal pregnancy has been reported.

Instructions for Items 30-22 to 30-24: Match the type of ectopic pregnancy with its definition.

  a. Tubouterine pregnancy
  b. Tuboabdominal pregnancy
  c. Tubo-ovarian pregnancy

30-22. Fimbrial implantation that extends to the peritoneal cavity

30-23. Interstitial implantation that extends to uterine cavity

30-24. Fetal sac partially attached to both tube and ovary

30-25. Which of the following are "classical" signs or symptoms of a ruptured tubal pregnancy?

a. Sudden onset lower abdominal pain
b. Cul-de-sac bulging
c. Vasomotor symptoms
d. Shoulder or neck pain
e. Cervical motion tenderness
f. Tender, boggy adnexal mass

30-26. The shoulder or neck pain felt on inspiration in cases of ruptured tubal pregnancy occurs because of _____ .

30-27. Which of the following statements about pain in a ruptured tubal pregnancy is correct?

a. It is always unilateral.
b. It may be confined to the upper abdomen.
c. Pain is proportional to the amount of intra-abdominal blood.
d. Abdominal tenderness occurs with hemorrhage exceeding 1,000 mL.

30-28. Which of the following conditions rules out the presence of a ruptured tubal pregnancy?

a. A reported menstrual period
b. Profuse vaginal bleeding
c. A negative pregnancy test
d. A normal blood pressure and pulse rate
e. Leukocytosis

30-29. Which of the following clinical measurements is appropriate to detect significant hypovolemia before hypovolemic shock develops?

a. Blood pressure in supine and upright positions
b. Pulse rate in supine and upright positions
c. Urine output

30-30. What type of anemia may be identified soon after a ruptured tubal pregnancy?

30-31. Regarding pregnancy tests in the diagnosis of ectopic pregnancy, which of the following statements are true?

a. Ectopic pregnancy cannot be diagnosed without a positive pregnancy test
b. Urinary pregnancy tests of the latex agglutination inhibition slide variety have a sensitivity of generally 500 to 800 mIU/mL
c. Tube tests for the identification of ectopic pregnancy generally are able to detect human chorionic gonadotropin (hCG) in the range of 150 to 250 mIU/mL
d. ELISA testing generally has a sensitivity of about 50 mIU/mL
e. Serum radioimmunoassay is the most sensitive and precise method for diagnostic pregnancy testing and can virtually diagnose any pregnancy with a sensitivity range of 5 to 10 mIU/mL

30-32. List the conditions most commonly included in the differential diagnosis of a ruptured tubal pregnancy.

30-33. Which of the following suggest salpingitis rather than a ruptured tubal pregnancy?

a. History of abnormal bleeding
b. Bilateral pain and tenderness
c. Unilateral pelvic mass
d. Temperature in excess of 38°C
e. Negative pregnancy test

30-34. Which of the following statements regarding the differentiation of a ruptured tubal pregnancy from abortion of an intrauterine pregnancy is correct?

a. In tubal pregnancy rupture, vaginal bleeding tends to be more profuse.
b. In tubal pregnancy rupture, shock from hypovolemia is usually in proportion to the extent of vaginal hemorrhage.
c. The pain from uterine abortion is less severe.
d. Endometrial biopsy is a reliable diagnostic tool to differentiate the two situations.
e. The shed decidua of a tubal pregnancy can be mistaken for the products from an intrauterine pregnancy.

30-35. The identification of products of conception in the cervical canal or vagina eliminates the possibility of an ectopic pregnancy.

a. True
b. False

30-36. Kadar and associates described four clinical possibilities based on quantitative hCG determinations and ultrasound findings in early pregnancy. Which of the following are among these possibilities?

a. When the β-CG is above 6,000 mIU/mL and an intrauterine gestational sac is seen using abdominal sonography, normal pregnancy is certain.
b. When the β-hCG is above 6,000 mIU/mL and there is an empty uterine cavity with sonography, ectopic pregnancy is likely.
c. When the β-hCG is less than 6,000 mIU/mL and a definite intrauterine ring is seen on sonography, ectopic pregnancy is assured.
d. When the β-hCG is less than 6,000 mIU/mL and there is an empty uterus on sonography, no definitive diagnosis can be made.

30-71. Which of the following statements about ovarian pregnancy is correct?

a. The usual termination is early rupture.
b. A tumor may originate from an unruptured pregnancy that has undergone degeneration.
c. Ovarian pregnancy can easily be distinguished from tubal pregnancy.
d. Oophorectomy is the procedure of choice for all cases.

30-72. Cervical pregnancy occurs when the ovum implants _____.

30-73. Which of the following statements about cervical pregnancy is correct?

a. Painless bleeding is the most common characteristic.
b. Cervical pregnancy usually proceeds to term.
c. Attempts to remove the placenta can result in heavy bleeding.
d. Hysterectomy is commonly the procedure of choice for treatment of cervical pregnancy.

31. DISEASES AND ABNORMALITIES OF THE PLACENTA AND FETAL MEMBRANES

Instructions for Items 31-1 to 31-3: Match the placental abnormality with the corresponding description.

a. Placenta bipartita
b. Placenta duplex
c. Placenta triplex
d. Placenta succenturiata

31-1. Presence of a small accessory lobe
31-2. Incomplete division into lobes (vessels extend from one lobe to the other)
31-3. Presence of two separate lobes (vessels remain distinct)

31-4. If, on examination of the placenta, defects in the membranes are noted a short distance from the placental margin, retention of a _____ should be suspected.

31-5. The incidence of a succenturiate lobe is approximately _____ percent.

a. 1
b. 3
c. 6
d. 12

31-6. Which of the following abnormalities is associated with postpartum hemorrhage?

a. Placenta bipartita
b. Placenta duplex
c. Placenta succenturiata
d. Placenta triplex

31-7. A ring-shaped placenta is associated with

a. Fetal growth retardation
b. Congenital malformations
c. Antepartum bleeding
d. Postpartum bleeding
e. Prematurity

31-8. Which of the following statements about placenta membranacea is correct?

a. All of the fetal membranes are covered by functioning villi.
b. The placenta develops as a thin membranous structure occupying the entire periphery of the chorion.
c. The nutrition of the fetus is compromised.
d. Serious bleeding is rare.
e. During the third stage of labor, the placenta may not separate.

31-9. What is a fenestrated placenta?

31-10. In an extrachorial placenta, the chorionic plate (fetal side) is smaller than the basal plate (maternal side).

a. True
b. False

Instructions for Items 31-11 to 31-15: Match the type of extrachorial placenta with the appropriate description.

a. Circumvallate placenta
b. Marginate placenta

31-11. Fetal surface presents a central depression surrounded by a thickened, grayish white ring
31-12. Ring coincides with the placental margin
31-13. Ring is composed of a double fold of amnion and chorion with degenerated decidua and fibrin in between
31-14. Chorion and amnion are raised at the margin by interposed decidua and fibrin
31-15. Associated with antepartum hemorrhage and fetal malformations

31-16. The normal term placenta weighs about _____ g.

a. 250
b. 500
c. 750
d. 1,000

31-17. Which of the following conditions is associated with an enlarged placenta?

a. Erythroblastosis fetalis
b. Sickle cell disease
c. Epilepsy
d. Syphilis
e. Gonorrhea

31–18. A placental polyp is formed from _____ .

31–19. What etiologic factors do degenerative lesions (e.g., placental infarct) of the placenta have in common?

31–20. Which histopathologic findings are characteristic of placental infarcts?

a. Calcification
b. Ischemic infarction from spiral artery occlusion
c. Fibrinoid degeneration of trophoblasts
d. Marked cellular hyperplasia

31–21. Which of the following statements about placental infarcts is correct?

a. Placental infarcts are the most common lesions of the placenta.
b. The degenerative changes due to trophoblast aging and impairment of the uteroplacental circulation make the term placenta an essentially dying organ.
c. Marginal infarcts occur at the edges of the central cotyledons of the placenta and may be quite extensive.
d. The frequencies of placental infarcts in normal term pregnancies and in pregnancies complicated by hypertension are almost identical.
e. Syncitial degeneration begins during the latter half of pregnancy.

31–22. Which of the following statements about placental calcification is correct?

a. Calcification of the placenta occurs in less than 10 percent of pregnancies.
b. The amount of calcium deposited decreases as the pregnancy progresses.
c. Calcification of the placenta may be detected by sonography.
d. Discovery of placental calcification is an indication for immediate delivery and can be used grossly as a predictor of fetal lung maturity.

31–23. Thrombosis of a fetal villous stem artery produces discrete areas of avascularity.

a. True
b. False

31–24. Enlargement of chorionic villi is associated with

a. Erythroblastosis (hydropic type)
b. Diabetes
c. Sickle cell disease
d. Fetal congestive heart failure
e. Rheumatic fever

31–25. Placental abnormalities detected by electron microscopy indicate

a. When a third or more of the placental villi are involved with syncytial knots, it is considered abnormal.
b. In prolonged pregnancy there is a marked number of syncytial knots.
c. Cytotrophoblast cells continue to proliferate throughout pregnancy.
d. Diabetes mellitus and erythroblastosis fetalis both demonstrate significantly decreased numbers of cytotrophoblastic cells when compared with term to a normal pregnancy.

Instructions for Items 31–26 to 31–29: Match the abnormality of umbilical cord length with the problem with which it has been associated.

a. Short cord
b. Long cord

31–26. True knots
31–27. Umbilical cord prolapse
31–28. Abruptio placentae
31–29. Rupture with intrafunicular hemorrhage

31–30. Which of the following statements about abnormalities of the umbilical cord (funis) is correct?

a. A single umbilical artery is associated with an increased incidence of fetal malformations.
b. A battledore placenta occurs when the umbilical cord inserts at the placental margin.
c. Velamentous insertion occurs in almost all cases of triplets and in about 1 percent of singleton pregnancies.
d. Vasa previa occurs when a velamentous insertion crosses the internal os.
e. Vasa previa is associated with an increased risk of maternal exsanguination.
f. Vasa previa may be identified by the demonstration of nucleated red blood cells in a patient with antepartum hemorrhage.

31–31. Which of the following statements about impeded blood flow in the umbilical cord is correct?

a. Nuchal cord is a common cause of fetal death.
b. Extreme degrees of torsion in the cord commonly cause fetal demise.
c. Cord stricture is associated with a focal deficiency of Wharton jelly.
d. True cysts of the cord are derived from remnants of the umbilical vesicle or the allantois.

31–32. Hydatidiform moles are _____ .

31-33. The villi of an invasive mole may

   a. Invade the uterus
   b. Metastasize to distant organs

31-34. Choriocarcinoma consists of neoplastic trophoblast _____ stroma.

   a. With
   b. Without

31-35. Choriocarcinoma occurs when _____ .

Instructions for Items 31-36 to 31-37: Match the type of neoplastic trophoblasts with the correct synonym.

   a. Invasive mole
   b. Choriocarcinoma

31-36. Chorioadenoma destruens
31-37. Chorionepithelioma

31-38. Hydatidiform moles may occupy the

   a. Uterine cavity
   b. Oviduct
   c. Ovary

31-39. Describe the features of a complete hydatidiform mole.

Instructions for Items 31-40 to 31-46. Match the type of hydatidiform mole with the appropriate description.

   a. Complete hydatidiform mole
   b. Partial hydatidiform mole

31-40. Chromosomal composition mostly 46, XX
31-41. Karyotype is typically triploid
31-42. Chromosomes are of paternal origin
31-43. Presence of focal trophoblastic hyperplasia
31-44. Absence of fetus and amnion
31-45. Risk of choriocarcinoma is slight
31-46. Associated with ovarian theca lutein cysts

31-47. What is molar degeneration?

31-48. Careful histologic scrutiny of hydatidiform moles can identify those which will eventually give rise to choriocarcinoma.

   a. True
   b. False

31-49. Which of the following statements about theca lutein cysts is correct?

   a. They are exclusively associated with hydatidiform moles.
   b. The cysts are lined with lutein cells.
   c. Torsion, infarction or hemorrhage may occur in large cysts.
   d. Extensive cystectomy or oophorectomy is usually necessary.
   e. After molar evacuation, the ovaries may enlarge before they regress.

31-50. The incidence of hydatidiform mole is approximately _____ .

31-51. The demographic groups at greater risk for the development of hydatidiform mole include women

   a. Of European origin
   b. Less than 20 years old
   c. With a history of a previous mole
   d. Who have had a previous multifetal pregnancy
   e. With a history of ovarian cysts

31-52. Early in its development, hydatidiform mole is difficult to distinguish from a normal pregnancy.

   a. True
   b. False

31-53. Which of the following aid in the diagnosis of hydatidiform mole?

   a. Bleeding
   b. Uterine size
   c. Fetal activity
   d. Hypertension
   e. Disturbed thyroid function

31-54. The outstanding clinical sign of hydatidiform mole is _____ .

31-55. Which of the following statements about bleeding with hydatidiform mole is correct?

   a. Bleeding always begins just before abortion.
   b. Bleeding is always profuse.
   c. Iron deficiency anemia is a relatively common finding.
   d. Hemorrhage may be concealed as well as external.

31-56. In about one-half the cases of hydatidiform mole, the uterus is _____ than normal for gestational age.

   a. Larger
   b. Smaller

31-57. In molar pregnancy, the ovaries are often enlarged due to the presence of _____ .

31-58. Which of the following statements about the clinical course of hydatidiform mole is correct?

a. Survival of a fetus in the presence of hydatidiform mole is impossible.
b. Pregnancy-induced hypertension is frequently associated with hydatidiform mole.
c. Hypertension before 24 weeks strongly suggests chronic hypertension rather than a molar pregnancy.
d. Embolization of trophoblastic tissue typically progresses to maternal death.

31-59. In case of hydatidiform mole, the levels of free thyroxine may be elevated due to the effects of

a. Estrogen
b. Human chorionic gonadotropin
c. Thyroid-stimulating hormone

31-60. Spontaneous expulsion of a hydatidiform mole is most likely to occur around which month of pregnancy?

a. Third
b. Fourth
c. Fifth
d. Sixth

31-61. Which of the following must be ruled out in determining the presence of a hydatidiform mole?

a. Myomata
b. Multifetal pregnancy
c. Hydramnios
d. Error in determining gestational age

31-62. The diagnostic technique of choice for determining the presence of hydatidiform mole is

a. An amniogram
b. Ultrasonography
c. Physical examination
d. Urinary chorionic gonadotropin levels
e. Flat plate x-ray of abdomen

31-63. Which of the following statements about the use of human chorionic gonadotropin (hCG) in the diagnosis of hydatidiform mole is correct?

a. Serum assays are more reliable than urine assays.
b. Levels far above normal for a certain stage of pregnancy are definitively diagnostic.
c. High values early in pregnancy are particularly characteristic of hydatidiform mole.
d. Rising levels after 100 days of pregnancy are strong evidence for abnormal trophoblastic growth.

31-64. Which of the following is a diagnostic clinical feature of complete hydatidiform mole?

a. Continuous or intermittent bloody vaginal discharge from about 12 weeks' gestation
b. Uterine enlargement out of proportion to the gestational age
c. Absence of fetal parts on palpation and fetal heart sounds on auscultation
d. Characteristic ultrasonographic pattern
e. Very high hCG level in serum 100 days or more after LMP
f. Preeclampsia–eclampsia developing before 24 weeks' gestation

31-65. The maternal mortality from hydatidiform mole is about _____ percent.

31-66. What percent of hydatidiform moles progress to choriocarcinoma?

a. 10
b. 40
c. 70
d. 100

31-67. Which of the following statements about the treatment of hydatidiform mole is correct?

a. If a fetus and a hydatidiform mole coexist, it is necessary to treat the mole to the exclusion of concern for the fetus.
b. Prophylactic chemotherapy reduces the incidence of uterine perforation and hemorrhage at the time of molar evacuation.
c. Molar evacuation should be undertaken with at least 4 units of compatible whole blood available.
d. Intravenous oxytocin should be administered as the uterus is emptied by vacuum aspiration.
e. Uterine relaxation induced by anesthesia reduces intraoperative complications.

31-68. What is the purpose of obtaining a separate sharp curettage specimen at the time molar evacuation is performed?

31-69. The possibility of uterine trauma and/or uncontrollable hemorrhage at the time of molar evacuation necessitates immediate availability of facilities to perform _____ .

Instructions for Items 31-70 and 31-71. Match the treatment method for molar pregnancy with its potential negative effect.

a. Incomplete evacuation
b. Hemorrhage

31-70. Oxytocin
31-71. Prostaglandin

31-72. In women over 40 years of age, hysterectomy is a more logical treatment for hydatidiform mole than vacuum aspiration.

a. True
b. False

31-73. What is the prime objective of follow-up after treatment of hydatidiform mole?

31-74. Serial measurement of _____ is the most important component of follow-up after hydatidiform mole.

31-75. Which of the following statements about the evaluation and treatment of persistent trophoblastic disease is correct?

a. Rising hCG titers indicate persistent trophoblastic disease requiring treatment.
b. Estrogen–progestin contraceptives should be given in the first year posttreatment to prevent subsequent pregnancy.
c. Chest x-rays should be obtained at the first posttreatment visit.
d. Treatment with methotrexate, actinomycin D or other tumoricidal agents is indicated until hCG levels return to normal.
e. Once hCG levels have returned to normal after chemotherapy, no further evaluation is required.

Instructions for Items 31-76 to 31-78: Match the clinical circumstance with the appropriate treatment.

a. Hysterectomy
b. Curettage
c. Chemotherapy

31-76. Rising hCG levels, no disease beyond the uterus, further childbearing desired
31-77. Rising hCG levels, no disease beyond the uterus, no further childbearing desired
31-78. Rising hCG levels, presence of a lung lesion

31-79. Which of the following is a part of the recommended follow-up for persistent trophoblastic disease?

a. Prevent pregnancy
b. Perform urine pregnancy tests weekly
c. Use medical therapy for any patient desiring further childbearing
d. Follow for 1 year after hCG levels return to normal
e. Evaluate and treat rising or plateau levels of hCG

31-80. Choriocarcinoma is equally likely to develop from a normal pregnancy as from hydatidiform mole.

a. True
b. False

31-81. Which of the following statements about the pathology of choriocarcinoma is correct?

a. It is classified as a moderately malignant lesion.
b. The main factor involved in the malignant transformation of the trophoblast is the previous use of steroidal contraceptives.
c. The characteristic gross picture of choriocarcinoma is a slowly growing mass spreading through the uterine endometrium.
d. Choriocarcinoma is characterized by the absence of a villous pattern.
e. Only cytotrophoblast is involved in choriocarcinoma.
f. Metastases in choriocarcinoma are generally carried by the lymphatic system.
g. The most common metastatic site for choriocarcinoma is the vagina.

31-82. Theca lutein cysts of the ovary occur in about _____ percent of cases of choriocarcinoma.

a. 10
b. 30
c. 50
d. 70
e. 90

31-83. Which of the following clinical circumstances suggest the possibility of choriocarcinoma?

a. Irregular bleeding after pregnancy termination
b. Bloody cough
c. Uterine subinvolution
d. Vaginal tumor

31-84. The most common cause of death from choriocarcinoma is infection associated with lymphatic system blockage.

a. True
b. False

31-85. Which of the following statements about the diagnosis of choriocarcinoma is correct?

a. All cases of hydatidiform mole should be followed for the appearance of choriocarcinoma.
b. The best method to evaluate unusual bleeding after a term pregnancy or abortion is by curettage.
c. Elevated hCG levels in the absence of pregnancy are indicative of trophoblastic neoplasia.
d. Malignant tissue may be inaccessible to routine surgical diagnostic techniques.

31-86. The overall cure rate for persistent gestational trophoblastic disease is approximately _____ percent.

a. 10
b. 30
c. 50
d. 70
e. 90

31–87. Which of the following statements about the treatment of choriocarcinoma is correct?

a. Methotrexate and actinomycin D are effective in the treatment of choriocarcinoma.
b. Hysterectomy is usually not necessary for successful treatment.
c. Patients in the low-risk category have an overall cure rate approaching 100 percent.
d. Cerebral metastases may respond to high-voltage radiation and combination chemotherapy.

31–88. List the criteria for low-risk (good prognosis) cases of choriocarcinoma.

31–89. What treatment modality should be used for low-risk choriocarcinoma patients?

a. Combination chemotherapy
b. Single agent chemotherapy
c. Radiation

31–90. Which of the following statements about invasive mole (chorioadenoma destruens) is correct?

a. The incidence is markedly greater than that of choriocarcinoma.
b. It is locally invasive.
c. Trophoblastic elements penetrate the myometrium.
d. Methotrexate may be curative when used alone.

31–91. Which of the following statements about chorioangioma (hemangioma) of the placenta is correct?

a. They are most likely hamartomas of primitive chorionic mesenchyme.
b. Large tumors may be associated with antepartum hemorrhage or hydramnios.
c. Fetal malformations are common complications.
d. Infants tend to be large for gestational age.
e. Fetal to maternal hemorrhage may occur.

31–92. What is the most common tumor metastatic to the placenta?

31–93. Which of the following statements about diseases of the amnion is correct?

a. Meconium staining of the amnion is always associated with significant fetal distress.
b. Chorioamnionitis is characterized by mononuclear and polymorphonuclear infiltration of the chorion.
c. Amnion nodosum is associated with multiple congenital abnormalities.
d. Amnionic bands are associated with intrauterine amputations.

31–94. What is hydramnios?

31–95. Which of the following statements about hydramnios is correct?

a. Most hydramnios is of gradual onset.
b. Moderate hydramnios (2 to 3 liters) is rather common.
c. The diagnosis of hydramnios rests primarily on clinical evaluation and ultrasonographic estimation of the amount of amnionic fluid.
d. Hydramnios severe enough to be symptomatic occurs in about 0.1 percent of singleton pregnancies.

31–96. Which of the following conditions is highly associated with hydramnios?

a. Multifetal pregnancy
b. Esophageal atresia
c. Maternal diabetes
d. Anencephaly
e. Erythroblastosis fetalis, hydropic variety
f. Cleft lip and palate
g. Intrauterine growth retardation
h. Maternal hypertension
i. Spina bifida

31–97. Hydramnios may be associated with

a. Maternal dyspnea
b. Edema of the lower extremities
c. Oliguria
d. Pain
e. Premature labor

31–98. List the signs and symptoms that are helpful in diagnosing hydramnios.

31–99. Which of the following complications are commonly associated with hydramnios?

a. Placental abruption
b. Uterine dysfunction
c. Postpartum hemorrhage
d. Abnormal presentation

31–100. Which of the following is an effective treatment method for hydramnios?

a. Diuretics
b. Salt restriction
c. Water restriction
d. Removal of excess fluid

Instructions for Items 31–101 to 31–104: Match the complication with the method of extracting excess amnionic fluid.

    a. Transcervical
    b. Transabdominal

31–101. Infection
31–102. Prolapsed cord
31–103. Placental abruption
31–104. Fetal vessel injury

31–105. Which of the following statements about oligohydramnios is correct?

    a. Oligohydramnios is most often associated with postmature or prolonged pregnancy.
    b. Oligohydramnios is associated with fetal renal agenesis or obstruction of the fetal urinary tract.
    c. Fetal distress is no more common with oligohydramnios than in a pregnancy with a normal amount of amnionic fluid.
    d. There is increased risk of fetal amnionic band amputation with oligohydramnios.
    e. Pulmonary hypoplasia is associated with oligohydramnios.
    f. Esophageal atresia is associated with oligohydramnios.

31–106. Oligohydramnios may be the cause of serious fetal musculoskeletal deformities.

    a. True
    b. False

32. CONGENITAL MALFORMATIONS AND INHERITED DISORDERS

32–1. What percentage of newborn infants have a recognizable anomaly?

    a. Less than 1 percent
    b. Three to 5 percent
    c. Nearly 10 percent
    d. Twenty-five percent

Instructions for Items 32–2 to 32–6: Match the etiologic category of birth defect with its appropriate descriptor.

    a. Genetic–chromosomal and single gene defects
    b. Fetal infections
    c. Maternal diseases
    d. Drugs and medications
    e. Multifactorial or unknown
    f. Diethylstilbestrol
    g. Marijuana
    h. Birth asphyxia

32–2. Accounts for the majority of fetal damage
32–3. Blamed for many malformations on a medico-legal basis, probably contribute less than 1 percent of malformations
32–4. 20 to 25 percent of malformations
32–5. Toxoplasmosis, cytomegalovirus, syphilis
32–6. Diabetes, alcohol abuse, seizures, and others

32–7. Regarding induced fetal malformations, which of the following statements are true?

    a. The susceptibility of an embryo to a teratogen depends solely on the length of the exposure to the teratogen in utero.
    b. In general all teratogens act on the same aspect of cellular metabolism.
    c. The genotype influences to a degree the reaction to a teratogen.
    d. Agents causing malformation also usually cause an increase in embryonic mortality.
    e. Teratogens often show no effect on the maternal organism.

32–8. In the science of teratology which of the following statements is true?

    a. The embryonic period is the most critical with regard to malformations as it encompasses organogenesis.
    b. Drugs ingested in late pregnancy are most often associated with limb reduction defects.
    c. Some agents are harmful only if given in sufficient amounts over prolonged periods.
    d. In some instances teratogenicity is not apparent for years.

Instructions for Items 32–9 to 32–14: Match the category of drug with the corresponding correct definition.

    a. Category A
    b. Category B
    c. Category C
    d. Category D
    e. Category E
    f. Category G
    g. Category PG 13
    h. Category R
    i. Category X

32–9. Drugs with proven fetal risk that clearly outweigh any benefits
32–10. Drugs for which no adequate studies, either animal or human are available
32–11. Drugs for which animal or human studies have not demonstrated a significant risk
32–12. Drugs for which there is evidence of fetal risk, but benefits are thought to outweigh risks
32–13. Drugs for which controlled studies in humans have demonstrated no fetal risk
32–14. Describes a movie you would not let your 12-year-old see

32-15. Of nearly 1,600 drugs tested in animals, probably half cause teratogenic effects, although there are only 30 documented human teratogens.

   a. True
   b. False

32-16. The best time to counsel a diabetic about drug usage and glucose control in pregnancy would be

   a. Before she gets pregnant
   b. The first trimester
   c. The early second trimester
   d. The third trimester
   e. After delivery when glucose control is not so essential

32-17. Acyclovir should be used in pregnancy for any attack of genital herpes.

   a. True
   b. False

32-18. Which of the following statements regarding the use of cardiac medications in pregnancy is true?

   a. Digoxin rapidly crosses the placenta and has shown to be harmful to the fetus 25 percent or more of the time.
   b. Propranolol has been shown to cause neonatal bradycardia and hypoglycemia but is not contraindicated in pregnancy.
   c. Nifedipine, although used for preterm labor as well as cardiac indications, may decrease uteroplacental perfusion.
   d. Quinine has never shown any adverse fetal effect.

32-19. Which of the following statements regarding the use of antihypertensive medications in pregnancy is true?

   a. Diuretics for hypertension are contraindicated in pregnancy.
   b. Most are class C drugs.
   c. Methyldopa is widely used for the treatment of chronic hypertension in pregnancy.
   d. Atenolol is widely used in the United Kingdom for treatment of hypertension complicating pregnancy.

Instructions for Items 32-20 to 23-24: Match the letter of the drug or medication with the most appropriate descriptor

   a. Heparin
   b. Coumarin
   c. Terbutaline
   d. Trimethadone
   e. Valproic acid

32-20. Associated with neural tube defects and microcephaly
32-21. Does not cross the placenta
32-22. Anticoagulant of choice in pregnancy

32-23. Used to treat asthma and widely used in pregnancy
32-24. Thought to cause defects similar to hydantoin syndrome

32-25. Regarding the use of antiemetics in pregnancy, which of the following statements is true?

   a. Until recently antiemetics were probably the most widely prescribed drugs in pregnancy.
   b. Bendectin was removed from the market solely because of litigation reasons, not because it was proven harmful.
   c. Phenothiazines prescribed in early pregnancy show no harmful fetal effects.
   d. Most emetics in pregnancy have been shown to have distinctly harmful effects.

32-26. The use of alcohol in pregnancy

   a. Has been associated with fetal maldevelopment
   b. Has been associated with growth retardation
   c. Has been associated with increased perinatal mortality
   d. When chronic or severe, may effect as many as 30 to 40 percent of fetuses

32-27. Regarding illicit drug use in pregnancy

   a. Seldom is it of harm to the fetus
   b. Often it is complicated by a lack of prenatal care
   c. Methadone use in pregnancy may be associated with neonatal withdrawal symptoms worse than those of heroin
   d. To date cocaine has not been implicated with adverse perinatal outcomes.
   e. Marijuana is not associated with any adverse effects in the human fetus.

32-28. The use of psychotropic drugs in pregnancy has shown

   a. Chlordiazepoxide is associated with a fourfold increase in severe congenital anomalies.
   b. Lithium is a cardiac teratogen when given in early pregnancy.
   c. Amitriptyline, nortriptyline, and imipramine have not been associated with increased incidence of congenital anomalies.
   d. No antipsychotic medications are safe for use in pregnancy.

32-29. Aspirin in pregnancy

   a. Is used by about 60 percent of women during pregnancy
   b. Is a category C drug
   c. Does not affect maternal or fetal platelets
   d. Has been associated with prolonged gestation

32-30. Most antineoplastic drugs should be considered capable of inducing teratogenic changes in the fetus.

   a. True
   b. False

32-31. Regarding the use of oral contraceptives in pregnancy, which of the following statements are true?

   a. They have been shown to have little association with fetal birth defects.
   b. They are associated with the same vaginal adenosis as are other estrogenic compounds.
   c. They can be used with clomiphene for ovulation induction to inhibit multifetal gestation.
   d. They are a class X drug.

Instructions for Items 32-32 to 32-37: Match the appropriate lettered item with its best descriptor.

   a. Lead
   b. Methylmercury
   c. Agent orange
   d. Radiation
   e. 5 rads

32-32. In small doses not teratogen, in larger doses associated with microcephaly and mental retardation

32-33. Associated with a negligible risk of fetal malformation

32-34. Although widely thought of as a teratogens, there have been no studies to support this claim

32-35. Excessively high levels may be embryotoxic, cord levels in excess of 10 ug dL have been associated with subnormal infant development

32-36. Associated with cerebral palsy and microcephaly in up to 6 percent of children born to women ingesting this substance

32-37. Results in Yusho

32-38. The incidence of chromosomal abnormalities in liveborn infants has been estimated to be

   a. 1 in 5
   b. 1 in 10 to 20
   c. 1 in 50 to 200
   d. 1 in 500 to 1,000

Instructions for Items 32-39 to 32-43: Match the appropriate letter item with its corresponding descriptor.

   a. Nondisjunction
   b. Mosaicism

32-39. Having cells of two or more chromosomal constitutions

32-40. Failure of the gamete to split equally during meiosis

32-41. Possibly responsible for trisomy

32-42. May be confusing to differentiate unless many cells are karyotyped

32-43. Produces individuals with cells that are chromosomally equal but with an abnormal increase in chromosomal number

32-44. Which of the following statements is true regarding Down syndrome?

   a. Most common as trisomy of chromosome 18
   b. Identified in about 1 of every 800 liveborn infants
   c. May be undetectable on physical examination of the newborn
   d. Using a bone marrow aspirate a karyotype may be available within a few hours

32-45. Paternal age does not appear to be an important risk factor for Down syndrome, but paternal age does play a role in the development of autosomal dominant genetic disease.

   a. True
   b. False

32-46. Which of the following is true regarding abnormalities of sex chromosomes?

   a. Most (45,X) fetuses abort
   b. Fragile X syndrome is the most common cause of inherited mental impairment
   c. Autism is commonly associated with Klinefelter syndrome (47,XXY)
   d. The most common chromosomal abnormality of the sex chromosomes is Fragile X

32-47. In relation to single gene defects, which of the following statements is true?

   a. In the dominant form of inheritance, no generation will be skipped.
   b. All dominant genes have 100 percent penetrance.
   c. In sex-linked recessive inheritance, the affected individuals are almost always female.
   d. Pedigree information in sex-linked recessive inheritance will be of use generally only from the maternal side of the family.

32-48. Which of the following is classified as an inborn error of metabolism?

   a. Down syndrome
   b. Turner syndrome
   c. Phenylketonuria
   d. Fragile X syndrome

32–49. Regarding multifactorial inheritance which of the following statements is true?

    a. Also called polygenic inheritance
    b. Usually seen in about 1 percent of newborns
    c. Include cleft lip, pyloric stenosis, spina bifida, and congenital hip dislocations
    d. The risk of a first child being malformed is about 1 percent, the second child's risk if a previous sibling has a malformation increases to 5 percent.

32–50. In dealing with an anatomically abnormal fetus, it must be remembered that isolated defects are unusual, and that other anomalies frequently coexist.

    a. True
    b. False

32–51. Which of the following statements regarding neural tube defects is true?

    a. The incidence seems to be increasing.
    b. About 70 percent of anencephalic fetuses are male.
    c. Elevated levels of α-fetoprotein in the amniotic fluid or maternal serum reliably predict open and closed neural tube defects.
    d. The results of intra-amnionic shunt placements in the treatment of hydrocephalus have been very promising.

32–52. Omphalocele is associated with other anomalies in about _____ percent of cases.

    a. Less than 1
    b. 25
    c. 40
    d. 70

32–53. Umbilical hernias are found more commonly in black than white infants.

    a. True
    b. False

32–54. Genetic counseling

    a. Is usually best done in a retrospective fashion
    b. Allows the examiner at the completion of the history to identify with certainty the pattern of inheritance
    c. Is usually simple enough so that most practitioners could perform it without consultation
    d. Often allows identification of risks for the fetus

32–55. In the evaluation of a malformed infant who dies, which of the following statements is true?

    a. A detailed history of events from before the time of conception through delivery should be obtained.
    b. Photographs should be made of the face, the body, and all anomalies.
    c. Chromosomal analysis can be carried out on 3 mL of blood, sterile skin, umbilical cord, amnion, or lung.
    d. The value of routine autopsy is questionable at best and should not be encouraged.

32–56. Regarding prospective genetic counseling, which of the following statements is true?

    a. The ideal time for counseling is in the first trimester.
    b. Known carriers will have the greatest risk of passing genes that will affect the offspring.
    c. Screening programs are now in existence to allow identification of some of the more common autosomal recessive disorders such as sickle cell anemia and Tay-Sachs disease.
    d. α-Fetoprotein testing before pregnancy is one of the newer and more successful screening programs.

32–57. Which of the following statements regarding sonography is true?

    a. The role of sonography in detection of fetal anomalies cannot be overestimated.
    b. Down syndrome can be identified in some cases from a thickened nuchal fold on sonography.
    c. Sabbagha and associates have reported predictive values of abnormal and normal studies to be 95 and 99 percent, respectively.
    d. Dangerous levels of radiation are reported with some prolonged obstetrical scanning.

32–58. Which of the following are indications for amniocentesis?

    a. Pregnancies in women over 30 years old
    b. A previous pregnancy with a chromosomally abnormal fetus
    c. Down syndrome in a sibling
    d. An abnormal sonogram
    e. Fetal sex determination in a woman with an autosomal dominant hereditary disorder

32–59. Amniocentesis to detect an open neural tube defect is best accomplished at which stage of gestation?

    a. As early as possible in the pregnancy
    b. 10 to 14 weeks' gestation
    c. 16 to 20 weeks' gestation
    d. During the third trimester

32–60. Amnionic fluid acetylcholinesterase activity is increased with

 a. Neural tube defects
 b. Congenital nephritis
 c. X-linked recessive disorders
 d. Tay-Sachs syndrome

32–61. An abnormally low α-fetoprotein concentration in maternal serum may be indicative of a

 a. Healing neural tube defect
 b. Closed neural tube defect
 c. Chromosomally abnormal fetus
 d. Celtic heritage
 e. Down syndrome

32–62. Which of the following statements is true regarding chorionic villi sampling?

 a. It was developed in the early 1970s.
 b. It has become a widely accepted alternative to amniocentesis in determination of fetal chromosomal anomalies.
 c. The major advantage is that diagnosis can take place with less fear of spontaneous abortion than other techiques.
 d. The technique can be performed either transvaginally or transabdominally.

Instructions for Items 32–63 to 32–71: Match the lettered item with its corresponding correct description.

 a. Gene
 b. Messenger RNA
 c. Transcription
 d. Translation
 e. Mutation
 f. Purine and pyrimidine bases
 g. A probe
 h. Restriction endonuclease
 i. Restriction fragment length polymorphisms

32–63. An alternation of sequencing passed onto future progeny
32–64. The total sequence combinations that specify amino acid sequence for a single polypeptide chain
32–65. Generates a single stranded RNA identical in sequence with one strand of the DNA helix
32–66. Genetic information is transcribed onto this carrier in the nucleus
32–67. May not allow identification of a mutant gene but can locate a known gene or marker gene found closely linked to the mutant gene
32–68. Forms a template in the nucleus to be used for ribosomal synthesis to occur in the cytoplasm
32–69. Converts the RNA nucleotide sequence into the amino acid sequence that constitutes a protein

32–70. Complementary DNA that when radiolabeled using reverse transcriptase allows for very specific detection of cell types
32–71. Cleaves a specific sequence of base pairs

33. DISEASES, INFECTIONS, AND INJURIES OF THE FETUS AND NEWBORN INFANT

33–1. What is the function of the surfactant synthesized by the type II pneumocytes of the fetal lung?

33–2. What are the characteristics of respiratory distress that develops in the neonate?

 a. Formation of hyaline membrane in the distal bronchioles and alveoli
 b. Cardiopulmonary shunting of blood
 c. Hypoxia
 d. Metabolic and respiratory alkalosis

33–3. Which of the following statements about hyaline membrane disease is correct?

 a. It is more common in female than in male newborns.
 b. It is more common in black than in white newborns.
 c. It accounts for about 1 to 2 neonatal death per 1,000 live births in the United States.

33–4. Hyaline membrane disease

 a. Requires that the newborn exert more effort to overcome the low compliance of its atelectatic lungs
 b. Is characterized by an increased respiratory rate
 c. Is associated with a grunting tachypnea
 d. Is often associated with poor peripheral circulation and systemic hypotension
 e. Is identified by an x-ray pattern of diffuse reticulogranular infiltrates throughout the lung fields and an air-filled tracheobronchial tree

33–5. Which of the following causes of respiratory insufficiency may be confused with idiopathic respiratory distress (hyaline membrane disease)?

 a. Pneumonia
 b. Sepsis
 c. Aspiration
 d. Pneumothorax
 e. Diaphragmatic hernia
 f. Heart failure
 g. Patent ductus arteriosus
 h. Primary myocardial disease

33-6. Which of the following statements about the treatment of hyaline membrane disease is correct?

a. An arterial PO_2 of less than 40 mm Hg indicates the need for oxygen therapy.
b. Humidified oxygen should be administered to maintain an arterial PO_2 tension of 50 to 70 mm Hg.
c. It is important to keep the neonate warm to reduce oxygen consumption.
d. The administration of oxygen-rich air under pressure prevents the collapse of unstable alveoli.

33-7. The establishment of appropriately staffed and equipped neonatal intensive care units has served to dramatically reduce the number of deaths from idiopathic respiratory distress, even in very small infants.

a. True
b. False

Instructions for Items 33-8 to 33-11: Match the complication associated with the treatment of hyaline membrane disease with the appropriate cause.

a. Persistent hyperoxia
b. Prolonged endotracheal intubation
c. Prolonged high oxygen tension therapy

33-8. Neonatal pulmonary hypertension
33-9. Retrolental fibroplasia
33-10. Tracheal abrasion
33-11. Bronchopulmonary dysplasia

33-12. Regarding the surfactant used in the treatment of neonatal respiratory distress syndrome, which of the following statements are true?

a. Studies to date seem to show that the administration of surfactant will ameliorate lung disease.
b. Surfactant has been prepared from animal lung extracts, human amnionic fluid, and artificially synthesized.
c. Surfactant is composed of phospholipids.
d. Surfactant is now widely available and used in the United States.

33-13. Which of the following statements about meconium aspiration is correct?

a. Aspiration of small amounts of meconium is a normal event that occurs in most pregnancies.
b. Aspiration causes both mechanical obstruction of the airways and chemical pneumonitis.
c. Aspiration may be associated with atelectasis, consolidation, pneumothorax, and pneumomediastinum.
d. It often occurs as a consequence of fetal distress.

33-14. In the newborn who has suffered meconium aspiration, the initial chest x-ray is useful for predicting outcome.

a. True
b. False

33-15. List the steps that should be taken at the time of delivery when meconium is identified in the amniotic fluid.

33-16. At present, the largest single cause of blindness in the United States is retrolental fibroplasia.

a. True
b. False

33-17. Retrolental fibroplasia

a. Occurs when air enriched with more than 30 percent oxygen is administered to a newborn
b. Results from vascular damage to the developing eye with subsequent adhesion, scar formation, and retinal detachment
c. May be prevented by the administration of vitamin E

33-18. In the hours after delivery, neonatal hematocrit values may

a. Rise
b. Fall

33-19. Which of the following statements about intraventricular hemorrhage is true?

a. These lesions are usually seen in infants born before 34 weeks' gestation.
b. Most hemorrhages develop within 72 hours of birth.
c. These intraventricular hemorrhages are almost always secondary to intrapartum birth events.
d. The main pathological event appears to be hemorrhage into the germinal matrix of the brain.

33-20. About half of all infants born before 34 weeks' gestation will suffer intraventricular hemorrhage.

a. True
b. False

33-21. In most cases, intracranial hemorrhage secondary to birth trauma results in a rapidly deteriorating clinical status that begins just after birth.

a. True
b. False

33-22. Prophylactic cesarean section has been shown to prevent intraventricular hemorrhage in infants.

a. True
b. False

33-23. Cerebral palsy is a specific clinical syndrome arising solely from birth injury/asphyxia.

    a. True
    b. False

33-24. Which of the following statements about ABO incompatibility is correct?

    a. The major blood group factors A and B are the most common, although not the most serious, cause of hemolytic disease.
    b. About 20 percent of infants have an ABO incompatibility that results in some degree of hemolytic disease.
    c. There are no racial differences in the incidence or severity of hemolytic disease associated with ABO incompatibility.
    d. Like Rho(D) disease, the stillbirth rate is increased in the presence of ABO isoimmune disease.
    e. ABO-associated isoimmune disease is very rarely seen in primigravidas.
    f. ABO disease is likely, but not certain, to recur.

33-25. Which of the following statements regarding ABO blood group incompatibility between fetus and mother is *untrue*?

    a. The major blood group antigens A and B are the most common.
    b. Although 20 percent of infants have a maternal ABO incompatibility, only 5 percent of them show overt hemolytic disease.
    c. Black infants are less likely than white infants to develop ABO disease.
    d. There is no adequate antenatal method of diagnosis to detect ABO incompatibility.

33-26. List the usual criteria utilized for the diagnosis of hemolysis associated with ABO incompatibility.

33-27. Which of the following statements about the evaluation and treatment of ABO incompatibility is correct?

    a. There are no adequate antenatal diagnostic methods.
    b. Like Rho(D) disease, the Coombs' antiglobulin test is always positive in ABO isoimmune disease.
    c. Infants affected by ABO isoimmune disease deal with their residual bilirubin more efficiently than do infants with Rho(D) isoimmune disease.
    d. Simple or exchange transfusion with group O blood is the basic treatment of choice.

33-28. Rho(D) incompatibility and ABO heterospecificity are the causes of about 98 percent of all hemolytic neonatal disease.

    a. True
    b. False

33-29. Which of the following statements about fetal to maternal bleeding is correct?

    a. The severely anemic fetus may demonstrate an ominous heart rate pattern.
    b. A large fetal to maternal hemorrhage is usually due to a placental lesion.
    c. Placental abruption commonly leads to severe fetal to maternal hemorrhage.
    d. A large fetal to maternal hemorrhage may cause a transfusion reaction in the mother.
    e. The majority of stillbirths are caused by a massive in utero fetal to maternal hemorrhage.

33-30. Why does severe hemolytic disease occur in only a few pregnancies when the potential exists in a great many more?

33-31. Which of the following statements about Rh antigens is correct?

    a. They are usually inherited independently from other blood group antigens.
    b. The distribution of Rh antigens varies with regard to sex.
    c. American Indians and Asiatics are almost all Rho(D) positive.
    d. Black and white Americans both average about 25 percent Rho(D) negative.
    e. Most Rh antigens are moderately to strongly immunogenic.

33-32. All pregnant women should be routinely tested for the presence or absence of Rho(D) antigens.

    a. True
    b. False

33-33. Which of the following statements about the factors influencing the perinatal mortality rate in cases of Rho(D) hemolytic disease is correct?

    a. The number of perinatal deaths from Rho(D) hemolytic disease has dropped dramatically in recent times.
    b. Pregnant women who are Rho(D) negative and possess antibody to Rho(D) antigen can be readily identified.
    c. It is difficult to accurately determine hemolysis in the fetus of a Rho(D)-negative woman.
    d. Administration of Rho(D) immune globulin to the Rho(D)-negative woman during or immediately after pregnancy has eliminated most, but not all, cases of isoimmunization.

33–34. Rho(D) immune globulin should be administered to previously unsensitized Rho(D)-negative women in which of the following situations?

a. Abortion
b. Ectopic pregnancy
c. Hydatidiform mole
d. Amniocentesis
e. Vaginal bleeding during pregnancy

33–35. Rho(D)-negative women who receive transfusions of blood or blood products should be given Rho(D) immune globulin only if there is evidence of maternal hemolysis.

a. True
b. False

33–36. As a general rule, when in doubt about whether or not to administer Rho(D) immune globulin, the rule of thumb should be to give it.

a. True
b. False

33–37. Describe the recommended procedure for treating the Rho(D)-negative nonsensitized pregnant woman with immune globulin.

33–38. The administration of prophylactic Rho(D) immune globulin to an Rho(D)-negative woman will, in about 90 percent of cases, result in a weakly positive direct Coombs test on cord and infant blood.

a. True
b. False

33–39. Which of the following statements about maternal–fetal bleeds is correct?

a. A maternal–fetal bleed must have occurred sometime before the clamping of the umbilical cord for an Rho(D)-negative woman to have become sensitized in utero to Rho(D) antigen.
b. A major blood group incompatibility does not offer appreciable protection against Rho sensitization.
c. Studies suggest that about 2 percent of Rho(D)-negative women with Rho(D)-positive mothers will have been sensitized in utero.
d. Rho(D) immune globulin prophylaxis should be instituted for all Rho(D)-negative female neonates born to Rho(D)-positive mothers.

33–40. When an acid elution test is performed, fetal red cells are _____ stained and maternal red cells are _____ stained.

a. Darkly
b. Lightly

33–41. In cases of fetal to maternal hemorrhage, sensitization of the mother can be prevented by injecting sufficient Rho(D) immune globulin intramuscularly to provide demonstrable free antibody in the maternal serum.

a. True
b. False

33–42. In the absence of intervention, the perinatal mortality in the case of a Rho(D)-negative sensitized woman with an Rho(D)-positive fetus will be about _____ percent.

a. 10
b. 30
c. 50
d. 70
e. 90

33–43. Optimal outcome of cases involving Rho(D) isoimmunization requires the individualization of management based on information about what factors?

33–44. Which of the following statements about the use of antibody measurement in the management of the Rho(D)-negative sensitized mother is correct?

a. An indirect Coombs' test is utilized to assess antibody titer.
b. A titer no higher than 1:64 almost always assures that the fetus will not die in utero from hemolytic disease.
c. A titer higher than 1:64 assures that severe, often fatal, hemolytic disease will occur in utero.
d. If the fetus is Rho(D) negative, the titer will never be above 1:16.

33–45. Appropriately timed amniocentesis is indicated when an antibody titer of _____ is found in suspected cases of Rho(D) isoimmunization.

a. 1:8
b. 1:16
c. 1:32
d. 1:64

33–46. For any gestational age, the intensity of hemolytic disease correlates well with the absorbance of amnionic fluid supernatant at a wavelength of 450 nm.

a. True
b. False

Instructions for Items 38-47 to 38-49: Match the severity of the hemolytic disease as determined by absorbance of amnionic fluid at 450 nm (Liley zones) with the appropriate prognosis.

    a. Zone 1
    b. Zone 2
    c. Zone 3

33-47. Fetus will be unaffected or will have mild hemolytic disease

33-48. Fetal death will most likely occur within 10 days

33-49. Prognosis inaccurate; requires further measurements to determine trends

33-50. Which of the following statements about hemolytic disease of the newborn associated with Rho(D) isoimmunization is correct?

    a. Antibodies to fetal Rho(D)-positive erythrocytes produced by the Rho(D)-negative mother are both adsorbed onto fetal red cells and exist free in the infant's serum.
    b. The adsorbed antibodies act as hemolysins, accelerating the rate of red cell destruction.
    c. Maternal antibodies in the infant circulation disappear by 3 weeks after birth.
    d. An indirect Coombs' test will definitively determine whether antibodies are adsorbed on infant red cells.
    e. The severity of Rho(D) isoimmune hemolytic disease depends on the duration of exposure to antibodies and the intensity of the immunologic reaction.

33-51. Some clinicians have shown that the Liley curve may not be an accurate predictor of the severity of anemia as measured from fetal cord blood.

    a. True
    b. False

33-52. Which of the following statements about immune hydrops is correct?

    a. Hydrops fetalis is characterized by the accumulation of ascites, both subcutaneous and effusive, in the serous cavities.
    b. The diagnosis of hydrops fetalis can only be made by examining the infant after delivery.
    c. Immune hydrops is associated with a small, atrophic placenta and chronic uteroplacental insufficiency.
    d. Extramedullary hematopoiesis is a common finding.
    e. Heart failure associated with severe fatal anemia is the main cause of the ascites seen in immune hydrops.
    f. Ascites and hepatosplenomegaly may be severe enough to cause dystocia.
    g. Hydropic infants usually survive until after birth.

33-53. Intrauterine transfusion of blood into the fetal peritoneal cavity for the management of Rho(D) isoimmunization

    a. Should be limited to cases between 23 and 32 weeks of gestation, where the likelihood of in utero death is high
    b. Is associated with a 20 percent overall survival rate
    c. Is more likely to be successful if the fetus is not hydropic
    d. Is associated with an approximately 75 percent incidence of mild to moderate neurologic disease

33-54. Which of the following modalities has proved to be an acceptable method to minimize fetal hemolysis?

    a. Plasmapheresis
    b. Promethazine (Phenergan) in large doses
    c. Rho(D)-positive erythrocyte membrane in enteric capsules
    d. Corticosteroids

33-55. A sinusoidal fetal heart rate and repetitious decelerations in the presence of Rh isoimmunization is often indicative of severe fetal anemia.

    a. True
    b. False

33-56. Cesarean delivery should be employed in all cases of hemolytic disease caused by Rh isoimmunization.

    a. True
    b. False

33-57. Which of the following statements about exchange transfusion for hemolytic disease of the newborn is correct?

    a. If the infant is overtly anemic, the initial exchange should be carried out promptly.
    b. If the infant is not overtly anemic, the rate of bilirubin increase, the maturity of the infant, and the presence of other complications determine whether an exchange transfusion should be performed.
    c. Excluding moribund, hydropic, and kernicteric infants, the mortality rate for exchange transfusions is about 15 percent.

33-58. What are the clinical signs of kernicterus?

33-59. Which of the following factors may contribute to the development of kernicterus?

    a. A level of unconjugated bilirubin above 18 to 20 mg/dL
    b. Hypoxia and acidosis
    c. Hyperthermia
    d. Hyperglycemia
    e. Sepsis

33-60. Administration of which of the following drugs may contribute to or cause hyperbilirubinemia/kernicterus?

a. Sulfonamides
b. Salicylates
c. Sodium benzoate in injectable diazepam
d. Furosemide
e. Gentamicin
f. Vitamin K analogs

33-61. Breast milk jaundice

a. May be caused by the presence in breast milk of the steroid pregnane-3 (alpha), 20 (beta)-diol, which blocks bilirubin conjugation
b. May be caused by the inability of milk from certain mothers to block bilirubin reabsorption
c. Is associated with bilirubin levels that rise from the fourth day to the 15th day, and then slowly decline over the next few weeks
d. Will persist in all cases if breast feeding is continued
e. Results in kernicterus and encephalopathy in about 5 percent of cases

33-62. Which of the following statements about neonatal physiologic jaundice is correct?

a. It is the most common form of unconjugated nonhemolytic jaundice.
b. In mature infants, bilirubin increases to levels of about 10 mg/dL and then falls rapidly.
c. Jaundice is often more prolonged and severe in premature infants.
d. It almost never requires therapy, since the resolution is usually rapid.

33-63. The mechanisms involved in physiologic jaundice of the newborn include a

a. Normally increased rate of erythrocyte destruction and bilirubin production
b. Decreased rate of uptake of free bilirubin by hepatic cells
c. Decreased rate of bilirubin conjugation in the liver
d. Reduced conversion of bilirubin to urobilinogen by intestinal bacteria

33-64. Which of the following statements about the treatment of hyperbilirubinemia in the neonate is correct?

a. Exchange transfusion is indicated in severe cases.
b. The sole mechanism by which phototherapy decreases hyperbilirubinemia is through the photo-oxidation of unconjugated bilirubin.
c. Serum bilirubin levels should continue to be monitored for at least 24 hours after the phototherapy is discontinued.
d. Phenobarbital may increase the conjugation and excretion of bilirubin through an increase in liver microenzymes.

33-65. Nonimmune hydrops fetalis occurs _____ frequently than hydrops fetalis associated with isoimmune fetal red cell destruction.

a. More
b. Less

33-66. Which of the following statements regarding nonimmune hydrops fetalis is true?

a. It can be a transient phenomenon.
b. Many cases of nonimmune hydrops are associated with fetal cardiac abnormalities.
c. Up to one-third of these cases are associated with chromosomal abnormalities.
d. The most useful tool for diagnosis and follow-up of this entity is with ultrasound.

33-67. Which of the following is characteristic of hemorrhagic disease of the newborn?

a. Spontaneous internal or external bleeding
b. Hypoprothrombinemia
c. Low levels of vitamin K-dependent coagulation factors
d. Bleeding usually beginning 2 to 6 hours after birth
e. Prolonged prothrombin and partial thromboplastin times

33-68. Which diseases are included in the differential diagnosis of hemorrhagic disease of the newborn?

33-69. The physiologic hypoprothrombinemia in the neonate is a consequence of poor placental transport of vitamin K_1 to the fetus.

a. True
b. False

33-70. Hemorrhagic disease of the newborn may be treated

a. Prophylactically by the intramuscular injection of 1 mg of vitamin K_1 just after birth
b. By intravenous administration of vitamin K_1
c. With intravenous heparin
d. By breast feeding the affected infant

Instructions for Items 33-71 to 33-76: Match the type of immune thrombocytopenia with the appropriate statement.

a. Autoimmune (idiopathic) thrombocytopenia purpura
b. Isoimmune thrombocytopenia

33-71. Antiplatelet IgG transferred from mother to fetus
33-72. Maternal isoimmunization exists against fetal platelet antigens
33-73. Infant but not maternal thrombocytopenia is present
33-74. Treatment includes corticosteroid therapy for the infant

33-75. Treatment includes transfusion of maternal platelets to the infant

33-76. Cesarean delivery is of benefit to the fetus and of little added risk to the mother

33-77. Which of the following statements about polycythemia and hyperviscosity syndrome is correct?

a. The viscosity of neonatal blood rises remarkably as the hematocrit reaches 50.
b. Polycythemia and hyperviscosity are associated with the various transfusion syndromes and with chronic hypoxia.
c. Signs and symptoms include plethora, cyanosis, and neurologic aberrations.
d. Laboratory findings include hyperbilirubinemia, thrombocytosis, erythrocyte fragmentation, and hypoglycemia.
e. Partial exchange transfusion with plasma is the immediate treatment.

33-78. Which of the following statements about neonatal staphylococcal infection is correct?

a. Penicillin-sensitive staphylococcal disease, although uncommon, represents a significant but usually preventable neonatal infection
b. Infection may become epidemic when contamination from infected or carrier staff or from infant to infant occurs.
c. The risk of infection may be eliminated by careful handwashing and child handling by nursery staff.
d. Continuous epidemiologic surveillance in the nursery is only necessary when there has been an outbreak of infection within the past 6 months.
e. Routine care of the umbilical cord with the use of triple dye is important to prevent infection.

33-79. Currently, gram-negative organisms are the most common neonatal pathogens.

a. True
b. False

33-80. Which of the following are associated with drug addiction in pregnancy?

a. Higher risks of infection
b. Accelerated fetal lung maturation
c. Fetal withdraw
d. Child abuse

33-81. Which of the following statements about infections in the newborn is correct?

a. Active immunologic capacity is impaired in the neonate as compared with an older child.
b. Passive immunity is temporarily provided by maternal IgM transferred across the placenta.
c. Early infection in the neonate may be difficult to recognize because the signs are often vague and nonspecific.
d. In general, infection occurring within 72 hours of birth was acquired in utero.
e. Infection manifesting after 72 hours was most likely acquired after birth.

Instructions for Items 33-82 to 33-84: Match the organism to the time period when it was the major cause of neonatal infection in the United States.

a. Group A β-hemolytic streptococci
b. Group B β-hemolytic streptococci
c. Staphylococci

33-82. 1930s to 1940s
33-83. 1950s
33-84. 1970s

33-85. Susceptible women should be vaccinated against rubella as part of their routine medical and gynecological care.

a. True
b. False

33-86. Which of the following statements about the diagnosis of rubella is correct?

a. Absence of maternal rubella antibodies indicates the absence of immunity.
b. The presence of maternal rubella antibody in a nonvaccinated woman indicates that rubella infection has occurred within the last 6 to 8 months.
c. A woman with rubella antibodies has little chance of infection if exposed to rubella while pregnant.
d. Peak antibody levels are seen 1 to 2 weeks after the onset of rash, and 2 to 3 weeks after the onset of viremia.
e. An antibody titer done 10 days after the onset of a rash can differentiate between the presence of the disease and a previously acquired immunity.
f. The presence of specific IgM indicates a primary infection has occurred within the previous month.

33-87. Rubella occurring in the first month of pregnancy probably causes serious defects in about _____ percent of infants who survive; in the second month the incidence of defects is _____ percent, and in the third month the incidence is _____ percent.

33–88. List the abnormalities that may form part of the congenital rubella syndrome.

33–89. There maybe a relationship between congenital rubella and juvenile diabetes.

a. True
b. False

33–90. Rubella vaccine is an attenuated live virus, which can cross the placenta and cause fetal infection and defects.

a. True
b. False

33–91. Which of the following statements about cytomegalovirus infection is correct?

a. It is the most common type of congenital infection, occurring in about 0.5 to 2.0 percent of births.
b. Fifty percent of infected infants will be permanently affected.
c. Infection may lead to abortion or to a wide variety of abnormalities, some of which are fatal.
d. Specific IgM antibody is present in all affected infants.
e. There is no effective treatment.

33–92. Which of the following neonatal abnormalities can be associated with cytomegalovirus infection?

a. Microcephaly
b. Hydrocephaly
c. Mental retardation
d. Cerebral palsy
e. Epilepsy
f. Deafness
g. Chorioretinitis
h. Blindness
i. Hemolytic anemia
j. Thrombocytopenia
k. Hepatosplenomegaly

33–93. In the mnemonic TORCH, what do the letters stand for?

33–94. The use of the TORCH screening test series has proven to be of significant value in reducing neonatal morbidity and mortality.

a. True
b. False

33–95. Which of the following statements about *Chlamydia trachomatis* infection is correct?

a. *Chlamydia trachomatis* has been cultured from the cervices of up to 13 percent of pregnant women.
b. Neonates can acquire infection, including conjunctivitis and pneumonia, from transvaginal delivery.
c. Erythromycin is effective for treatment of maternal but not neonatal infections.
d. Chlamydial infection is a major cause of spontaneous abortion and premature labor.

33–96. List ways that humans may be infected by *Toxoplasma gonadii*.

33–97. Which of the following statements about toxoplasmosis is correct?

a. For congenital toxoplasmosis to occur, the mother must have acquired the infection during pregnancy.
b. Maternal toxoplasmosis is always characterized by fatigue, muscle pain, and lymphadenopathy.
c. Virulence of the fetal infection is increased if it occurs late in pregnancy.
d. Chorioretinitis occurs in those infants who develop symptoms in the neonatal period but not in those who develop neurologic disease later in life.
e. The Sabin-Feldman dye test, IgM fluorescent antibody test, and the indirect fluorescent antibody test are screening blood tests for toxoplasmosis.

33–98. The reduction of birth injuries in recent years is in large part the result of what changes in obstetrical practice?

33–99. Which of the following statements about intracranial hemorrhage is correct?

a. Most case of intracranial hemorrhage are the result of inappropriate obstetric management.
b. Severe molding is sometimes associated with rents in the veins entering the sagittal sinus from the cortex.
c. Essentially all intracranial hemorrhages occur in the subarachnoid area.
d. Compression of the fetal skull may be associated with tears in the vein of Galen and/or tentorial stretching.

33–100. In most cases, intracranial hemorrhage secondary to birth trauma results in a rapidly deteriorating clinical status that begins just after birth.

a. True
b. False

33-101. Which of the following signs and symptoms may be associated with neonatal intracranial hemorrhage?

a. Drowsiness
b. Apathy
c. Feeble cry
d. Pallor
e. Dyspnea
f. Cyanosis
g. Vomiting
h. Convulsions

33-102. List the conditions that are included in the differential diagnosis of intracranial hemorrhage in the newborn.

33-103. What sites of intracranial hemorrhage are more common in premature infants?

33-104. Which of the following statements about the management of intracranial hemorrhage in the newborn is correct?

a. Oxygen should be administered to correct associated dyspnea and cyanosis.
b. Sedation is administered to control associated convulsions.
c. Needle aspiration of the accumulated blood to relieve intracranial pressure should be performed in all types of intracranial hemorrhage.
d. Plasma-clotting factors should be infused to decrease bleeding.
e. Intramuscular injection of vitamin K is indicated for all newborn infants.

Instructions for Items 33-105 to 33-109: Match the clinical condition with the appropriate description.

a. Caput succedaneum
b. Cephalohematoma

33-105. The effusion consists of blood
33-106. Fluid accumulation overlies the periosteum
33-107. Fluid accumulation lies under the periosteum
33-108. Is at maximum size at birth, and subsequently grows smaller
33-109. Appears after birth and grows larger

33-110. Extensive cephalohematoma warrants evaluation of the newborn for coagulation defects and the possibility of extensive intracranial injury.

a. True
b. False

Instructions for Items 33-111 to 33-116: Match the type of brachial plexus injury with the appropriate statement.

a. Duchenne's or Erb's paralysis
b. Klumpke's paralysis

33-111. Arises from injury to the upper roots of the brachial plexus
33-112. Arises from injury to the lower roots of the brachial plexus
33-113. Paralysis of the arm excluding the fingers
33-114. Paralysis of the hand
33-115. Results from pulling on the head, sharply flexing it toward a shoulder
33-116. Has an incidence of about 1 in 500 births

33-117. Which of the following statements about brachial plexus injuries at birth is correct?

a. Brachial plexus injury is always associated with difficult deliveries.
b. Brachial plexus injury in a cephalic presentation is usually associated with an unusually large fetus.
c. To prevent brachial plexus injury in breech presentations, the extension of the arms over the head should be prevented.
d. With appropriate physiotherapy, the prognosis for most brachial plexus injuries is good.

33-118. Facial paralysis is almost always associated with forceps deliveries.

a. True
b. False

33-119. Which of the following statements about neonatal fractures at the time of birth is correct?

a. Fractures of the clavicle are usually associated with shoulder dystocia.
b. Fractures of the humerus are much less common than fractures of the clavicle.
c. Fractures of the femur at uncommon and usually associated with vaginal breech delivery.
d. Crepitation or unusual irregularity on palpation of the bony skeleton is an indication for further evaluation by x-ray.
e. Fracture of the skull is usually associated with forcible attempts at delivery.

33-120. As a child grows, progressive turning of the head toward the side of the sternocleidomastoid muscle that was injured at birth is called _____ .

33–121. Which of the following statements about constricting bands and congenital amputations is correct?

    a. Focal constrictions of the extremities are relatively common.

    b. Premature rupture of the amnion with subsequent formation of tough, adherent bands may cause constriction of an extremity.

    c. Actual amputation of an extremity by an amniotic band is quite rare.

    d. Lesser degrees of constriction may result in edema.

33–122. Which of the following deformities may result from oligohydramnios and the presence of a small, inappropriately shaped uterine cavity?

    a. Talipes

    b. Scoliosis

    c. Hip dislocation

    d. Limb reduction

    e. Polydactyly

    f. Body wall deficiency

33–123. Maternal trauma is relatively unlikely to result in trauma to the fetus because of _____ .

33–124. In cases of severe maternal trauma, the major risks to the fetus are indirect, through the effect of the maternal injuries on maternal cardiac output, maternal blood oxygenation, and uteroplacental perfusion.

    a. True

    b. False

34. MULTIFETAL PREGNANCY

34–1. List the complications common to multifetal pregnancy.

34–2. Two infants who resulted from the division of one fertilized zygote are referred to as _____ twins.

    a. Monozygotic

    b. Dizygotic

34–3. Monozygotic twins are always "identical."

    a. True

    b. False

Instructions for Items 34-4 to 34-10: Match the type of monozygotic twin pregnancy with the appropriate statement.

    a. Diamnionic, dichorionic

    b. Diamnionic, monochorionic

    c. Monoamnionic, monochorionic

    d. Conjoined

34–4. Division after the amnion has become established

34–5. Division of the fertilized ovum before the inner cell mass is formed

34–6. Division after cells destined to become chorion have differentiated

34–7. Division after the embryonic disc has formed

34–8. Two embryos within a common amnionic sac

34–9. Two embryos, two amnions, and two chorions

34–10. Two amnionic sacs covered by a single chorion

34–11. In which type of monozygotic twinning do two distinct placentas or a single fused placenta develop?

    a. Diamnionic, dichorionic

    b. Diamnionic, monochorionic

    c. Monoamnionic, monochorionic

    d. Conjoined

34–12. The frequency of monozygotic twins is approximately _____ .

34–13. Which of the following factors strongly influences the incidence of monozygotic twins?

    a. Race

    b. Heredity

    c. Maternal age

    d. Parity

    e. Therapy for infertility

34–14. Which of the following factors strongly influences the incidence of dizygotic twins?

    a. Race

    b. Heredity

    c. Maternal age

    d. Parity

    e. Therapy for infertility

34–15. Which of the following statements about factors influencing the frequency of twins is correct?

    a. Once twinning occurs, delivery of viable twins is the most likely outcome.

    b. Paternal and maternal genotypes are equally important in determining the probability of twinning.

    c. Twinning is inversely proportional to maternal age and parity.

    d. There is a higher rate of dizygous twinning in women who conceive within 1 month after discontinuing oral contraceptives.

    e. The induction of ovulation is associated with the release of multiple ova.

    f. In humans, the percentage of male conceptuses increases as the number of fetuses per pregnancy increases.

35-57. In preeclampsia, symptoms such as headache or visual disturbance tend to occur _____ the development of hypertension or proteinuria.

a. Before
b. After

35-58. Which of the following statements about blood pressure measurements in preeclampsia is correct?

a. A rise in blood pressure is the most dependable warning sign of preeclampsia.
b. The systolic pressure is a more reliable prognostic sign than the diastolic pressure.
c. A persistent diastolic pressure of 90 or above is generally considered abnormal.
d. Diastolic blood pressures between 90 and 100 are not considered abnormal in edematous or obese patients.

35-59. Which of the following statements about the clinical presentation of preeclampsia is correct?

a. Incipient preeclampsia should be suspected if a patient gains 2 pounds or more in a given week or 6 pounds or more in a given month.
b. In both mild and severe preeclampsia, proteinuria manifests simultaneously with weight gain and hypertension.
c. Frontal headache is common in all preeclamptic patients.
d. Epigastric or right upper quadrant pain is often indicative of imminent convulsions.
e. Visual disturbances such as blurring or blindness usually carry a poor prognosis for return to normal vision.

35-60. The prognosis for the fetus in a pregnancy complicated by pregnancy-induced hypertension is solely dependent on its gestational age.

a. True
b. False

35-61. List the factors predisposing to preeclampsia which warrant careful attention in the antepartum period.

35-62. Which of the following steps should be taken by the health care provider to detect early evidence of pregnancy-induced hypertension?

a. Weigh patient at each visit.
b. Monitor blood pressure at each visit.
c. Instruct patient to immediately report symptoms of PIH.
d. Immediately evaluate patients reporting symptoms of PIH.

35-63. The development of pregnancy-induced hypertension can be controlled by limiting weight gain during pregnancy to 20 pounds or less.

a. True
b. False

35-64. What are possible effects of the routine use of diuretics during pregnancy?

a. Reduced incidence of pregnancy-induced hypertension
b. Decreased renal perfusion
c. Reduced uteroplacental perfusion
d. Increased incidence of fetal thrombocytopenia

35-65. There is some current evidence that the daily administration of very small doses of aspirin during the third trimester of pregnancy might help in the prevention of preeclampsia.

a. True
b. False

35-66. Which of the following statements about the treatment of pregnancy-induced hypertension is correct?

a. The sole objective in the treatment of PIH is the survival of the fetus.
b. Most women with PIH can be successfully managed as outpatients.
c. Hospitalized patients should have oral fluids limited.
d. Hospitalized patients should be sedated with phenobarbital.

35-67. The systematic hospital management of mild preeclampsia includes

a. Daily clinical evaluation for the development of symptoms
b. Weight measurement every other day
c. Urine test for proteinuria at least every 2 days
d. Blood pressure measurements every 4 hours around the clock
e. Measurement of plasma creatinine
f. Measurement of hematocrit, platelets, and SGOT
g. Frequent evaluation of fetal size clinically or by serial ultrasonography
h. Bed rest throughout much of the day

35-68. The correct management of a pregnancy complicated by preeclampsia depends on what factors?

35-69. Regarding the use of antihypertensive agents in pregnancy, which of the following statements is true?

a. Thiazide diuretics do not seem to improve pregnancy outcome and may increase risks to the mother.
b. β-Blockers have shown some effect in lowering the mean arterial pressure of gravida with preeclampsia but may worsen fetal growth retardation.
c. Antihypertensives have not been successfully shown to prolong gestation when used in the treatment of preeclampsia.
d. Magnesium shows a significant antihypertensive effect allowing prolongation of gestation.

35-70. Which of the following statements about the management of worsening or severe preeclampsia is correct?

a. Blood pressure in excess of 160/110, edema, and proteinuria are signs of imminent eclampsia.
b. Oliguria is a sign of impending eclampsia.
c. All women in labor who have severe preeclampsia or eclampsia should be treated with magnesium sulfate.
d. Hydralazine (Apresoline) in small intermittent doses can be safely used for the control of blood pressure.
e. In severe cases of preeclampsia, the risk to the fetus even if remote from term may be less if delivery is accomplished than if the pregnancy is allowed to continue.

35-71. Which of the following is an argument against using glucocorticoids to enhance fetal lung maturation in severe preeclampsia or eclampsia?

a. Risk to the mother
b. Risk to the fetus
c. Rarity of severe respiratory distress in infants from pregnancies complicated with severe PIH

35-72. Which of the following assessments of fetal well-being and placental function provide unique information for the management of a pregnancy complicated by pregnancy-induced hypertension?

a. Serial plasma estriol
b. Serial urinary estriol
c. Placental lactogen
d. Fetal biophysical profile
e. Contraction stress test

35-73. In cases of pregnancy-induced hypertension, failure of the fetus to grow is an ominous sign of fetal jeopardy.

a. True
b. False

35-74. Which of the following statements about the postpartum period in cases of severe preeclampsia or eclampsia is correct?

a. The mother's condition usually improves rapidly after delivery.
b. Anticonvulsant medication should be continued for at least 24 hours postpartum.
c. Patients should remain hospitalized until they are normotensive.
d. Patients should be discharged on oral antihypertensive medication.
e. Pregnancy-induced hypertension is a contraindication to later use of oral contraceptives.

35-75. Regarding the management of preeclampsia, which of the following statements is true?

a. It is malpractice to manage as an outpatient any patient with preeclampsia.
b. There are no controlled studies demonstrating that the outpatient management of preeclampsia is either safe or effective.
c. Up to 90 percent of women initially hospitalized for elevated blood pressure who subsequently become normotensive and are discharged will again develop hypertension.
d. Hospital treatment of this distress has never been shown to be cost-effective.

35-76. Which of the following statements about eclampsia is correct?

a. Eclampsia is most serious when it occurs postpartum.
b. Eclampsia is almost always preceded by preeclampsia.
c. Convulsions begin in the lower extremities and ascend throughout the body.
d. During the eclamptic convulsion, the diaphragm is fixed.
e. The patient has no memory of the convulsion.
f. There is a "refractory period" of about 6 minutes after a convulsion when another seizure cannot occur.

35-77. Which of the following are grave signs in association with eclampsia?

a. Pulmonary edema
b. Coma
c. Fever of >39.5°C
d. Increased urinary output
e. Blindness

35-78. Define and describe intercurrent eclampsia.

35-79. What is the significance of sustained hypertension after delivery in a patient with severe preeclampsia or eclampsia?

35–80. The differential diagnosis of eclampsia includes

a. Epilepsy
b. Ruptured cerebral aneurysm
c. Hysteria
d. Acute porphyria
e. Encephalitis
f. Meningitis
g. Cerebral tumor

35–81. All pregnant women with convulsions should be considered to be eclamptic until proven otherwise.

a. True
b. False

35–82. List the essential components in the treatment of eclampsia.

35–83. Which changes arising from eclampsia generally tend to be permanent?

a. Central nervous system
b. Kidney
c. Liver
d. Thrombocytopenia
e. Hemolysis

35–84. Summarize the Parkland Hospital regimen for treatment of eclampsia.

35–85. Magnesium sulfate

a. Arrests and prevents convulsions in eclampsia
b. Is not effective as an antihypertensive agent
c. Is initially administered intravenously and intramuscularly
d. Is administered in subsequent doses when patellar reflexes are present, respirations are not decreased, and urine output is 100 cc/4 hours
e. Intoxication is avoided by rapid renal clearance

Instructions for Items 35–86 to 35–88: Match the level of magnesium sulfate with the appropriate effect.

a. 12 mEq/L
b. 8 to 10 mEq/L
c. 4 to 7 mEq/L

35–86. Convulsions prevented
35–87. Loss of patellar reflex
35–88. Respiratory depression and arrest

35–89. What is the drug of choice to treat respiratory depression due to magnesium sulfate toxicity?

35–90. The goal of intermittent intravenous hydralazine therapy in preeclampsia and eclampsia is to maintain diastolic blood pressure at about 90, thus decreasing the risk of intracranial hemorrhage while not compromising uteroplacental perfusion.

a. True
b. False

Instructions for Items 35–91 to 35–94: Match the antihypertensive drug with its possible side effects.

a. Diazoxide
b. Sodium nitroprusside

35–91. Cyanide poisoning in the fetus
35–92. Arrest of labor
35–93. Maternal and neonatal hyperglycemia
35–94. Increased intracranial pressure

35–95. Why should diuretics and hyperosmotic agents not be used to treat eclampsia?

a. They constrict maternal blood volume.
b. They compromise uteroplacental perfusion.
c. They are not needed as postpartum diuresis occurs naturally.
d. Hyperosmotic agents cause edema in vital organs.
e. There is a lack of documented efficacy with their use.

35–96. Which of the following statements about fluid therapy in eclampsia is correct?

a. Five percent dextrose in water is the intravenous solution of choice.
b. Administration of large volumes of fluid may enhance the maldistribution of extracellular and intracellular fluids.
c. A significant postpartum fall in hematocrit after delivery is usually due to the relief of vasospasm.
d. A significant decrease in blood pressure just after delivery most often is related to excessive blood loss.
e. On a regimen of limited fluid therapy, postpartum dialysis for renal failure is usually not required.

35–97. The severely preeclamptic patient cannot be treated appropriately without the use of invasive hemodynamic monitoring.

a. True
b. False

35–98. At Parkland Hospital, which of the following is the anesthesia of choice for vaginal delivery of eclamptic patients?

a. General anesthesia
b. Demerol with promethazine
c. Epidural
d. Spinal
e. Pudendal or local

35–99. What are potential risks from the use of conduction anesthesia for delivery of eclamptic patients?

    a. Splanchnic blockade (hypotension)
    b. Danger from pressor agents
    c. Danger from the large volumes of fluid needed to correct hypotension
    d. Edema formation (cerebral, pulmonary, laryngeal)

35–100. Which of the following statements about magnesium sulfate use in the treatment of preeclampsia and eclampsia is correct?

    a. Magnesium sulfate is associated with depressed myometrial contractility.
    b. Magnesium sulfate is not transferred across the placenta.
    c. In high doses, magnesium sulfate may be associated with neonatal depression.
    d. Magnesium sulfate acts both centrally and peripherally in the nervous system.

35–101. Which of the following statements about treatment of eclampsia is correct?

    a. Diazepam is a well-documented substitute for magnesium sulfate.
    b. Most sedatives including morphine can be used to manage eclampsia with minimal risk.
    c. Heparin has not been shown to be effective in the treatment of eclampsia.
    d. Eclampsia should be considered one of the hypertensive encephalopathies in planning appropriate treatment mechanisms.

35–102. What percent of eclamptic patients will be eclamptic in a subsequent pregnancy?

    a. <5
    b. 15 to 20
    c. 40 to 50
    d. 75 to 80

35–103. Women who had eclampsia associated with a multifetal pregnancy are at no greater risk for future health problems than nulliparous eclamptics.

    a. True
    b. False

35–104. Preeclampsia probably neither causes residual hypertension nor aggravates preexisting hypertension.

    a. True
    b. False

35–105. Which of the following statements about the diagnosis of chronic hypertension in pregnancy is correct?

    a. Hypertension appearing late in repeated pregnancies may signal latent hypertensive vascular disease.
    b. In most women with chronic hypertension, elevated blood pressure is the only abnormal finding.
    c. Heredity, obesity, and age play a role in chronic hypertension.
    d. The incidence of placental abruption is increased in women with chronic hypertension.
    e. Babies of hypertensive mothers tend to be large for gestational age.

35–106. Which of the following statements about the treatment of chronic hypertension in pregnancy is correct?

    a. Treatment with antihypertensive agents reduces the risk of superimposed preeclampsia.
    b. The administration of antihypertensive medications significantly reduces the perinatal mortality rate.
    c. The use of alpha methyldopa is associated with significant fetal abnormalities.
    d. Perinatal mortality is unacceptably high unless antihypertensive medication are begun in the first trimester.
    e. Captopril should not be used in pregnancy.

35–107. Describe the typical manifestation of pregnancy-aggravated hypertension.

36. OBSTETRICAL HEMORRHAGE

36–1. Obstetrical hemorrhage is most likely to be fatal for the mother when _____ .

36–2. In pregnancies complicated by bleeding during the second and third trimesters, the rates of premature delivery and preinatal mortality are at least quadrupled.

    a. True
    b. False

36–3. Which of the following statements about blood loss at the time of delivery is correct?

    a. Postpartum hemorrhage is defined as the loss of 500 mL or more of blood.
    b. About 1 out of 10 women who are delivered vaginally fulfill the criteria for postpartum hemorrhage.
    c. One-half of women who undergo cesarean section fulfill the criteria for postpartum hemorrhage.
    d. Blood loss at delivery may approach the amount added during pregnancy without a significant decrease in hematocrit.

36–4. The woman who develops a normal degree of pregnancy induced hypervolemia usually increases her blood volume by _____ mL.

36-5. Life-threatening obstetrical hemorrhage is confined to the third trimester of pregnancy.

a. True
b. False

36-6. List the causes of obstetrical hemorrhage related to abnormal placental implantation or development.

36-7. List the causes of obstetrical hemorrhage related to trauma during labor or delivery.

36-8. List the causes of obstetrical hemorrhage related to uterine atony.

36-9. List the causes of obstetrical hemorrhage related to small maternal blood volume.

36-10. List the causes of obstetrical hemorrhage related to conditions predisposing to impaired coagulation.

36-11. The term "third trimester bleeding" is useful for distinguishing those patients who are to be managed aggressively from those to be managed conservatively.

a. True
b. False

36-12. Which of the following statements about bleeding from the placental site is correct?

a. The mechanism of hemostasis at the placental implantation site depends on intrinsic vasospasm and formation of local blood clots.
b. Hemostasis after placental separation depends on contraction of the myometrium.
c. Hemostasis at the implantation site may be hindered by large blood clots or placental fragments.
d. Postpartum hemorrhage occurs with a hypotonic uterus in the presence of normal maternal coagulation mechanisms.
e. Postpartum hemorrhage occurs with a well-contracted uterus if the blood coagulation mechanism is impaired.

36-13. Following delivery of an intact placenta, hemorrhage that persists in the presence of a contracted uterus usually indicates bleeding from lacerations of the genital tract.

a. True
b. False

36-14. Oxytocic drugs and uterine massage are ineffective in controlling hemorrhage that does not originate from a hypotonic uterus.

a. True
b. False

36-15. The presence of what three major causes of postpartum hemorrhage must be identified in cases of excessive blood loss?

32-16. Which of the following is needed in the management of obstetrical hemorrhage?

a. Intravenous infusion system(s)
b. Available operating room
c. Surgical team
d. Anesthesiologist

36-17. Which techniques provide a precise measurement of the amount of blood loss in cases of obstetrical hemorrhage?

a. Visual estimate
b. Vital signs
c. "Tilt test"
d. Urine flow
e. Blood volume measurements

36-18. Which of the following statements about estimating the degree of obstetrical hemorrhage is correct?

a. Visual estimates of blood loss are usually low.
b. A normal blood pressure precludes the possibility of dangerous hypovolemia.
c. The "tilt test" is most useful in patients who are hypotensive when recumbent.
d. The rate of urine flow reflects renal perfusion even during the use of potent diuretics.
e. The total absence of urine flow through an indwelling catheter is an indication for diuretic therapy.

36-19. What potential harm can arise from administration of diuretics in cases of obstetrical hemorrhage?

36-20. Administration of oxytocin in an isotonic electrolyte solution to a hemorrhaging woman is likely to cause severe oliguria.

a. True
b. False

36-21. Which of the following is a reason that blood volume measurements have not been widely used in cases of obstetrical hemorrhage?

a. The ideal blood volume for a given woman is not known.
b. The size of the intravascular compartment changes drastically at delivery.
c. In cases of severe hemorrhage, the blood volume measurement obtained is invalid by the time it has been determined.

36-22. Which of the following statements about fluid replacement in obstetrical hemorrhage is correct?

    a. Lactated Ringer's is a preferred intravenous replacement solution.
    b. Packed cells are more effective therapy than whole blood.
    c. Urine flow should be maintained at a minimum of 30 ml per hour.
    d. The hematocrit should be maintained at about 30 percent.
    e. The best method to monitor central venous pressure is through a catheter in the subclavian vein.

36-23. Fresh whole blood is better for the treatment of hypovolemia than stored blood because _____ .

36-24. Which of the following statements about the replacement of blood fractions is correct?

    a. An adequate substitute for whole blood is packed red cells plus normal saline.
    b. Infusion of large volumes of normal saline results in a drop in the colloid oncotic pressure.
    c. Use of reconstituted blood increases the risk of blood-transmitted infection.
    d. Infusion of many units of stored blood may result in generalized bleeding due to thrombocytopenia or low levels of Factors V and VIII.

Instructions for Items 36-25 and 36-26: Match the appropriate treatment with the problem arising from blood replacement therapy.

    a. Administration of platelets from donors with same blood type as recipient
    b. Administration of fresh frozen plasma

36-25. Development of thrombocytopenia after administration of stored whole blood

36-26. Low levels of Factors V and VIII after administration of stored whole blood

36-27. Which of the following coagulation factors is markedly increased in pregnancy?

    a. I (fibrinogen)
    b. V
    c. VII
    d. VIII
    e. IX
    f. X
    g. Platelets

Instructions for Items 36-28 to 26-31: Match the clinical circumstance with the proposed mechanism of activation of the blood coagulation system.

    a. Activation of extrinsic pathway
    b. Activation of intrinsic pathway
    c. Direct activation of Factor X
    d. Induction of procoagulant activity

36-28. Bacterial toxins
36-29. Collagen exposure due to loss of endothelial integrity
36-30. Thromboplastin released at sites of tissue destruction
36-31. Protease activity in neoplasias

36-32. How do fibrin degradation products contribute to defective hemostasis?

36-33. The laboratory identification of possible stigmas of intravascular coagulation are indications for the prompt use of heparin, fibrinogen, or ε-amino caproic acid.

    a. True
    b. False

36-34. ε-Amino caproic acid is the treatment of choice for comsumptive coagulopathy in pregnancy.

    a. True
    b. False

36-35. Excessive bleeding from sites of modest trauma is an inaccurate and uninformative sign of defective hemostasis.

    a. True
    b. False

36-36. In preeclampsia thrombin time may be prolonged even in the face of normal levels of coagulant factors and platelets.

    a. True
    b. False

36-37. Which statement about uterine bleeding before delivery is correct?

    a. Slight bleeding through the vagina is common during labor.
    b. Placenta previa and abruptio placentae cause bleeding from a site above the cervix.
    c. Vasa previa is a rare cause of uterine bleeding.
    d. If uterine bleeding ceases, the pregnancy is not considered at higher risk than if bleeding had not occurred at all.
    e. The origin of uterine bleeding from above the cervix is often difficult to identify.

36-38. Which of the following terms are synonomous?

    a. Abruptio placentae
    b. Ablatio placentae
    c. Accidental hemorrhage
    d. Premature separation of the normally implanted placenta
    e. Placenta previa

Instructions for Items 36–39 to 36–41: Match the type of bleeding from placental abruption with the appropriate statement.

    a. External hemorrhage
    b. Concealed hemorrhage

36–39. Blood escapes through the cervix.

36–40. Blood is retained between the detached placenta and the uterus

36–41. It carries a greater risk of intense consumptive coagulopathy.

36–42. Which of the following statements about the frequency and significance of abruptio placentae is correct?

    a. The variability of reported frequencies of abruptio placentae is a function of the different diagnostic criteria in use.
    b. The reported frequency is between 1 in 75 and 1 in 100 deliveries.
    c. The perinatal mortality rate is approximately 5 percent.
    d. In recent years, abruptio placentae has become a relatively rare cause of stillbirths as compared to other causes.
    e. Maternal mortality from abruptio placentae is common.
    f. If the fetus survives, the newborn is at greater risk for morbidity and mortality.

36–43. Suggested causes of abruptio placentae include

    a. Trauma
    b. Maternal hypertension
    c. Sudden uterine decompression
    d. Short cord syndrome
    e. Uterine anomaly
    f. Uterine tumors
    g. Hydramnios
    h. Multifetal pregnancy
    i. Dietary deficiency

36–44. Severe placental abruption is _____ to be associated with maternal hypertension than are lesser degrees of abruption.

    a. More likely
    b. Less likely

36–45. In women with a previous placental abruption, the risk of placental abruption in a subsequent pregnancy is higher than is the risk for the general population.

    a. True
    b. False

36–46. Which of the following are consistently useful in identifying imminent abruptio placentae?

    a. Urinary estriol levels
    b. Nonstress test
    c. Contraction stress test
    d. Ultrasonography

36–47. Which of the following statements about the pathology of abruptio placentae is correct?

    a. Placental abruption begins with hemorrhage into the decidua basalis, with the resulting decidual hematoma affecting separation of the placenta from its implantation site.
    b. All abruptio placentae are symptomatic.
    c. Spiral artery rupture is a cause of retroplacental hematoma formation.
    d. Decidual spiral artery rupture always results in severe vaginal bleeding.

36–48. In which of the following situations is a concealed hemorrhage likely to occur?

    a. Placental margins remain adherent
    b. Membranes are attached to uterine wall
    c. Blood enters into amnionic cavity
    d. Fetal head is closely applied to lower uterine segment

36–49. What is chronic placental abruption?

36–50. Severe hemorrhage from fetus to mother is common with placental abruption.

    a. True
    b. False

36–51. The intensity of the symptoms of abruptio placentae are _____ to the severity of the abruption.

    a. Directly proportional
    b. Inversely proportional
    c. Unrelated
    d. Variably related

36–52. Which of the following statements about the diagnosis of abruptio placentae is correct?

    a. A normal ultrasound excludes life-threatening abruption.
    b. Common symptoms include vaginal bleeding and uterine tenderness.
    c. Fetal demise is more common than fetal distress.
    d. The intensity of shock is out of proportion to the extent of maternal blood loss.
    e. Either hypotension or anemia is always associated with placental abruption.

36–53. Signs and symptoms of abruptio placenta that occur in more than 50 percent of cases include

a. Premature labor
b. Vaginal bleeding
c. Fetal demise
d. Fetal distress
e. Uterine hypertonus
f. Uterine tenderness or back pain
g. High frequency contractions.

36–54. Painful uterine bleeding is usually associated with abruptio placentae, whereas painless uterine bleeding is usually associated with placenta previa.

a. True
b. False

36–55. The presence of painful uterine bleeding in the third trimester is always indicative of placental abruption.

a. True
b. False

36–56. The most common cause of consumptive coagulopathy in pregnancy is _____ .

36–57. Which of the following statements about placental abruption and consumptive coagulopathy is correct?

a. Significant coagulation derangements are relatively uncommon in cases in which the fetus survives.
b. The coagulation defect arises principally from induction of intravascular coagulation.
c. Levels of fibrin degradation products are higher in serum from the uterine cavity than in peripheral blood.
d. At the outset, thrombocytopenia is found as frequently as hypofibrinogenemia.

36–58. Which of the following statements about renal failure and placental abruption is correct?

a. Acute renal failure usually occurs with any degree of placental abruption.
b. The most common renal lesion is acute tubular necrosis.
c. Major etiologic factors probably include impaired renal perfusion and coexistent hypertension.
d. Renal dysfunction may be avoided by the treatment of hemorrhage with blood and fluids.
e. Proteinuria is only rarely seen in placental abruption.

36–59. Describe the characteristics of uteroplacental apoplexy (Couvelaire uterus).

36–60. The Couvelaire uterus must be treated by hysterectomy to prevent severe postpartum uterine hemorrhage.

a. True
b. False

Instructions for Items 36–61 to 36–63: Match the clinical circumstance with the indicated management in third trimester bleeding.

a. Administration of whole blood and electrolyte solution
b. Procrastination and close observation
c. Prompt delivery

36–61. Massive external bleeding
36–62. Blood loss at a slow rate with no evidence of fetal distress
36–63. Evidence of fetal distress

36–64. Failure to identify a blood clot in the uterine cavity by sonography excludes the possibility of serious placental abruption.

a. True
b. False

36–65. List the major causes of fetal distress from abruptio placentae.

36–66. Which of the following is recommended in cases of uterine hypertonicity associated with fetal distress and placental abruption?

a. Magnesium sulfate
b. Ritodrine
c. Other β-receptor agonists

36–67. If placental abruption is suspected, facilities for immediate cesarean delivery should be continuously available.

a. True
b. False

36–68. Which of the following statements about placental abruption and vaginal delivery is correct?

a. If fetal death occurs, vaginal delivery is usually preferable.
b. Coagulation defects may be more troublesome in an abdominal delivery than in a vaginal delivery.
c. Postpartum stimulation of the myometrium pharmacologically and with uterine massage can prevent hemorrhage from the implantation site.
d. Postcesarean bleeding may accumulate as troublesome hematomas.

36–69. There is definite evidence that early amniotomy in cases of abruptio placentae decreases bleeding from the implantation site and reduces thromboplastin entry into the maternal circulation.

a. True
b. False

36-70. Which of the following statements about labor in cases of placental abruption is correct?

a. With mild degrees of abruption, labor contractions appear normal.
b. Uterine hypertonus characterizes severe cases of placental abruption.
c. Failure of the cervix to dilate in the presence of definite effacement should be considered as a lack of progress.
d. In severe cases, it is often difficult to determine by palpation if the uterus is contracting and relaxing.

36-71. Delivery of the infant within 6 hours of the diagnosis of placental abruption maximizes fetal and maternal outcome.

a. True
b. False

36-72. In what aspects does the basic management of obstetrical hemorrhage differ from the optimal method of treating placental abruption?

a. Use of blood
b. Types of intravenous fluid administered
c. Amount of intravenous fluid administered
d. Hematocrit goal
e. Urine output goal
f. Use of furosemide

36-73. Which of the following statements about the treatment of coagulation defects associated with abruptio placentae is correct?

a. If the clot observation test reveals a small or absent clot, coagulation studies will be grossly abnormal.
b. The platelet count will always fall abruptly and in parallel with the fibrinogen level in severe abruptio placentae.
c. Microangiopathic hemolysis is very common in severe abruptio placentae.
d. Transfusion with packed platelets is indicated in cases of severe thrombocytopenia.
e. Coagulation defects (factors plus low platelets) will usually return to normal levels within a few days of delivery.
f. Intravenous heparin administration to block DIC is not effective and should be avoided.
g. The use of ϵ-aminocaproic acid will aid in controlling fibrinolysis.

36-74. What is the major problem arising from the use of lyophilized fibrinogen in cases of severe hypofibrinogenemia?

36-75. In the presence of coagulation defects due to placental abruption, supracervical hysterectomy is the best prophylactic measure available.

a. True
b. False

36-76. What are causes of consumptive coagulopathy in the newborn?

a. Placental abruption
b. Sepsis
c. Prematurity
d. Trauma
e. Hypoxia

36-77. What is a placenta previa?

Instructions for Items 36-78 to 36-81: Match the type of placenta previa with the correct description.

a. Total placenta previa
b. Partial placenta previa
c. Marginal placenta previa
d. Low-lying placenta previa

36-78. The edge of the placenta is at the margin of the internal os.
36-79. The internal os is partially covered by the placenta.
36-80. The placental edge is in close proximity to the internal os.
36-81. The internal os is completely covered by the placenta.

36-82. The degree of a placenta previa is independent of cervical dilation.

a. True
b. False

36-83. Which of the following statements about placenta previa is correct?

a. As labor progresses, the degree of placenta previa becomes greater.
b. Digital palpation is the most accurate method of monitoring the changing relationship between placental edge and cervical os.
c. As the lower uterine segment forms, some degree of placental separation invariably occurs.

36-84. What are the possible outcomes of a zygote implanting very low in the uterine cavity?

a. Abortion
b. Placenta previa
c. Placental migration

36-85. Placenta previa is _____ placental abruption.

a. More common than
b. About as common as
c. Less common than

36-86. Which of the following factors are associated with placenta previa?

a. Multiparity
b. Previous cesarean delivery
c. Advancing maternal age
d. Erythroblastosis
e. Multiple fetuses
f. Placenta accreta
g. Defective vascularization of the decidua

36-87. The most characteristic event in placenta previa is

_____ .

36-88. Which of the following statements about bleeding with placenta previa is correct?

a. The initial bleeding episode is usually fatal to the fetus and often fatal to the mother.
b. Hemorrhage may be better controlled as labor ensues.
c. Excessive bleeding after delivery may be expected.
d. Consumptive coagulopathy is rarely associated with placenta previa.

36-89. Which of the following statements about the diagnosis of placenta previa is correct?

a. The diagnosis of placenta previa can seldom be made without palpation of the placenta through the cervical os.
b. Vaginal examination for placenta previa should only be conducted in the operating room after full preparation for delivery is made.
c. Vaginal examination should be withheld in women with an immature fetus.
d. Ultrasound localization of the placenta is reasonably reliable in the diagnosis of placenta previa.
e. Placentas seen to lie low or over the os in early pregnancy will, in the majority of cases, lie above the lower uterine segment in advanced pregnancy.

36-90. A woman with placenta previa who has no vaginal bleeding and a premature fetus must always be hospitalized.

a. True
b. False

36-91. Aside from fetal lung maturation, what benefits are possible with delayed delivery in cases of placenta previa?

Instructions for Items 36-92 to 36-94: Match the mode of delivery with its advantages in the management of placenta previa.

a. Cesarean
b. Vaginal

36-92. Allows for immediate delivery and consequent uterine contraction to halt hemorrhage

36-93. Tamponade of bleeding vessels
36-94. Avoids cervical lacerations

36-95. Which of the following statements about cesarean delivery for placenta previa is correct?

a. It is the accepted method of delivery in practically all cases.
b. Cesarean delivery may be indicated for a dead fetus if done for the welfare of the mother.
c. With anterior placenta previa, a transverse uterine incision is optimal.
d. With placenta accreta, a vertical uterine incision will avoid the need for hysterectomy.

36-96. The preferred compression (tamponade) method for vaginal delivery in cases of placenta previa is _____ .

36-97. Which of the following statements concerning the outcome of cases of placenta previa is correct?

a. Cesarean section and adequate transfusion have improved maternal outcome.
b. Perinatal outcome has been improved by expectant management for pregnancies remote from term.
c. Labor or hemorrhage may force delivery of a premature fetus.
d. Perinatal mortality is higher in cases of placenta previa for a given fetal weight than for the general population.
e. Serious fetal malformations are more common in cases of placenta previa.

36-98. The primary mode of management of intrauterine fetal demise is ''watchful waiting'' until spontaneous labor ensues.

a. True
b. False

36-99. What factors have contributed to a more aggressive management of the patient whose fetus has died?

a. Psychologic stress on mother
b. Dangers of blood coagulation defects
c. Advent of effective methods of labor induction

36-100. The majority of pregnancies with a fetal demise will deliver within

a. 24 hours
b. 72 hours
c. 1 week
d. 2 weeks

36-101. Which of the following statements about consumptive coagulopathy after fetal demise is correct?

    a. Marked disruption of maternal coagulation rarely occurs in less than 1 month after fetal death.
    b. If the fetus is retained more than 1 month, approximately 25 percent of cases develop changes in the coagulation mechanism.
    c. Thrombocytopenia precedes severe hypofibrinogenemia.
    d. Coagulation defects are always irreversible until delivery occurs.

36-102. In women with delayed delivery of a dead fetus, heparin can be used to correct coagulation defects if the maternal circulatory system is intact.

    a. True
    b. False

36-103. Death of a fetus in a multifetal pregnancy remote from term warrants immediate cesarean delivery to avoid the risks of consumptive coagulopathy.

    a. True
    b. False

36-104. In the presence of coagulation defects, serious hemorrhage that occurs as the dead products of conception are being expelled should be treated by

    a. Heparin
    b. ϵ-Aminocaproic acid
    c. Fibrinogen
    d. Blood
    e. Lactated Ringer's solution

36-105. Which of the following is useful in cases of fetal death requiring pregnancy termination?

    a. Oxytocin
    b. Laminaria
    c. Hypertonic saline
    d. Prostaglandin E_2 suppositories.

Instructions for Items 36-106 to 36-109: Match the means used to terminate pregnancy with its possible complication.

    a. Oxytocin
    b. Laminaria
    c. Prostaglandin E_2
    d. Hypertonic saline

36-106. Nausea, vomiting, and diarrhea
36-107. Water intoxication
36-108. Infection
36-109. Coagulation defects

36-110. List the conditions essential to the development of an amnionic fluid embolism.

36-111. Amnionic fluid embolism is characterized by

    a. Respiratory distress
    b. Circulatory collapse
    c. Hemorrhage
    d. Coagulation defects

36-112. Which of the following statements about amnionic fluid embolism is correct?

    a. The lethality of intravenously infused amnionic fluid appears related to the particulate matter it contains.
    b. The clot-accelerating activity of amnionic fluid is greater at term than early in the third trimester.
    c. Amnionic fluid embolism can be confirmed by the widespread appearance of amnionic fluid debris in pulmonary vessels.
    d. Successful treatment is dependent upon vigorous antibiotic therapy.
    e. The benefits of the use of fibrinogen outweigh its risks in cases of amnionic fluid embolism.

36-113. In what circumstances may coagulopathy develop as a consequence of abortion?

    a. Prolonged retention of a dead fetus
    b. Sepsis
    c. Intrauterine instillation of hypertonic saline
    d. Medical induction with prostaglandins
    e. Use of instrumentation to terminate a pregnancy

36-114. In an abortion induced by hypertonic saline, thromboplastin may be released from the

    a. Placenta
    b. Fetus
    c. Decidua

36-115. In cases of septic abortion, disruption of coagulation is always associated with intravascular hemolysis.

    a. True
    b. False

36-116. Severe hemorrhage may itself induce coagulation defects.

    a. True
    b. False

36-117. Which of the following can be associated with consumptive coagulopathy?

    a. Eclampsia
    b. Diabetes
    c. Barlow syndrome
    d. Severe preeclampsia

37. ABNORMALITIES OF THE REPRODUCTIVE TRACT

37-1. Which of the following statements about inflammation of the Bartholin glands is correct?

a. An abscess may result in a puerperal infection.
b. Drainage should be accomplished at the time of delivery.
c. The principal organism found in Bartholin gland abscesses is *Neisseria gonorrhoeae*.
d. Oral antibiotics may be as effective as drainage of an abscess.

37-2. A Bartholin duct cyst is best excised under the anesthetic used for delivery.

a. True
b. False

37-3. Which of the following should be surgically excised during pregnancy?

a. Periurethral abscess
b. Periurethral cyst
c. Urethral diverticula

37-4. Human papillomaviruses are

a. Sexually transmitted
b. Incurable
c. Always precancerous
d. A cause of vulvar varices

37-5. Large vulvar varicosities usually decrease in size and become asymptomatic after delivery.

a. True
b. False

37-6. What events during pregnancy predispose to the development of cystocele or rectocele?

37-7. Which of the following statements about cystocele and rectocele is correct?

a. Rectocele and cystocele always coexist in the same patient.
b. Large symptomatic cystoceles and rectoceles are now relatively uncommon.
c. Surgical repair should not be carried out in the antepartum or intrapartum periods.
d. Use of cesarean delivery and episiotomy have contributed to the increased incidence of cystoceles and rectoceles.

37-8. The development of stress incontinence during pregnancy is due to the progressive lengthening of the urethra.

a. True
b. False

37-9. Most vaginal cysts are derived from _____ .

37-10. Due to their malignant potential, all vaginal cysts should be excised soon after diagnosis.

a. True
b. False

37-11. Which of the following statements about cervical neoplasia during pregnancy is correct?

a. Pregnancy has a small but measurable tendency to increase the rate of progression of cervical dysplasia.
b. Fungating or ulcerating lesions should be evaluated by biopsy or colposcopy.
c. All degrees of dysplasia identified by pap smear must be biopsied as soon as possible.
d. Directed focal biopsy of the cervix is safe to perform in pregnancy.
e. There is an association between cervical cancer and human papillomavirus types 16, 18, and 31.

37-12. Possible problems associated with conization in pregnancy include

a. Risk of membrane rupture
b. Inability to obtain an adequate tissue sample
c. Appreciable blood loss
d. Risk of abortion or premature delivery

37-13. If care is taken, endocervical curettage should be performed in all pregnant patients with cervical dysplasia.

a. True
b. False

37-14. Patients previously treated for cervical dysplasia should

a. Avoid pregnancy
b. Be encouraged to conceive as quickly as possible
c. Be followed for recurrence of the dysplasia

37-15. Staging errors in pregnant women with invasive cervical carcinoma tend to _____ the extent of the tumor.

a. Underestimate
b. Overestimate

37-16. Which of the following statements about invasive cervical carcinoma in pregnancy is correct?

a. Staging is more difficult.
b. The type of delivery (vaginal or abdominal) does not significantly affect maternal survival.
c. Survival rates are relatively similar for pregnant and nonpregnant women with a given disease stage.
d. During the first half of pregnancy, treatment for invasive carcinoma should be initiated immediately.

Instructions for Items 37-17 to 37-20: Match the degree of cervical neoplasia with the appropriate treatment.

 a. Vaginal delivery and follow-up with colposcopy and biopsy
 b. Cesarean hysterectomy
 c. Radiation therapy
 d. (Cesarean) radical hysterectomy and pelvic lymphadenectomy

37-17. Severe cervical dysplasia
37-18. Carcinoma in situ
37-19. Cervical carcinoma—stage 1
37-20. Extensive cervical carcinoma

37-21. Which of the following is common in pregnancy?

 a. Endometrial carcinoma
 b. Uterine myoma
 c. Tubal carcinoma
 d. Ovarian cancer

37-22. List the groups of developmental abnormalities of the female reproductive tract.

Instructions for Items 37-23 to 37-26: Match the type of uterus with the appropriate description.

 a. Single
 b. Septate
 c. Bicornuate
 d. Double
 e. Single hemiuterus

37-23. Two hemiuteri, each with a distinct cervix
37-24. Y-shaped, forked uterus; single cervix
37-25. Externally the uterus appears normal; internally the uterine cavity is divided into two or more compartments
37-26. Normal, symmetrical uterus

37-27. List and describe the four types of cervix.

37-28. A longitudinally septate vagina occurs when ____ (1) and a transversely septate vagina results from ____ (2) .

37-29. Most major obstetric difficulties related to abnormalities of the reproductive tract are associated with anomalies of the

 a. Vagina
 b. Cervix
 c. Uterus

37-30. A hemiuterus that fails to dilate and hypertrophy during pregnancy can lead to

 a. Abortion
 b. Premature birth
 c. Abnormal presentation
 d. Uterine dysfunction
 e. Uterine rupture

37-31. Women with minor uterine abnormalities may be expected to have relatively normal deliveries.

 a. True
 b. False

37-32. All anatomic abnormalities of the female reproductive tract must be confirmed using some form of radiologic imaging technique.

 a. True
 b. False

37-33. Anomalies of the reproductive tract are frequently associated with anomalies of the ____ tract.

37-34. What obstetric outcomes are more common in women with major anatomic abnormalities of the uterus?

 a. Cesarean delivery
 b. Low-birthweight infants
 c. Perinatal loss
 d. Abortion

37-35. Which of the following therapies have been found to be beneficial in improving pregnancy outcomes in patients with major anatomic abnormalities of the reproductive tract?

 a. Progestational agents
 b. β-Mimetic drugs
 c. Metroplasty
 d. External podalic version
 e. Cerclage

37-36. What type of chemical compound is stilbesterol (diethyl stilbesterol)?

37-37. Which of the following statements about stilbesterol use during pregnancy is correct?

 a. It prevents most forms of pregnancy wastage.
 b. In utero exposure increases the risk of clear cell adenocarcinoma of the vagina.
 c. Lower conception rates have been reported in women who were exposed to stilbesterol in utero.
 d. One in ten women exposed in utero exhibit structural anomalies of the reproductive tract.
 e. Structural abnormalities in exposed women are confined to the cervix and vagina.

37-38. Which of the following statements about uterine malposition is correct?

a. Extreme anteflexion of the uterus in early pregnancy is uncommon but associated with an increased incidence of spontaneous abortion.
b. Retroversion of the uterus probably has no adverse effects on early pregnancy.
c. Incarceration of a retroverted uterus first manifests in abdominal discomfort and paradoxic incontinence.
d. Sacculation will often occur if the uterus remains incarcerated.
e. Pregnancy associated with a partially prolapsed uterus usually proceeds without problems, with the uterus "rising" as the pregnancy advances.

37-39. Sacculation of the uterus is characterized by _____ .

37-40. What therapies are appropriate for treatment of uterine prolapse during pregnancy?

a. Expectant management
b. Use of a pessary
c. Bed rest
d. Attention to careful hygiene

37-41. Cystocele and rectocele may prolapse even though the uterus is in normal position.

a. True
b. False

37-42. Why is primary acute inflammation of the tubes and ovaries rarely, if ever, seen in pregnancy?

37-43. The rare situation where there is a continuous loss of clear fluid, often believed to represent a persistent amniorrhea following rupture of the membranes, is termed

_____ .

37-44. Endometriosis is a frequent cause of

a. Premature labor
b. Uterine dysfunction
c. Third trimester bleeding
d. Preeclampsia

38. PRETERM AND POSTTERM PREGNANCY AND INAPPROPRIATE FETAL GROWTH

38-1. Determination of the appropriateness of fetal growth depends on knowledge of what important factor?

Instructions for Items 38-2 to 38-4: Match the term with the appropriate interval following the LMP (when ovulation and fertilization occurred 2 weeks later).

a. Fetus (infant) at term
b. Preterm infant
c. Premature infant
d. Postterm infant

38-2. An infant born before the 38th week
38-3. An infant born between the 38th week and 42nd weeks
38-4. An infant born at or after 42 completed weeks

Instructions for Items 38-5 to 38-7: Match the term with the correct definition.

a. Appropriately grown, preterm fetus
b. Growth-retarded, term fetus
c. Growth-retarded, preterm fetus

38-5. A shortened gestation and an impaired rate of growth
38-6. A shortened gestation and a normal rate of growth
38-7. A gestation of normal duration and an impaired rate of growth

38-8. An infant whose birthweight is below the _____ $_{(1)}$ percentile is defined as small for gestational age, while an infant above the _____ $_{(2)}$ percentile is categorized as large for gestational age.

38-9. It is useful in obstetric practice to exactly equate fetal size with level of fetal maturity.

a. True
b. False

38-10. In utero fetal growth is somewhat retarded in infants who are born prematurely.

a. True
b. False

38-11. Which of the following factors influences birthweight in term pregnancies?

a. Sex of the infant
b. Parity
c. Race
d. Maternal age

38-12. The mean birthweight in the United States at 40 weeks of gestation is reported as _____ $_{(1)}$ g with a range of _____ $_{(2)}$ g.

38-13. According to Hendricks, the mean daily fetal growth in grams during the previous week of gestation increases until about the _____ week and then begins to decline.

a. 31st
b. 34th
c. 37th
d. 40th

38-14. High-risk pregnancy refers to a situation where the fetus may not be liveborn, may not survive after birth, or may suffer physical, intellectual, or emotional impairment as the consequence of a hostile antepartum, intrapartum, or neonatal environment.

a. True
b. False

38-15. Fetal distress refers to the acute situation where compromise of the fetal unit is discovered by electronic fetal monitoring or direct blood gas sampling.

a. True
b. False

38-16. Which of the following statements about intensive neonatal care is correct?

a. Advances in intensive care have lowered the neonatal death rate by nearly 100 percent in the last quarter century.
b. All hospitals providing maternity care should have all facilities for neonatal intensive care available.
c. Maternal or infant transportation to well-equipped intensive care facilities are equally acceptable in terms of cost, safety, and logistics.
d. With modern neonatal care facilities, there are no demonstrable differences in long-term outcome of term and preterm infants (excluding infants with congenital anomalies or severe birth trauma).
e. Most infants weighing more than 1000 g or born after 27 weeks of gestation and who are not malformed will survive with appropriate intensive care.
f. Much of the cost of prematurity could be avoided by appropriate levels of antepartum care.

38-17. In comparing fetal survival rates by birthweight at Parkland Hospital in 1985, the most striking improvement in survival occurs once the infant has reached what weight?

a. 500 to 750 g
b. 751 to 1,000 g
c. 1,001 to 1,250 g
d. 1,251 to 1,500 g

38-18. What is the first question to be answered when preterm labor is diagnosed?

38-19. Until term, the intrauterine environment is safer for the fetus than extrauterine existence, unless the mother is mortally ill.

a. True
b. False

Instructions for Items 38-20 and 38-21: Match the term with the correct definition.

a. Preterm rupture of the membranes
b. Premature rupture of the membranes

38-20. Rupture of the membranes at any time before the onset of labor

38-21. Rupture of the membranes remote from term

38-22. In most cases, premature rupture of the membranes is followed within a few days by labor and delivery.

a. True
b. False

38-23. Describe the management of rupture of the membranes remote from term that is used at Parkland Memorial Hospital.

38-24. Prolonged rupture of the membranes is defined as _____ .

38-25. Prophylactic antibiotics should be administered to infants in all cases of prolonged rupture of the membranes.

a. True
b. False

38-26. In which of the following situations is there the possibility of accelerated surfactant production in an infant remote from term?

a. Maternal chronic renal or cardiovascular disease
b. Sickle cell disease
c. Heroin addiction
d. Hyperthyroidism
e. Chorioamnionitis
f. Placental infarction

38-27. Even though rupture of the membranes remote from term is associated with accelerated fetal lung maturation, the risk of infection makes deliberate delay in delivery poor obstetric practice.

a. True
b. False

38-28. Glucocorticoid therapy for preterm rupture of the membranes

a. Has been clearly shown to accelerate the production of pulmonary surfactant
b. Has a transient effect of about 7 days in humans
c. Is associated with an increased risk of maternal and fetal infection
d. May intensify the metabolic derangements of diabetes and worsen severe pregnancy-induced hypertension
e. May result in long-term risks for the fetus-infant

38-29. Which of the following statements about conditions that predispose to preterm labor is correct?

a. The onset of labor remote from term is commonly preceded by rupture of the membranes.
b. Cervical incompetency is a common predisposing factor to preterm labor.
c. Uterine anomalies are a relatively rare predisposing factor.
d. Overdistention of the uterus, as with severe hydramnios or multifetal pregnancy, is associated with an increased incidence of preterm labor.
e. Anomalies of the fetus or placenta predispose to preterm labor.
f. Faulty placentation is associated with preterm labor.

38-30. A woman who previously gave birth to a preterm infant is at no higher risk for a subsequent delivery remote from term than the general population.

a. True
b. False

38-31. What are the signs generally used to identify preterm labor?

38-32. In essentially all cases of preterm labor, the good of the fetus requires that an attempt be made to inhibit the labor.

a. True
b. False

38-33. Which of the following statements about the management of preterm labor and delivery is correct?

a. The more premature the fetus, the greater the risk, especially in the breech position.
b. Significant birth passage resistance is uncommon in preterm labor.
c. Cord compression is relatively common with premature rupture of the membranes.
d. The fragile preterm head is best protected during vaginal delivery by the application of outlet forceps.
e. A liberal episiotomy is advantageous in the vaginal delivery of a preterm infant.

38-34. For any gestational age, as weight decreases below the _____ percentile, the risk of fetal death increases greatly.

a. 10th
b. 20th
c. 30th

38-35. Which of the following statements about the treatment of preterm labor is correct?

a. Bed rest alone never provides a satisfactory outcome.
b. The administration of progestational agents (especially 17α-hydroxyprogesterone or Delalutin) has proven effective in inhibiting labor.
c. Ethanol inhibits endogenous oxytocin formation, which results in successful inhibition of labor.

38-36. Which of the following statements about the use of magnesium sulfate in the treatment of preterm labor is correct?

a. Ionic magnesium in high enough concentrations alters myometrial activity.
b. Magnesium is presumed to act as an antagonist of calcium in the process of muscle contraction.
c. Magnesium toxicity can be a problem for the mother but not for the fetus-infant.
d. The possibility of hypermagnesemia is monitored by checking the patellar reflex and monitoring respiration.
e. Magnesium sulfate is clearly an effective long-term inhibitor of preterm labor.

Instructions for Items 38-37 and 38-38: Match the β-receptor with the appropriate cell type.

a. β_1 receptor
b. β_2 receptor

38-37. Heart and intestine
38-38. Myometrium, blood vessels, bronchioles

38-39. Which of the following statements about the use of β-adrenergic receptor stimulants in the treatment of preterm labor is correct?

a. Epinephrine in low doses is an effective and long-acting depressant of myometrial activity.
b. β-Adrenergic agonists act by coupling with adrenergic receptors located on the myometrial cell membrane, ultimately resulting in the reduction of intracellular calcium ions.
c. The ideal β-agonist would stimulate only β-adrenergic receptors on myometrial cells without stimulation of β-receptors on other cell types.
d. None of the compounds similar in structure to epinephrine that have been evaluated to date has been found to be ideal in the inhibition of preterm labor.

38-40. Which of the following β-adrenergic agonists is approved for use by the FDA?

a. Isoxuprine
b. Ritodrine
c. Terbutaline
d. Salbutamol
e. Fenoterol

Instruction for Items 38-41 to 38-43: Match the β-adrenergic receptor stimulant with its significant potential side effects.

    a. Isoxuprine
    b. Ritodrine
    c. Terbutaline
    d. Salbutamol
    e. Fenoterol

38-41. Maternal pulmonary edema
38-42. Maternal tachycardia and hypotension
38-43. Hypoglycemia in the infant after delivery

38-44. Which of the following statements about the management of preterm labor is correct?

    a. Combined therapy with ritodrine and magnesium sulfate has proved especially effective in refractory cases.
    b. While some antiprostaglandins seem to be effective in the arrest of preterm labor, their use is discouraged because they may cause cardiovascular problems such as premature closure fo the ductus arteriosus.
    c. Narcotics and sedatives have little efficacy in inhibiting preterm labor and they may depress the preterm infant.
    d. Diazoxide is safe and effective because its side effects are uncomfortable but not dangerous.

38-45. Fifteen percent of all pregnancies eventually become postterm.

    a. True
    b. False

38-46. The reported incidence of postterm pregnancies may be inaccurate because of _____ .

38-47. Postterm pregnancy is associated with

    a. Anencephaly
    b. A history of previous postterm pregnancy
    c. A history of previous preterm pregnancy
    d. Placental sulfatase activity
    e. Extrauterine pregnancy
    f. Multifetal pregnancy

38-48. The in utero postterm fetus

    a. May continue to grow, with an increased risk of fetopelvic disproportion
    b. May suffer an arrest of growth
    c. May experience umbilical cord compression and fetal distress, especially when there is associated oligohydramnios
    d. Is often at increased risk for meconium defecation and aspiration

38-49. Outline the management of postterm pregnancy utilized at Parkland Hospital.

38-50. What are the most dangerous times for the postterm fetus?

38-51. A cesarean delivery should be strongly considered in a woman in early labor who has hypotonic uterine dysfunction and thick meconium in her amnionic fluid.

    a. True
    b. False

38-52. There is no convincing evidence that the serial use of either nonstress or contraction stress tests improves the outcome in postterm pregnancies.

    a. True
    b. False

38-53. The presence of scant amnionic fluid is the most ominous sign of impending fetal distress in postterm pregnancy.

    a. True
    b. False

38-54. Which of the following situations is associated with fetal growth retardation?

    a. Chronic maternal vascular disease complicated by superimposed preeclampsia and proteinuria
    b. Late occurring pregnancy-induced hypertension
    c. Chronic maternal renal disease
    d. Maternal anemia of any cause
    e. Maternal cyanotic heart disease
    f. Smoking
    g. Alcoholism
    h. Maternal residence at high altitude
    i. Cytomegalic inclusion disease
    j. Rubella

Instruction for Items 38-55 to 38-59: Match the placental abnormality with the likelihood of fetal growth retardation.

    a. Commonly associated with fetal growth retardation
    b. Not commonly associated with fetal growth retardation

38-55. Chronic focal placental abruption
38-56. Extensive placental infarction
38-57. Placenta previa
38-58. Chorioangioma
38-59. Circumvallate placenta

38-60. Fetal growth retardation is usually not a repetitive event.

    a. True
    b. False

38-61. Growth retardation is common with

a. Multifetal pregnancy
b. Chronic fetal infection
c. Prolonged pregnancy
d. Extrauterine pregnancy
e. High maternal hemoglobin concentrations

38-62. A careful medical history including factors predisposing to fetal growth retardation and careful serial measurements of uterine fundal height reinforced by ultrasonography are sufficient to diagnose fetal growth retardation in essentially all cases of singleton pregnancy.

a. True
b. False

38-63. The Ponderal index is

a. Derived from ultrasonic measurements
b. A means of identifying fetal growth
c. A ratio comparing the weight in grams to the cube of the fetal length in centimeters × 100
d. A ratio of fetal arm circumference to fetal head circumference

38-64. Prompt delivery is the best management for a severely growth retarded fetus at or near term.

a. True
b. False

38-65. Which of the following statements about the management of fetal growth retardation remote from term is correct?

a. The risk of preterm labor is virtually eliminated by strict bed rest.
b. The demonstration of an L/S ratio <2 means that respiratory distress will most likely occur upon delivery.
c. Worsening maternal disease that has contributed to the growth retardation is an indication for delivery only if the L/S ratio is >2.
d. When the estimated fetal weight is below the 10th percentile for a given gestational age and remains static, continued intrauterine time does not decrease mortality.

38-66. Problems associated with intrauterine growth retardation include

a. Relative shoulder dystocia
b. Polycythemia
c. Hyperviscosity
d. Slowed growth rates after birth

38-67. Delayed head growth in utero has been associated with slowed intellectual development.

a. True
b. False

38-68. Compared with a normal infant, the growth retarded infant is

a. At increased risk of being born hypoxic
b. More likely to require cesarean delivery
c. More likely to show intrapartum evidence of uteroplacental insufficiency
d. More susceptible to hypothermia
e. More likely to become hyperglycemic

Instructions for Items 38-69 to 38-71: Match the following situations with the subsequent development of the growth retarded infant.

a. Likely to attain normal growth and/or to catch up
b. Likely to remain small or slow growing

38-69. Symmetrical growth retardation
38-70. Asymmetrical growth retardation
38-71. Normal length at birth

38-72. In most cases, growth retardation is associated with subsequent neurologic and intellectual problems.

a. True
b. False

38-73. Which of the following statements about the types of fetal growth retardation is correct?

a. In asymmetrical growth retardation, the head is of relatively normal size.
b. Symmetrical growth retardation is often difficult to distinguish from erroneous determination of gestational age.
c. Sonographic measurement of the biparietal diameter and head circumference at the level of the third ventricle will detect both symmetrical and asymmetrical growth retardation.
d. Normally, the head and abdominal circumferences are about equal between 32 and 36 weeks of gestation.
e. After 36 weeks of gestation, the head circumference normally exceeds the abdominal circumference.

39. MEDICAL AND SURGICAL ILLNESSES COMPLICATING PREGNANCY

39-1. Which of the following statements about the presence of medical disease during pregnancy is correct?

a. Essentially all diseases that affect the nonpregnant woman may be contracted during pregnancy.
b. The presence of most diseases does not prevent conception.
c. Normal pregnancy affects the signs, symptoms, and laboratory values in most diseases.
d. A disease may be misdiagnosed if the possibility of pregnancy is not considered.
e. There must be a strong justification to deviate from accepted therapy simply because a patient is pregnant.

39-2. The definition of anemia may be complicated by which of the following factors?

a. Altitude
b. Sex
c. Race
d. Pregnancy

39-3. At low altitudes, which of the following hemoglobin levels may be considered to constitute anemia?

a. <12 g/dL in a nonpregnant woman
b. <10 g/dL in a pregnant woman
c. <10 g/dL immediately postpartum

39-4. During pregnancy, the volume of plasma expansion is _____ than the increase in hemoglobin mass and erythrocyte volume.

a. Greater
b. Less

39-5. Which of the following statements about anemia in pregnancy is correct?

a. Anemia is more common among indigent patients.
b. Laboratory error may contribute to the misdiagnosis of anemia.
c. A decreased hemoglobin mass is normal in pregnancy.
d. Women who take iron supplements are likely to have higher hemoglobin levels than women who do not receive supplements.

39-6. What are the two most common causes of anemia during pregnancy and the puerperium?

Instructions for Items 39-7 to 39-10: Match the quantity of iron with its utilization in pregnancy.

a. 200 mg
b. 300 mg
c. 500 mg
d. 800 mg
e. 1200 mg

39-7. Total maternal need for iron in pregnancy
39-8. Amount of iron needed for fetus and placenta
39-9. Amount of iron needed to expand maternal hemoglobin mass
39-10. Amount of iron shed through the gut, urine, and skin

39-11. The newborn infant of a severely anemic mother does not usually suffer from iron deficiency anemia.

a. True
b. False

39-12. Which of the following statements about the identification of iron deficiency anemia is correct?

a. The serum iron binding capacity is the best single diagnostic indicator.
b. Examination of the bone marrow is usually necessary to diagnose iron deficiency.
c. Hematologic response to iron may be first detected in a peripheral blood smear.
d. Pregnancy is known to depress erythropoiesis and hemoglobin formation.
e. Evidence of Plummer–Vinson syndrome is rarely seen in pregnancy.
f. In severe iron deficiency anemia during pregnancy, erythrocytes demonstrate hypochromia and microcytosis.

39-13. Which of the following may be appropriate for the evaluation of moderate anemia in a pregnant woman?

a. Hemoglobin concentration
b. Hematocrit
c. Red cell indices
d. Peripheral blood smear
e. Sickle cell preparation
f. Serum ferritin level

39-14. What is the preferred therapy for simple iron deficiency anemia in pregnancy?

a. Parenteral iron
b. Blood transfusion
c. Oral iron

39-15. Which of the following statements about oral iron therapy is correct?

a. Therapy should provide 200 mg of iron daily.
b. Oral therapy should be discontinued as soon as the anemia has been corrected.
c. Patients receiving iron and folic acid do considerably better than those receiving only iron.
d. Ferrous sulfate is a better iron source than ferrous fumarate or ferrous gluconate.
e. Iron preparations totally free of adverse effects are likely to be poorly absorbed.

39-16. What type of transfusion is an effective way of raising the hemoglobin concentration of severely anemic women without inducing circulatory overload?

39-17. Which of the following statements about acute blood loss anemia is correct?

a. It is more likely in the puerperium than during the pregnancy.
b. Acute hemorrhage may have little immediate effect on hemoglobin concentration.
c. Immediate blood replacement with whole blood is indicated.
d. Once stable, the patient can be satisfactorily treated with oral iron.

39-18. Which of the following statements about anemia with chronic disease in pregnancy is correct?

a. Erythrocytes are usually normocytic or slightly microcytic.
b. Bone marrow cytology is typically bizarre.
c. There is decreased erythropoiesis and slightly increased destruction of erythrocytes.
d. The anemia of infection, renal disease, and malignancy is not corrected with iron, folic acid, or vitamin B_{12}.
e. Iron and folate therapy is not worthwhile in pregnancy where anemia with chronic disease is present.

39-19. Which of the following statements about megaloblastic anemia in pregnancy is correct?

a. It is a common complication of pregnancy in the United States.
b. It is usually found in pregnant women who consume neither fresh vegetables nor animal protein.
c. It is most commonly due to vitamin B_{12} deficiency.
d. The earliest morphologic finding in cases of folate deficiency is hypersegmentation of neutrophils.
e. Severe cases of folate deficiency may be accompanied by thrombocytopenia and leukopenia.
f. The fetus of a mother who is anemic due to severe folate deficiency will also be severely anemic.
g. Megaloblastic anemia tends to recur in subsequent pregnancies.

39-20. Which of the following statements about the treatment of folic acid deficiency in pregnancy is correct?

a. One mg of oral folic acid per day produces a significant response.
b. The rate of hemoglobin increase is tempered by the expanding blood volume of pregnancy.
c. Iron as well as folic acid should usually be supplemented.

39-21. Pernicious anemia

a. Caused by the failure to absorb vitamin B_{12} is rare in women of reproductive age
b. If left untreated, may result in infertility
c. Should not be treated during pregnancy

39-22. Breast fed infants of mothers who suffer vitamin B_{12} deficiency may develop megaloblastic anemia during infancy.

a. True
b. False

39-23. Which of the following statements about acquired hemolytic anemia in pregnancy is correct?

a. Pregnancy may accelerate hemolysis in women with autoimmune acquired anemia.
b. In autoimmune hemolytic anemia, both the indirect and direct Coombs' test are positive.
c. Pregnancy-induced hemolytic anemia is a rare but treatable disease.
d. The most fulminant acquired hemolytic anemia during pregnancy is caused by the exotoxin of *Clostridium perfringens*.
e. Hemolysis may rarely be due to pregnancy-induced hypertension.
f. Pregnancy is a contraindication to the use of steroids for treatment of acquired hemolytic anemia.

39-24. Which of the following is a clinical aspect of paroxysmal nocturnal hemoglobinuria?

a. The hemoglobinuria only occurs at night.
b. There is a defect in the membranes of red cells, platelets, and granulocytes that makes them susceptible to lysis.
c. Heparin therapy has proven to be of considerable value.
d. The disease is familial, inherited as a sex-linked recessive trait.

39-25. Deficiency of glucose-6-phosphate dehydrogenase is an inherited enzymatic defect that accounts for drug-induced hemolysis in many black women.

a. True
b. False

39-26. Which of the following is characteristic of aplastic anemia in pregnancy?

   a. It is relatively rare.
   b. Anemia is coupled with thrombocytopenia and leukopenia.
   c. Bone marrow is markedly hypocellular.
   d. It is always congenital.
   e. It is never pregnancy related.
   f. Bone marrow transplantation is the most effective therapy.
   g. Antithymocyte globulin is the appropriate therapy for patients without a suitable bone marrow donor.

39-27. What are the two greatest risks to women with aplastic anemia during pregnancy?

39-28. List the most common sickle cell hemoglobinopathies.

39-29. Which of the following statements about sickle cell anemia is correct?

   a. Sickle cell crises are more common in pregnancy.
   b. Maternal and neonatal mortality rates are elevated in the presence of sickle cell anemia.
   c. Supplemental folic acid is indicated.
   d. Bone pain is best treated with heparin.
   e. Red cell transfusion after the onset of a painful crisis alleviates the pain dramatically.

39-30. Which of the following contraceptive techniques is probably contraindicated for women with sickle cell disease?

   a. Oral contraceptive
   b. Intrauterine device
   c. Diaphragm
   d. Condom
   e. Spermicidal jelly

39-31. Which of the following statements about sickle cell–hemoglobin C disease (SC) is correct?

   a. The gene for hemoglobin C is more common than the gene for hemoglobin S.
   b. In the nonpregnant woman, SC morbidity is lower and life span is longer than in the woman with sickle cell anemia.
   c. Attacks of bone pain and episodes of pulmonary dysfunction are increased during pregnancy and the puerperium.
   d. Perinatal mortality rates are as high for SC as for sickle cell anemia.
   e. Iron and folic acid supplementation is necessary.
   f. Prophylactic exchange transfusion may reduce maternal morbidity.

39-32. Perinatal morbidity and mortality in sickle cell–β-thalassemia is _____ (1) that in sickle cell–hemoglobin C disease and _____ (2) that in sickle cell anemia.

   a. Less than
   b. Similar to
   c. Greater than

39-33. Which of the following statements about prophylactic exchange transfusion for sickle hemoglobinopathies in pregnancy is correct?

   a. Transfusions should be initiated as soon as pregnancy is confirmed.
   b. Potential complications include hepatitis, iron overload, and alloimmunization.
   c. Reduction of potentially adverse reactions is beyond the scope of present technology.

39-34. Which of the following characterizes sickle cell trait?

   a. More S hemoglobin is produced than A hemoglobin.
   b. Erythrocytes usually appear normal.
   c. The frequencies of abortion and perinatal mortality are not increased.
   d. There is an association with asymptomatic bacteriuria.
   e. There is a higher incidence of pregnancy-induced hypertension.

Instructions for Items 39-35 to 39-38: Match the characteristic with the correct hemoglobin type.

   a. Hemoglobin C
   b. Hemoglobin E

39-35. Occurs in 2.5 percent of the black population
39-36. Presence of mild anemia
39-37. Folate and iron supplementation is needed in severe cases
39-38. Does not predispose to pathologic pregnancies

39-39. Hemolytic anemia characteristic of sickle cell anemia and sickle cell–hemoglobin C disease usually begins in utero.

   a. True
   b. False

39-40. If one parent has a hemoglobinopathy and the other parent has the trait, _____ (1) percent of their offspring will have the disease and _____ (2) percent will have the trait.

   a. 0
   b. 25
   c. 50
   d. 75
   e. 100

39-41. What techniques have been used to identify a fetus genetically destined to develop sickle cell disease?

   a. Fetoscopic collection of fetal red blood cells
   b. Enzymatic treatment of amniocytes
   c. Chorionic villus biopsy

39-42. Which of the following statements about hereditary spherocytosis is correct?

   a. It may be transmitted as an autosomal dominant with variable penetrance.
   b. Hemolysis depends on an intact, usually enlarged, spleen
   c. A previous normal pregnancy rules out the possibility of sudden anemia in a subsequent pregnancy.
   d. A newborn who has inherited spherocytosis may or may not develop hyperbilirubinemia and anemia in the neonatal period.

39-43. What are thalassemias?

Instructions for Items 39-44 to 39-48: Match the α-thalassemia with the appropriate hemoglobin composition where (+) means the presence of a functioning globin chain gene.

   a. Hemoglobin Bart disease
   b. Hemoglobin H disease
   c. α-Thalassemia minor
   d. Carrier state

39-44. $--/--$
39-45. $--/-+$
39-46. $-+/-+$
39-47. $--/++$
39-48. $-+/++$

39-49. Which of the following statements about α-thalassemia is correct?

   a. In the fetus with hemoglobin Bart disease there are four γ chains.
   b. Homozygous α-thalassemia results in the clinical picture of nonimmune hydrops fetalis.
   c. Hemoglobin H disease is incompatible with extrauterine life.
   d. α-Thalassemia minor is characterized by mild to moderate microcytic anemia.
   e. The simultaneous inheritance of sickle cell anemia and α-thalassemia results in a worse prognosis than that with sickle cell anemia alone.

39-50. Which of the following statements about β-thalassemia is correct?

   a. The rate of hemoglobin synthesis is unchanged and the rate of red blood cell destruction increases.
   b. β-Thalassemia minor is associated with intense hemolysis that is similar to that in the homozygous state.
   c. A woman with β-thalessemia major is often sterile.
   d. There is no specific therapy for β-thalassemia minor during pregnancy.
   e. β-Thalassemia intermedia is actually a variation of sickle-cell anemia.

39-51. Thrombocytopenia may be associated with

   a. Aplastic anemia
   b. Acquired hemolytic anemia
   c. Eclampsia–severe preeclampsia
   d. Consumptive coagulopathy
   e. Lupus erythematosus
   f. Megaloblastic anemia
   g. Infections

39-52. Which of the following is a feature of immune idiopathic thrombocytopenia?

   a. Presence of antiplatelet antibodies
   b. Familial occurrence
   c. Therapeutic response to splenectomy and/or corticosteroids
   d. Ameliorated by pregnancy
   e. Formation of IgG antibodies

39-53. Which of the following statements about the effects of maternal immune idiopathic thrombocytopenia on the fetus is correct?

   a. There is a strong correlation between maternal and fetal platelet counts.
   b. Administration of corticosteriods to the mother assures an adequate fetal platelet count.
   c. Intrapartum platelet counts on fetal scalp blood may aid in patient management.
   d. In a mother with severe thrombocytopenia, cesarean delivery is safest for both the mother and the fetus.

39-54. Which of the following may be an effective treatment for immune idiopathic thrombocytopenia?

   a. Polyvalent immunoglobulin therapy
   b. Danazol (a synthetic weak androgen)
   c. Estrogen plus progestin oral contraceptives

39-55. What are the principal findings in thrombotic microangiopathies?

39-56. Pregnancy has shown in most cases to worsen the prognosis for thrombotic microangiopathies.

   a. True
   b. False

39-57. What are effective treatment modalities for thrombotic thrombocytopenic purpura?

   a. Exchange transfusion
   b. Platelet transfusion
   c. Plasmapheresis
   d. Termination of pregnancy
   e. Dextran 70

39-58. Obstetrical hemorrhage is most commonly due to an inherited defect in the coagulation mechanism.

   a. True
   b. False

39-59. Which of the following is characteristic of hemophilia A?

   a. It is less common in women than in men.
   b. It is inherited as a sex-linked recessive trait.
   c. Bleeding is dependent on the level of circulating Factor VIII:C.
   d. Vaginal delivery is dangerous for the fetus with hemophilia A.
   e. Prenatal diagnosis using fetal plasma is possible near midpregnancy.

39-60. Antibodies to Factor VIII may be acquired and lead to life-threatening hemorrhage, especially in the puerperium.

   a. True
   b. False

39-61. Successful management of the pregnancy of a woman with hemophilia B requires the specific replacement of vitamin K.

   a. True
   b. False

39-62. Which of the following statements about von Willebrand's disease is correct?

   a. It is a distinct clinical entity.
   b. It is inherited only as an X-linked recessive trait.
   c. It is characterized by easy bruising, mucosal hemorrhage, and excessive bleeding with trauma or surgery.
   d. Bleeding time and partial thromboplastin time are prolonged.
   e. The level of Factor VIII is decreased.
   f. The hemostatic defects progressively worsen throughout pregnancy.

39-63. Which of the following is a relatively common disorder associated with pregnancy?

   a. Factor IX deficiency
   b. Familial hypofibrinogenemia
   c. Congenital afibrinogenemia
   d. Acquired hypofibrinogenemia

39-64. What are the two primary causes of cardiac disease in pregnancy?

   a. Rheumatic heart disease
   b. Myocarditis
   c. Congenital heart disease
   d. Kyphoscoliotic heart disease
   e. Hypertensive heart disease

39-65. Which of the following statements about cardiac disease in pregnancy is correct?

   a. It occurs in about 10 percent of pregnancies.
   b. Prognosis is independent of the psychologic and socioeconomic situation of the patient and her family.
   c. Cardiac decompensation seldom occurs after the 32nd week.
   d. Cardiac failure can occur during the puerperium.

39-66. What physiologic changes of pregnancy may mask cardiac disease?

   a. Systolic murmurs
   b. Dyspnea
   c. Changes simulating cardiac enlargement
   d. Edema

39-67. Which of the following is confirmatory evidence for the diagnosis of heart disease in pregnancy?

   a. Diastolic murmur
   b. Continuous murmur
   c. Cardiac enlargement
   d. Severe arrhythmia
   e. Loud, harsh systolic murmur associated with a thrill

Instructions for Items 39-68 to 39-71: Match the New York Heart Association classification with the corresponding limit on physical activity.

   a. Class I
   b. Class II
   c. Class III
   d. Class IV

39-68. Less than ordinary physical activity causes excessive fatigue
39-69. There is angina at rest
39-70. No limitation on physical activity
39-71. Ordinary physical activity causes dyspnea

39-72. Which of the following conditions may be especially hazardous for the pregnant patient with cardiac disease?

   a. Excessive weight gain
   b. Anemia
   c. Abnormal retention of blood
   d. Pregnancy-induced hypertension
   e. Hypotension

39-73. Which of the following statements about the management of class I and class II cardiac disease in pregnancy is correct?

  a. Most patients may be allowed to go through pregnancy.
  b. Maximum rest and minimum work are important.
  c. Cardiac failure can be precipitated by infection.
  d. Vaginal delivery is associated with greater morbidity and mortality than cesarean delivery.
  e. Hospitalization throughout pregnancy is necessary.

39-74. Which of the following are indications of heart failure during pregnancy?

  a. Increased vital capacity
  b. Persistent rales
  c. Dyspnea on exertion
  d. Hemoptysis
  e. Progressive edema
  f. Bradycardia

39-75. What is the major danger in the use of conduction anesthesia for delivery in a patient with cardiac disease?

39-76. Which of the following statements about the delivery of a patient with cardiac disease is correct?

  a. Relief from pain and apprehension are particularly important.
  b. The patient should be in the supine position.
  c. Anesthesia for cesarean delivery should avoid succinylcholine.
  d. Vital signs should be monitored more frequently in the second stage of labor than in the first stage.

39-77. At the first sign of cardiac failure during labor, delivery should be accomplished as quickly as possible.

  a. True
  b. False

39-78. Which of the following are important aspects of the medical treatment of heart failure in pregnancy?

  a. Morphine
  b. Oxygen
  c. Intramuscular digitalis preparation
  d. Oral diuretic
  e. Fowler position

39-79. Which of the following statements about the management of patients with the potential for cardiac failure is correct?

  a. Furosemide will reduce venous return and reduce pulmonary congestion.
  b. Use of Swan-Ganz catheter can aid in therapeutic decision making in cases of hypotension associated with cardiac failure.
  c. Postpartum decompensation only occurs in those patients who suffered cardiac failure intrapartum.
  d. In the absence of cardiac failure, breast feeding is not contraindicated.
  e. Postpartum sterilization should be performed as soon after delivery as possible.

39-80. Which of the following statements about class III cardiac disease in pregnancy is correct?

  a. Class III disease may be an indication for therapeutic abortion.
  b. Unless preventive measures are taken, about one-third of patients will decompensate during pregnancy.
  c. Hospitalization for the duration of pregnancy produces the best outcomes.
  d. Cesarean section is the most appropriate delivery method.
  e. Pregnancy has a long term deleterious effect on the condition.

39-81. Before performing a therapeutic abortion on a patient in cardiac failure, what must be done to stabilize the patient?

39-82. Mitral stenosis in pregnancy may be confused with

  a. Eisenmenger's syndrome
  b. Coarctation of the aorta
  c. Transposition of the great vessels
  d. Idiopathic peripartum cardiomyopathy

39-83. Severe maternal hypoxia predisposes to abortion, prematurity, and intrauterine death.

  a. True
  b. False

39-84. Which of the following statements about the effects of heart valve replacement on pregnancy is correct?

a. Valve replacements must not be done during pregnancy.
b. Women with artificial heart valves should take heparin during pregnancy.
c. Prolonged heparin administration during pregnancy may have adverse effects on the pregnancy outcome.
d. Complications with prosthetic valves include thrombosis and hemorrhage.
e. Spontaneous abortions and low-birthweight infants are more common in women with a prosthetic valve.
f. Combination estrogen–progestin birth control pills are the contraceptive of choice for women with prosthetic valves.

39-85. If a woman with an artificial heart valve is taking heparin, how soon before delivery should it be stopped?

39-86. In the patient with a patent ductus arteriosus and pulmonary hypertension, what abnormality may develop if systemic blood pressure drops?

39-87. In pregnant patients with a very high hematocrit, spontaneous abortion will be the most likely pregnancy outcome.

a. True
b. False

39-88. The maternal mortality with primary pulmonary hypertension has been reported to be as high as

a. 10 percent
b. 30 percent
c. 50 percent
d. 70 percent

39-89. In what circumstances should future pregnancy probably be avoided?

a. If coronary angiography indicates severe disease in a patient who has suffered a myocardial infarction
b. If there is persistent cardiomegaly and heart failure in a patient who has had periportal cardiomyopathy
c. In patients requiring antibiotic prophylaxis for the prevention of bacterial endocarditis
d. In a patient with a documented mitral valve prolapse
e. In a patient with coarctation of the aorta

39-90. Antimicrobial prophylaxis in labor should be given to women with

a. Valvular prostheses
b. Mitral valve prolapse
c. Coarctation of the aorta
d. Hypertension

39-91. Which of the following statements about kyphosis in pregnancy is correct?

a. Therapeutic abortion is indicated in women with marked degrees of kyphoscoliosis and markedly impaired pulmonary function.
b. Pelvic distortions may necessitate cesarean delivery.
c. Meperidine-induced respiratory depression is poorly tolerated.
d. Intermittent positive pressure breathing may be helpful.

39-92. Which of the following arrythmias is incompatible with a successful pregnancy outcome?

a. Complete heart block
b. Atrial fibrillation
c. Wolff–Parkinson–White syndrome
d. Supraventricular tachycardia

Instructions for Items 39–93 to 39–99: Match the parameter with its change in pregnancy from the nonpregnant state.

a. Increases
b. Decreases

39-93. Transverse thoracic diameter
39-94. Vertical chest diameter
39-95. Residual volume
39-96. Respiratory rate
39-97. Tidal volume
39-98. Plasma carbon dioxide
39-99. Oxygen consumption

39-100. Which type of pneumonia, if untreated, may result in a loss of ventilatory capacity that may pose significant problems for mother and fetus?

a. *Streptococcus pneumoniae*
b. *Mycoplasma pneumoniae*
c. Aspiration pneumonia
d. Viral pneumonitis

39-101. Thromboembolism and pulmonary infarction are both more common in the puerperium than during pregnancy.

a. True
b. False

39-102. Which of the following statements about asthma in pregnancy is correct?

a. An elevated P_{CO_2} is an ominous sign.
b. Pregnancy exacerbates all asthmatic conditions.
c. Therapy for asthma during pregnancy is markedly different than that which is effective in the nonpregnant woman.
d. Oxygen therapy should be instituted when the P_{O_2} is less than 70 mm Hg.
e. Iodine-containing medications may induce a fetal goiter.

39–103. What therapeutic modalities can be helpful in managing the pregnant patient with asthma?

    a. α-Adrenergic agents
    b. Steroids
    c. Theophyllines
    d. Hydration

39–104. Which of the following statements about tuberculosis in pregnancy is correct?

    a. Pulmonary resection for tuberculosis contraindicates future childbearing
    b. Chemotherapy that is effective when the woman is nonpregnant is also effective during pregnancy.
    c. All positive skin tests should be immediately treated with isoniazid.
    d. The infant should be isolated from a mother suspected of having acute disease.
    e. Pelvic tuberculosis is usually fatal to the mother.

39–105. When isoniazid is used for tuberculosis in pregnancy, what other medication should be given to prevent fetal harm?

39–106. Adult respiratory distress syndrome is best described as

    a. Pneumonia secondary to aspiration of gastric contents
    b. Lung injury with increased capillary membrane permeability, pulmonary edema, and reduced lung compliance
    c. Caused by *Mycoplasma*
    d. Streptococcal pneumonia

39–107. Corticosteroids should not be used to treat sarcoidosis in pregnancy.

    a. True
    b. False

39–108. Which of the following statements about cystic fibrosis and pregnancy is correct?

    a. Cystic fibrosis is transmitted as an autosomal recessive trait.
    b. The disease is more common in blacks than in whites.
    c. Most women who survive to adulthood are infertile.
    d. Pulmonary infection causes increased perinatal and maternal mortality.
    e. Nutrition may be compromised in pregnant women with cystic fibrosis.

39–109. Which of the following statements about hematologic disorders in pregnancy is correct?

    a. Pregnant women with leukemia may transmit the disease to their offspring.
    b. Pregnancy adversely affects the course of Hodgkin disease.
    c. Polycythemia during pregnancy is usually secondary and related to hypoxia from cardiac or pulmonary disease.
    d. Severe polycythemia is associated with poor pregnancy outcomes.
    e. Serum erythropoietin may be helpful in differentiating secondary polycythemia for polycythemia vera.

39–110. Pregnancy usually predisposes to the development or exacerbation of diseases of the urinary tract.

    a. True
    b. False

39–111. Which of the following statements about urinary tract infections in pregnancy is correct?

    a. Routine catheterization of the bladder at the time of delivery is recommended to prevent infection.
    b. Bacteriuria is present in about 35 percent of pregnant women at the time of the first prenatal visit.
    c. Asymptomatic bacteriuria need not be identified since it very rarely results in symptomatic urinary tract infections.
    d. Acute pyelonephritis in pregnancy is commonly an ascending infection from the bladder.
    e. Acute pyelonephritis is one of the most frequent complications of pregnancy.

39–112. Which of the following symptoms are typically associated with cystitis in pregnancy?

    a. Dysuria
    b. Urgency
    c. Frequency
    d. Fever
    e. Hematuria

39–113. Symptoms of frequency, urgency, dysuria, and pyuria without bacteriuria may be due to what common pathogen of the genitourinary tract?

    a. *Neisseria gonorrheae*
    b. *Escherichia coli*
    c. *Proteus mirabilis*
    d. *Chlamydia trachomatis*

39-114. Which of the following statements about acute pyelonephritis in pregnancy is correct?

a. It is most frequent during the second trimester.
b. If unilateral, the disease is more common on the left side.
c. Signs and symptoms are usually very subtle.
d. The body temperature is always sharply elevated.
e. The causative agent is usually a gram-negative bacteria.

39-115. The differential diagnosis of acute pyelonephritis includes

a. Labor
b. Placental abruption
c. Appendicitis
d. Infarction of a myoma
e. Cystitis

39-116. What factors predispose the bacteriuric pregnant woman to acute pyelonephritis?

39-117. Which of the following puerperal factors predispose to acute pyelonephritis?

a. Anesthetic effects on bladder sensitivity
b. Pelvic discomfort
c. Antidiuretic effect of oxytocin
d. Bladder overdistention
e. Bladder catheterization

39-118. What is ''asymptomatic bacteriuria?''

39-119. Which of the following statements about asymptomatic bacteriuria is correct?

a. The highest incidence is among black multiparas with sickle cell trait.
b. The condition is usually acquired in the second trimester.
c. A catheterized specimen is required to make the diagnosis.
d. Eradication of bacteriuria with antimicrobials prevents nearly all clinically evident infections.

39-120. Asymptomatic bacteriuria is not a prominent factor in the genesis of low birthweight or prematurity.

a. True
b. False

39-121. When should urologic evaluation be done in patients who do not respond to treatment of asymptomatic bacteriuria or who become reinfected after therapy?

a. As soon as possible
b. Immediately postpartum
c. After the puerperium

39-122. Which of the following statements about chronic pyelonephritis in pregnancy is correct?

a. It may be asymptomatic.
b. In advanced cases, the major symptoms are those of renal insufficiency.
c. Before symptomatic urinary infections can be documented in most patients.
d. Fetal prognosis is uniformly poor.
e. There is an increased risk of superimposed acute pyelonephritis.

39-123. Which of the following statements about the management of urinary tract infections in pregnancy is correct?

a. Gentamicin is usually the treatment of choice.
b. Asymptomatic bacteriuria should be treated with the patient hospitalized.
c. Patients with acute pyelonephritis are at risk for bacterial shock.
d. Therapy for acute pyelonephritis should be continued for at least 10 days.
e. It is unnecessary to repeat urine cultures after treatment of a urinary tract infection if the patient's symptoms have disappeared within 2 days.

Instructions for Items 39-124 to 39-130: Match the antimicrobial therapy used for urinary tract infections with its potential side effects.

a. Sulfonamide
b. Nitrofurantoin
c. Tetracycline
d. Chloramphenicol
e. Gentamicin

39-124. Ototoxicity
39-125. Maternal hemolysis
39-126. Maternal jaundice
39-127. Infant tooth discoloration
39-128. Kernicterus
39-129. Nephrotoxicity
39-130. Aplastic anemia

39-131. In severely ill pregnant women, what drug regimen provides effective treatment for urinary tract infections while culture and sensitivity results are pending?

a. Sulfonamides
b. Nitrofurantoin
c. Tetracycline
d. Chloramphenicol
e. Ampicillin/gentamicin

39-132. After antimicrobial treatment for urinary tract infection, absence of pyuria is adequate evidence for cure.

a. True
b. False

39–133. A history of renal tuberculosis is an absolute contra-indication to pregnancy.

a. True
b. False

39–134. Which of the following statements about urinary calculi during pregnancy is correct?

a. Pregnancy increases the risk of stone formation in women who have a history of renal stones.
b. There is an increased frequency of urinary tract infection among pregnant women with renal stones.
c. Surgical removal of stones should be accomplished as soon as they are discovered.
d. Renal calculi may be associated with hyperparathyroidism.

39–135. Which of the following statements about poststreptococcal glomerulonephritis in pregnancy is correct?

a. The condition is rare in pregnancy.
b. It may be clinically indistinguishable from preeclampsia.
c. Management should consist of expectant observation.
d. Some cases may turn into rapidly progressive glomerulonephritis.
e. Subsequent pregnancy is contraindicated.

39–136. Which of the following statements about chronic glomerulonephritis is correct?

a. It is characterized by progressive renal destruction.
b. Renal failure is almost always the first manifestation.
c. There is an increased rate of preeclampsia.
d. The prognosis for pregnancy outcome in cases of maternal azotemia or extreme hypertension is poor.
e. Renal plasma flow and glomerular filtration may increase during pregnancy.

39–137. Which of the following is found in nephrosis?

a. Edema
b. Massive proteinuria
c. Hypoalbuminemia
d. Hypercholesterolemia

39–138. When nephrotic syndrome complicates a pregnancy, the best predictor of maternal–fetal outcome is

a. The responsiveness of the gravida to steroid therapy
b. The degree of associated hypertension
c. The underlying cause of the disease and its resultant renal insufficiency
d. The ability to medically replace protein losses

39–139. The outcome of nephrotic syndrome in pregnancy is best summarized by the statement

a. The majority of women who are not hypertensive and do not have severe renal insufficiency will usually have a successful pregnancy outcome.
b. Interruption of the pregnancy is often indicated because of the severity of this disease.
c. As in other hypertensive states in pregnancy, the administration of glucocorticoids has been shown to have an adverse effect on maternal hypertension and should be avoided.
d. Plasmapheresis has been shown to be the most effective method of treatment in severe or recalcitrant cases and should be used in the face of rapidly deteriorating renal function.

39–140. Which of the following statements about acute renal failure in pregnancy is correct?

a. The most common cause is acute pyelonephritis.
b. Diuretics should be instituted as soon as oliguria is identified.
c. A urine:plasma creatinine ratio of greater than 30 is suggestive of prerenal azotemia.
d. In prerenal azotemia, sodium readsorption is low.

39–141. Which of the following statements about acute tubular necrosis (ATN) is correct?

a. It is largely preventable.
b. Hemodialysis is warranted in cases of azotemia and persistent oliguria.
c. It is a progresive disease.
d. Future pregnancies are contraindicated in women with ATN.

39–142. What measures can help prevent acute tubular necrosis?

a. Vigorous blood replacement
b. Termination of pregnancies in the presence of severe preeclampsia or eclampsia
c. Early identification and treatment of septic shock
d. Aggressive use of potent diuretics
e. Early use of vasoconstrictors in cases of hypotension

39–143. Which of the following statements about renal cortical necrosis is correct?

a. It is more common than acute tubular necrosis.
b. Most cases in pregnant women have occurred after placental abruption, preeclampsia/eclampsia, or bacterial shock.
c. The condition usually improves spontaneously without treatment.
d. Renal cortical necrosis can be clinically distinguished from acute tubular necrosis during the early phase of the disease.
e. The prognosis depends on the extent of the necrosis.

39–144. Which of the following is characteristic of postpartum hemolytic uremic syndrome?

a. Necrosis and endothelial proliferation in glomeruli
b. Necrosis, thrombosis, and intimal thickening in renal arterioles
c. Necrosis, thrombosis, and intimal thickening in pulmonary arterioles
d. Microangiopathic hemolysis
e. Thrombocytopenia

39–145. There may be a normal pregnancy outcome in which of the following situations?

a. After renal transplantation
b. After unilateral nephrectomy
c. Orthostatic proteinuria
d. Polycystic kidney disease
e. Renal failure requiring hemodialysis during pregnancy

39–146. Diabetes mellitus is _____ by pregnancy and $_{(1)}$ _____ the risk of a number of pregnancy complications. $_{(2)}$

a. Exacerbated
b. Improved
c. Increases
d. Decreases

39–147. Which of the following statements about diabetes in pregnancy is correct?

a. Before the discovery of insulin, diabetic women were most often too ill to conceive.
b. For most insulin dependent (type I) patients, there is no previous family history of diabetes.
c. Glycosuria usually reflects impaired glucose tolerance.
d. Lactose in the urine is definitive proof of diabetes.

39–148. The likelihood that a woman suffers from impaired carbohydrate metabolism is increased by

a. A strong family history of diabetes
b. The previous birth of a large infant
c. The presence of persistent glucosuria
d. An unexplained fetal loss

39–149. Which of the following statements is true regarding the use of a glucose tolerance test to identify diabetes during pregnancy?

a. Any abnormality of the test confirms diabetes.
b. Indications for testing are not uniform.
c. Any fasting value greater than 100 mg/dL should be treated with insulin.
d. It is universally recommended that all pregnant women should be screened with a glucose tolerance test.

39–150. Which of the following factors contributes to the final results of an oral glucose tolerance test?

a. Absorption of glucose from the intestinal tract
b. Uptake of glucose by tissues
c. Excretion of glucose in the urine.
d. Stimulation of pancreatic insulin production

39–151. Which of the following contributes to impaired insulin action in pregnancy?

a. Placental lactogen
b. Estrogen
c. Progesterone
d. Placental insulinase

39–152. Which of the following statements about the effects of pregnancy on diabetes is correct?

a. The worsening of diabetes seen during pregnancy usually disappears after delivery.
b. Nausea and vomiting during pregnancy may result in either insulin shock or insulin resistance.
c. Hypoglycemia may occur during labor, unless insulin levels are adjusted.
d. Pregnancy provides resistance to the ketoacidosis that might otherwise result from a severe infection.
e. There is less likelihood of developing metabolic acidosis during pregnancy complicated by diabetes than during normal pregnancy.

39–153. Which of the following are adverse maternal effects caused by diabetes during pregnancy?

a. Increased risk of preeclampsia–eclampsia
b. Greater frequency and severity of infections
c. Greater risk of maternal birth trauma from delivery of a large fetus
d. Risks from cesarean delivery
e. Risks from hydramnios and its effects
f. Increased frequency of postpartum hemorrhage

39–154. The potential adverse fetal effects resulting from maternal diabetes include an increased risk of

a. Perinatal death
b. Birth injury
c. Respiratory distress
d. Hypoglycemia
e. Hypocalcemia
f. Congenital anomalies
g. Diabetes

39–155. Inclusion of which of the following principles of management will result in the best outcome in cases of pregnancy complicated by diabetes?

a. Identification of the presence of abnormal carbohydrate metabolism
b. Control of blood sugar levels
c. Antepartum care by experienced providers
d. Perinatal and neonatal care by experienced providers

39–156. Which of the following statements about the management of gestational diabetes is correct?

a. The patients may usually be successfully managed by diet alone.
b. Delivery should be induced at 36 weeks.
c. An adequate diet should provide about 35 calories per kilogram per day.
d. Even with experienced health care providers, perinatal mortality is still about four times that in the general population.
e. Ten to 15 percent of class A diabetics develop overt diabetes during pregnancy.

39–157. Which of the following statements about the management of overt diabetes during pregnancy is correct?

a. Successful outcome is based solely on the control of blood sugar levels.
b. With proper care, perinatal mortality can approximate that in the general population.
c. Congenital malformations may be related to diabetes that was poorly controlled before conception and early in pregnancy.
d. Maternal glucose levels should be kept as close to normal as possible.
e. Pregnancy should always continue until pulmonary maturity is achieved.

39–158. Which of the following can help to achieve improved outcomes in pregnancies complicated by diabetes?

a. Frequent meals
b. Appropriate administration of insulin
c. Frequent measurement of plasma glucose levels
d. Precise knowledge of gestational age
e. Prenatal counseling

39–159. Insulin dosage in a pregnancy complicated by diabetes should be adjusted to eliminate glucosuria.

a. True
b. False

39–160. What management should follow the identification of acetonuria in a pregnancy complicated by diabetes?

39–161. Regarding the use of hemoglobin A1c, which of the following statements is true?

a. It is likely to be elevated in diabetics during pregnancy.
b. It correlates closely with fetal birthweight.
c. It correlates well with subsequent fetal hypoglycemia.
d. It bears no relationship to hemoglobins A1b or A1c.

39–162. Which of the following parameters presently offers the most information about fetal well-being near term in a woman with diabetes?

a. Twenty-four hour urinary estriol
b. Plasma estriol
c. Nonstress test/fetal heart reactivity test
d. Glycosylated hemoglobin A

39–163. What criteria must be met to safely begin induction of labor in a pregnancy complicated by diabetes?

a. The fetus must not be excessively large
b. The pelvis must not be contracted
c. Parity must not be great
d. The cervix must be favorable
e. There must be a vertex presentation
f. The presenting part must be fixed in the pelvis

39–164. Which of the following statements about delivery in a pregnancy complicated by diabetes is correct?

a. Cesarean delivery can avoid trauma to the fetus and the mother.
b. Long-acting insulin should be used on the day of delivery.
c. Plasma glucose levels should be checked frequently.
d. Postpartum insulin requirements are easily predictable based on maternal weight.
e. Postpartum starvation and infection pose significant maternal risks.

39–165. Which of the following are sources of significant perinatal morbidity in infants from pregnancies complicated by diabetes?

a. Congenital malformations
b. Hyperglycemia
c. Hypocalcemia
d. Hyperbilirubinemia
e. Idiopathic respiratory distress

39–166. In infants from pregnancies complicated by diabetes, organ system maturity is directly proportional to birthweight.

a. True
b. False

39–167. Which of the following reversible contraceptive methods is the best choice for women with overt diabetes?

a. Intrauterine device
b. Estrogen–progestin oral contraceptives
c. Contraception, barrier methods
d. Rhythm method

39–168. What normal pregnancy-induced changes mimic the signs and symptoms of thyroid dysfunction?

a. Increased cutaneous blood flow
b. Increased heart rate
c. Elevated free thyroxine
d. Increased thyroid uptake of radioiodine
e. Decreased thyroid-binding globulin

39–169. Which of the following is a helpful sign for identifying hyperthyroidism during pregnancy?

a. Excessive tachycardia
b. Elevated pulse rate during sleep
c. Enlarged thyroid gland
d. Exophthalmos
e. Failure to gain weight normally

39–170. Which of the following statements about the diagnosis of hyperthyroidism during pregnancy is correct?

a. The level of thyroxine in plasma is usually elevated.
b. The decreased uptake of triiodothyronine seen in normal pregnancy does not occur.
c. A normal plasma thyroxine level rules out hyperthyroidism.
d. A definitive diagnosis requires measuring thyroid uptake of radioactive iodine.
e. Management for a successful pregnancy outcome is primarily dependent on measurement of serial levels of thyroxine and triiodothyronine.

39–171. Which of the following statements about the medical treatment of hyperthyroidism in pregnancy is correct?

a. Medical management is primarily used to prepare the patient for definitive surgical treatment.
b. Fetal goiter and hypothyroidism may be induced by maternal ingestion of propylthiouracil.
c. Thyroid supplementation is often necessary when propylthiouracil is administered during pregnancy.
d. Propranolol is contraindicated during pregnancy.
e. Iodine should only be utilized for long-term therapy during pregnancy.

39–172. How is the proper dosage of propylthiouracil determined during pregnancy?

39–173. What adverse fetal effects may be associated with the use of propranolol for the treatment of hyperthyroidism during pregnancy?

a. Intrapartum fetal distress
b. Intrauterine growth retardation
c. Hypoglycemia
d. Hyperbilirubinemia
e. Low Apgar scores

39–174. Where drug therapy is toxic or the patient cannot adhere to the medical treatment plan, subtotal thyroidectomy after medical control has been achieved may be the treatment of choice for hyperthyroidism.

a. True
b. False

39–175. Propothiouracil is secreted in breast milk and, therefore, contraindicated in breast feeding mothers according to the American Academy of Pediatrics.

a. True
b. False

39–176. What mechanism causes a woman with Grave disease who is not hyperthyroid to give birth to an infant with manifestations of thyrotoxicosis?

39–177. A woman treated with propylthiouracil during pregnancy may give birth to an infant who is initially euthyroid but becomes hyperthyroid several days later.

a. True
b. False

39–178. Although thyroid storm may occur during pregnancy, women are resistant during the puerperium.

a. True
b. False

39–179. Which of the following statements about thyroid disease and pregnancy is correct?

a. The rates of infertility and spontaneous abortion are higher in women with hypothyroidism.
b. Untreated congenital hypothyroidism is associated with mental retardation.
c. Radioiodine is the best method to evaluate the thyroid in pregnancy.
d. Thyroid surgery is contraindicated in pregnancy.

39–180. Which of the following statements about parathyroid disease is correct?

a. Hyperparathyroidism in pregnancy is rare.
b. Neonatal tetany may be associated with maternal hyperparathyroidism.
c. Hypoparathyroidism is much more common than hyperparathyroidism.
d. Hypoparathyroidism usually leads to fetal demise.

39-181. Which of the following statements about adrenal dysfunction in pregnancy is correct?

   a. Due to advances in therapy, pregnancy has become more common in women with adrenocortical hypofunction.
   b. The level of steroid replacement required in patients with Addison disease approximately doubles each trimester.
   c. Pregnancy associated with Cushing disease is rare.
   d. Primary aldosteronism in pregnancy is usually life threatening for the mother.
   e. Pheochromocytoma in pregnancy is potentially associated with high fetal and maternal mortality rates.

39-182. Which of the following statements about pituitary disease in pregnancy is correct?

   a. Diabetes insipidus in pregnancy is rare.
   b. Pregnancies associated with diabetes insipidus should be terminated.
   c. A pituitary adenoma during pregnancy predisposes to fetal acromegaly.
   d. Bromocriptine in pregnancy has been shown to cause significant fetal skeletal deformities.

39-183. What are the physiologic changes in pregnancy related to liver function?

   a. Decreased serum albumin
   b. Increased plasma urea nitrogen
   c. Increased alkaline phosphatase activity
   d. Delayed excretion of sulfobromophthalein
   e. Palmar erythema
   f. Spider angiomata

39-184. What liver-related diseases are induced by pregnancy?

39-185. Which of the following are synonomous terms?

   a. Recurrent jaundice of pregnancy
   b. Idiopathic cholestasis of pregnancy
   c. Cholestatic hepatosis
   d. Icterus gravidarum

39-186. What are the two main clinical characteristics of intrahepatic cholestasis?

39-187. Which of the following statements about intrahepatic cholestasis is correct?

   a. It is more common in people of Asian extraction.
   b. Bile acids accumulate in the plasma.
   c. Ultrasonography may aid in establishing the diagnosis by ruling out the presence of gallstones.
   d. The use of cholestyramine is associated with the possibility of impaired coagulation.
   e. Intrahepatic cholestasis does not result in increased prematurity or pregnancy wastage.

39-188. What are the prominent histologic findings in acute fatty liver?

   a. Swollen hepatocytes
   b. Centrally placed hepatocyte nuclei
   c. Microvesicular fat droplets in hepatocyte cytoplasm
   d. Periportal sparing
   e. Liver necrosis

39-189. Which of the following statements about acute fatty liver is correct?

   a. The histology is similar to that seen in Reye syndrome.
   b. The most usual onset is in the second trimester.
   c. The onset of clinical symptoms is usually insidious.
   d. Delivery is essential for cure.
   e. Subsequent pregnancy should be avoided as the disease tends to recur in most cases.

39-190. What symptom signals potentially life-threatening liver involvement in pregnancy-induced hypertension?

39-191. Which of the following statements about hyperemesis gravidarum is correct?

   a. The differential diagnosis includes cholecystitis, hepatitis, peptic ulcer, gastroenteritis, and pyelonephritis.
   b. Jaundice and elevation of SGOT may result from hyperemesis.
   c. Social and psychological factors may play a contributing role.
   d. Treatment includes fluid and electrolyte replacement.
   e. Pregnancy termination is often necessary.

39-192. In rare circumstances, which of the following can result from hyperemesis?

   a. Weight loss
   b. Dehydration
   c. Starvation acidosis
   d. Alkalosis due to hydrochloric acid loss in vomitus
   e. Hypokalemia

39-193. Which of the following statements about viral hepatitis A is correct?

   a. Feces, secretions, and bed pans from hepatitis A patients should be handled while wearing gloves.
   b. The incubation period is from 2 to 7 weeks.
   c. Spread is by ingestion of contaminated water and blood.
   d. Diagnosis is confirmed by detection of IgM antibody to hepatitis A.
   e. Treatment should consist of a nutritious diet and sedentary living.
   f. Hepatitis A is teratogenic.
   g. Risk of transmission to the fetus is greater than 50 percent.

39-194. A pregnant woman who has been exposed to hepatitis A should not receive prophylactic gamma globulin.

a. True
b. False

39-195. Which of the following statements about hepatitis B is correct?

a. The disease is most often found among intravenous drug users, homosexuals, health care personnel, and individuals frequently treated with blood products.
b. It has been shown that routine screening for hepatitis B antigenemia in pregnancy could result in a net savings of more than $100 million per year.
c. The infectious state is characterized by the presence of e antigen.
d. The disease can be vertically transmitted.
e. An infant can obtain the virus through breast feeding.
f. Newborns can be effectively protected prophylactically with hepatitis B immune globulin and vaccine.

Instructions for Items 39-196 to 39-198: Match the type of hepatitis in pregnancy with its potential effects.

a. Hepatitis A
b. Hepatitis B

39-196. Disease course is not appreciably affected by pregnancy
39-197. There is an increased risk of prematurity
39-198. Antigenic screening of high-risk pregnant women should be carried out

39-199. What is the significance of the presence of e antigen in cases of hepatitis B during pregnancy?

39-200. Which of the following statements regarding delta hepatitis is true?

a. The virus must coinfect with hepatitis B.
b. Transmission is similar to hepatitis B.
c. Neonatal transmission is reported.
d. Vaccination may prevent this disease.

39-201. Immune serum globulin for prophylaxis against non-A–non-B hepatitis should be administered to the newborn of a mother with active disease.

a. True
b. False

39-202. Which of the following statements about chronic active hepatitis in pregnancy is correct?

a. The disease can progress to hepatic failure.
b. Fetal loss is increased.
c. There is no effective therapy.
d. Therapeutic abortion is usually necessary to save the mother.
e. There is a markedly increased rate of fetal malformations in those pregnancies that are maintained.

39-203. There is high morbidity and appreciable mortality in pregnancies complicated by cirrhosis of the liver.

a. True
b. False

39-204. Which of the following statements about the origin and management of gallbladder disease in pregnancy is correct?

a. There is usually incomplete emptying of the gallbladder during pregnancy.
b. The incidence of gallstones is higher than in the nonpregnant state.
c. Surgical management of gallbladder disease should be avoided during pregnancy.
d. Cholecystectomy is contraindicated during pregnancy.

39-205. What factors can mask the diagnosis of appendicitis in pregnancy?

39-206. Which of the following statements about appendicitis in pregnancy is correct?

a. Pregnancy predisposes to appendicitis.
b. Appendicitis has no effect on the likelihood of abortion or preterm labor.
c. The prognosis is worse if the disease occurs late in gestation.
d. Appendicitis-related mortality is most often related to surgical delay.
e. Cesarean delivery is usually indicated at the time of appendectomy.
f. Appendicitis is rare during the puerperium.

39-207. Which of the following statements about abdominal pain during pregnancy is correct?

a. Right upper quadrant pain or epigastric pain may be a sign of severe preeclampsia.
b. Peptic ulcer symptoms usually improve during pregnancy.
c. Unlike the nonpregnant patient, the pregnant patient with pancreatitis seldom has associated alcoholism.
d. Intestinal obstruction during pregnancy is most commonly associated with the presence of a malignancy.

39-208. Which of the following statements about chronic inflammatory bowel disease in pregnancy is correct?

a. Therapeutic abortion should be offered in most cases.
b. Pregnancy exacerbates regional enteritis.
c. Ulcerative colitis predisposes to congenital malformations.
d. Exacerbation of ulcerative colitis during pregnancy may be induced by psychogenic factors.

39-209. Which of the following statements regarding the use of parenteral nutrition during pregnancy is true?

a. The purpose is to provide calories, essential amino acids, vitamins, and minerals.
b. Jugular or subclavian catheterization is necessary to deliver hyperosmolar solutions.
c. Complications are seen in pregnant patients receiving parenteral nutrition in about 1/3 of the cases.
d. Sepsis and expense are two large drawbacks to this form of therapy.

39-210. Weight reduction during pregnancy should be recommended for the markedly obese patient.

a. True
b. False

39-211. For a successful pregnancy outcome after a patient has undergone gastric or jejunoileal bypass surgery for obesity, conception should be postponed until after the period of rapid postoperative weight loss.

a. True
b. False

39-212. List the criteria that may be used for the diagnosis of systemic lupus erythematosus.

39-213. A diagnosis of lupus may be made when _____ of the possible criteria are present, either serially or simultaneously.

a. 2
b. 4
c. 6
d. 8
e. 10

39-214. Which of the following statements about lupus in pregnancy is correct?

a. The major nonrenal manifestations of lupus are not induced by pregnancy unless immunosuppressive therapy is discontinued.
b. Renal function usually remains good during pregnancy.
c. An increase in the dosage of glucocorticosteriods and azathioprine may be advisable during labor and the puerperium.
d. Maternal diabetes may be a complication of steroidal therapy during pregnancy.

39-215. What laboratory tests are helpful in monitoring the activity of lupus during pregnancy?

a. Sedimentation rate
b. c3 and c4 Complement levels
c. Hematologic evaluations
d. Liver function tests
e. Renal function tests

39-216. What similar manifestations may occur in severe preeclampsia–eclampsia and systemic lupus erythematosus?

39-217. Which of the following are possible fetal effects of maternal systemic lupus erythematosus?

a. Stillbirth
b. Intrauterine growth retardation
c. Prematurity
d. Congenital heart block
e. Anemia
f. Transient discoid lupus
g. Positive LE factor in the infant's blood

39-218. Asymptomatic mothers of infants with isolated complete heart block should be evaluated for possible systemic lupus-erythematosus.

a. True
b. False

39-219. What is lupus anticoagulant and what is its significance for fetal outcome?

39-220. Regarding diseases of the skin in pregnancy, which of the following are true?

a. Telogen effluvium refers to an increased hair loss that may occur during pregnancy.
b. The most common pruritic dermatosis of pregnancy is called pruritic urticarial papules and plaques of pregnancy.
c. Herpes gestationis is a viral disease in pregnancy best treated with prednisone.
d. Women with burns over 50 percent or more of their body surfaces during pregnancy should be immediately delivered to decrease the likelihood of maternal mortality.

39-221. Which of the following statements about epilepsy in pregnancy is correct?

a. The condition of a woman with well-controlled seizures before conception will deteriorate significantly during pregnancy.
b. Anticonvulsant medication may not be absorbed as well in the pregnant patient.
c. Protein binding of drugs decreases in pregnancy.
d. Doses of phenytoin administered during pregnancy should be at least one-third higher than in the nonpregnant state.

39-222. What fetal anomalies have been associated with maternal ingestion of phenytoin during pregnancy?

    a. Craniofacial anomalies
    b. Distal limb dysmorphosis
    c. Mental deficiency
    d. Cleft lip/palate
    e. Congenital heart lesions
    f. Hemorrhagic disease of the newborn

Instructions for Items 39–223 to 39–226: Match the anticonvulsant medication with its potential fetal effects.

    a. Carbamazepine (Tegretol)
    b. Valproic acid

39-223. Craniofacial anomalies
39-224. Small head size
39-225. Neural tube defects
39-226. Facial, digital, and skeletal malformations

39-227. All women should cease taking anticonvulsant medications before conceiving.

    a. True
    b. False

39-228. What type of anemia has been reported to be aggravated by anticonvulsant medications?

39-229. Which of the following is true of cerebrovascular disease during pregnancy?

    a. Cerebrovascular accidents in pregnancy were responsible for five percent of nonabortion related maternal deaths from 1974–1978.
    b. The most common cause of cerebral emboli in pregnancy is the pelvic veins.
    c. A ruptured cranial aneurysm may be best managed in pregnancy by cesarean section and craniotomy with repair of the defect.

39-230. Which of the following statements about intracranial hemorrhage in pregnancy is correct?

    a. Hemorrhage can be readily identified by CT scan.
    b. There are minimal fetal risks from surgical repair.
    c. Therapeutic abortion may be indicated if the hemorrhage occurs early in pregnancy.
    d. All patients who survive the hemorrhage should undergo elective cesearean delivery.

39-231. Presence of which of the following paternal conditions may be an indication for therapeutic abortion?

    a. Ventriculoperitoneal shunt
    b. Maternal brain death
    c. Pseudotumor cerebri
    d. Spinal cord lesion
    e. Multiple sclerosis
    f. Guillain-Barre syndrome
    g. Myasthenia gravis
    h. Huntington chorea
    i. Chorea gravidarum
    j. Bell's palsy

39-232. Which of the following may complicate pregnancy in a woman with a spinal cord lesion?

    a. Urinary tract infections
    b. Pressure necrosis of the skin
    c. Autonomic hyperreflexia
    d. Painless, precipitous labor
    e. Prolonged second stage labor

39-233. Exacerbation of multiple sclerosis in the first few months postpartum is relatively common.

    a. True
    b. False

39-234. Which of the following statements about myasthenia gravis in pregnancy is correct?

    a. The primary therapy is thymectomy.
    b. Pregnancy and labor usually occur without difficulty.
    c. The second stage of labor may be prolonged because of impaired expulsive effects.
    d. The fetus seems to be protected against the disease while in utero.
    e. Neonatal myasthenia has been reported in greater than 90 percent of infants of myasthenic mothers.
    f. With proper treatment, neonatal myasthenia usually subsides completely within 5 to 6 weeks.

39-235. What characterizes neonatal symptomatic myasthenia gravis?

    a. Feeble cry
    b. Poor suckling
    c. Respiratory distress
    d. Response to parenteral neostigmine

39-236. What drugs may be potentially dangerous to patients with myasthenia gravis?

    a. Quinine
    b. Magnesium sulfate
    c. Kanamycin
    d. Gentamicin

39–237. Which of the following statements about the treatment of psychosis in pregnancy and the puerperium is correct?

  a. Electroshock therapy is incompatible with normal pregnancy outcome.
  b. The use of therapeutic lithium carbonate may be associated with fetal cardiac anomalies.
  c. Tricyclic antidepressants may be safely administered as they have no adverse fetal or neonatal effects.
  d. Bottle feeding is recommended when a woman is ingesting lithium carbonate.

39–238. Which of the following statements about varicella in pregnancy is correct?

  a. The disease is uncommon in adults.
  b. Varicella pneumonia may prove fatal.
  c. Acyclovir may be useful in preventing and treating varicella pneumonitis.
  d. Administration of immune globulin should be considered for exposed nonimmune pregnant women.
  e. Transplacental passage of the virus with fetal infection may occur.
  f. Exposure of the fetus during delivery may result in visceral and central nervous system disease.

Instructions for Items 39–239 to 39–245. Match the infection with the appropriate statement.

  a. Increases risk of abortion
  b. Increases risk of prematurity
  c. Vaccination during pregnancy is helpful
  d. Vaccination in pregnancy is contraindicated
  e. May result in pneumonia
  f. Pregnant women more susceptible to the infection

39–239. Mumps
39–240. Rubeola
39–241. Influenza
39–242. Common cold
39–243. Poliomyelitis
39–244. Typhoid fever
39–245. Malaria

39–246. Which of the following diseases indicates therapeutic abortion?

  a. Coxsackie virus
  b. Erysipelas
  c. Malaria
  d. Poliomyelitis
  e. Amebiasis
  f. Coccidioidomycosis
  g. Hansen's disease (leprosy)

39–247. Pregnancy makes the woman immune to several of the more common sexually transmitted diseases.

  a. True
  b. False

39–248. Which of the following is characteristic of syphilis?

  a. It is readily preventable.
  b. It is not susceptible to therapy.
  c. There is a 3-day incubation period.
  d. The primary lesion lasts from 1 to 5 weeks.
  e. Secondary syphilitic lesions may go unnoticed.

39–249. The raised lesions of secondary syphilis are known as _____ .

39–250. The first suggestion of syphilitic disease in many women is the birth of a stillborn infant or a liveborn infant with congenital syphilis.

  a. True
  b. False

39–251. Which of the following statements about the diagnosis of syphilis in pregnancy is correct?

  a. A VDRL screening test is a necessary part of the prenatal laboratory work-up.
  b. Serologic tests for syphilis are positive from 2 weeks of contracting the disease.
  c. A treponemal test is used to confirm a positive reagin test.
  d. For high-risk patients, repeat screening should be done in the third trimester and testing of cord blood is indicated.

Instructions for Items 39–252 to 39–258. Match the CDC recommended treatments of syphilis with the appropriate clinical situation.

  a. Benzathine penicillin G: 2.4 million units, IM
  b. Benzathine penicillin G: 2.4 million units weekly for 3 weeks, IM
  c. Crystalline penicillin G: 2 to 4 million units every 4 hours for 10 days, IV; then benzathine penicillin G: 2 to 4 million units weekly for 3 weeks, IM
  d. Erythromycin: 500 mg four times daily for 15 days, orally
  e. Tetracycline: 500 mg four times daily for 15 days, orally

39–252. Incubating syphilis
39–253. Culture proven gonorrhea present
39–254. Pregnant woman who is allergic to penicillin
39–255. Pregnant woman who is not allergic to penicillin
39–256. Persistent or recurrent signs of syphilis
39–257. Initial antibody titer is greater than 1:8
39–258. Neurosyphilis

39-259. If spinal fluid was positive for syphilis, at what intervals should repeat testing be done?

39-260. Which of the following statements about the treatment of syphilis in pregnancy is correct?

    a. For pregnant patients not allergic to penicillin, the optimal treatment is the same as for nonpregnant women.
    b. Women with a penicillin allergy can be desensitized.
    c. Tetracycline use during pregnancy can cause the staining of the child's permanent teeth.
    d. Women treated for syphilis should be monitored by monthly spinal fluid titers.
    e. The sexual partner of an infected woman should also be treated.

39-261. Which of the following statements about congenital syphilis is correct?

    a. Every infant suspected of having syphilis should have a cerebrospinal fluid examination before treatment.
    b. The drug of choice for symptomatic infants is erythromycin.
    c. Asymptomatic seropositive infants with a negative cerebrospinal fluid examination need not be treated.
    d. Infants born of mothers with erythromycin for syphilis during pregnancy should be treated as if they have congenital syphilis.

39-262. Why is gonococcal salpingitis not a problem after the third month of pregnancy.

39-263. Which organs of the lower genital tract may be affected by gonorrhea?

    a. Cervix
    b. Urethra
    c. Bartholin glands
    d. Periurethral glands

39-264. What clinical outcomes may result from gonorrhea in pregnancy?

39-265. Asymptomatic gonorrhea should be identified and treated during pregnancy.

    a. True
    b. False

39-266. Which of the following is recommended for the treatment of all forms of uncomplicated gonorrhea during pregnancy?

    a. Aqueous procaine penicillin plus probenecid
    b. Ampicillin
    c. Amoxicillin
    d. Spectinomycin
    e. Tetracycline

Instructions for Items 39-267 to 39-270: Match the treatment for gonorrhea during pregnancy with the appropriate situation.

    a. Erythromycin
    b. Spectinomycin
    c. Aqueous crystalline penicillin
    d. Ampicillin
    e. Tetracycline
    f. Aqueous procaine penicillin

39-267. Penicillinase-producing gonococci
39-268. Coexistent chlamydial infection
39-269. Disseminated gonococcal infection
39-270. Infants of mothers with gonorrhea

39-271. What three drugs are recommended in the treatment of penicillinase-producing gonococci?

39-272. How should gonococcal ophthalmia be treated?

39-273. Which of the following statements about chlamydial infections in pregnancy is correct?

    a. One specific serotype causes lymphogranuloma venereum.
    b. Culture techniques for *Chlamydia trachomatis* are readily available.
    c. The treatment of choice during pregnancy is tetracycline.
    d. There is no known deleterious effect of the disease on pregnancy.

39-274. Which of the following statements is true?

    a. Chlamydial infection causes preterm labor and delivery and low-birthweight infants.
    b. Ureaplasma and mycoplasma are found to coexist with *Chlamydia*.
    c. The role of *Chlamydia* in postpartum infections had been found to be minimal.
    d. Lymphogranuloma venereum may be characterized by long-standing infection unresponsive to multiple antimicrobial regimens.

39-275. Which type of herpes simplex virus is recovered almost exclusively from the genital tract?

39-276. Which of the following statements about herpes infection is correct?

    a. The incubation period for primary infections is 2 to 3 weeks.
    b. The cervix is the most common site of genital tract infection.
    c. Involvement of the cervix and the vagina is usually asymptomatic.
    d. Vulvar lesions are likely to be tender and easily traumatized.
    e. The virus is harbored in nerve ganglia.

39-277. Recurrent herpes infections can be prevented by treatment with acyclovir (Zovirax).

   a. True
   b. False

39-278. Which of the following statements about the identification of genital herpes is correct?

   a. Cervical smears usually contain large multinucleate cells with eosinophilic viral inclusion bodies.
   b. Monoclonal antibodies are available to identify herpes simplex virus.
   c. Women with herpes should undergo annual Pap smears to screen for cervical neoplasia.

39-279. Which of the following statements about herpes infection and the neonate is correct?

   a. The incidence of neonatal herpes has been slowly decreasing over the past 10 years.
   b. The morbidity rate, but not the mortality rate, is high in cases of neonatal herpes.
   c. The fetus is usually infected before rupture of the membranes.
   d. Infection in the newborn may be asymptomatic.
   e. Central nervous system and ocular involvement have been commonly reported in infected infants.

39-280. What is the rationale for advocating cesarean delivery for infants of mothers with suspected or documented herpes?

39-281. Which of the following statements about delivery and postpartum care in cases of maternal herpes is correct?

   a. All women with a history of herpes must undergo casarean delivery.
   b. If the membranes have already been ruptured, cesarean delivery provides no protection to the fetus.
   c. The neonate must be monitored more closely than usual.
   d. Breast feeding by infected mothers should not be allowed.

39-282. Regarding acquired immunodeficiency syndrome (AIDS), which of the following statements is true?

   a. The prevalence of asymptomatic infection in the United States in 1987 was estimated to be up to 1.5 million persons.
   b. The incubation period for asymptomatic viremia to the full-blown immunodeficiency syndrome can be as short as 2 months to as long as 2 years.
   c. About 10 percent of patients with serologic evidence of infection will develop clinical illness within 3 years.
   d. Currently used tests to identify human immunodeficiency virus antibodies consist first of a screen relying on enzyme immunoassay and a confirmatory test relying on an immunological reaction between an antibody and viral proteins.

39-283. Of the infants born to mothers with AIDS, it must be said that there is insufficient experience to ascertain the risk of fetal infection.

   a. True
   b. False

39-284. To prevent the transmission of AIDS, it may be said

   a. The same antepartum and peripartum measures as for hepatitis B should be applied.
   b. There is no prevention.
   c. Infants should not be suctioned using bulb techniques.
   d. Ventilatory support for preterm infants of AIDS mothers should not be given.

39-285. Human papilloma virus

   a. May be associated with genital dysplasia
   b. May be associated with laryngeal papillomatosis
   c. Should never be treated in pregnancy regardless of manifestations
   d. Should be considered serious enough in infants so that symptomatic gravidas undergo cesarean section

Instructions for Items 39-286 to 39-292: Match the infection with the appropriate statement.

   a. Chancroid
   b. Granuloma inguinale

39-286. Caused by *Haemophilus ducreyi*
39-287. Caused by *Donovania granulomata*
39-288. Painful nonindurated genital ulcers
39-289. Multiple, large, foul-smelling ulcerations
39-290. Painful inguinal lymphadenopathy
39-291. Diagnosis by culture of the infecting organism from lesions
39-292. Diagnosis by identification of Donovan bodies in smears

39-293. Which of the following statements about breast carcinoma in pregnancy is true?

   a. Therapeutic abortion improves prognosis.
   b. Breast cancer prognosis in pregnancy depends on fetal gestational age at the time of diagnosis.
   c. Mastectomy adversely affects subsequent pregnancy outcomes.
   d. Chemotherapy cannot be administered during pregnancy.

39-294. Regarding Hodgkin disease in pregnancy, which of the following is true?

a. It is the most common lymphoma encountered in pregnancy.
b. Neither standard radiotherapy nor chemotherapy in the second trimester appears to affect adversely the fetus or the neonate.
c. Pregnant women with this disease are very susceptible to infection.
d. More than half of women resume normal menses after treatment for this disease.

39-295. Leukemia during pregnancy makes it nearly impossible to induce satisfactory remission.

a. True
b. False

39-296. Which of the following statements regarding malignant melanoma in pregnancy is true?

a. It is the most common malignancy to metastasize to placenta.
b. Pregnancy has an adverse effect on the outcome of malignant melanoma.
c. Prognosis is solely dependent on the stage of the lesion.
d. Pregnancy is associated with an increased amount of melanocyte-stimulating hormone.

PART X REPRODUCTION IN WOMEN

40. ANATOMY OF THE REPRODUCTIVE TRACT OF WOMEN

40-1. Which one of the following does NOT mean the same as the others?

a. Vulva
b. External generative organs
c. Organs providing for ovulation, fertilization, and implantation
d. Pudenda

40-2. Which of the following is a part of the vulva?

a. Labia majora
b. Labia minora
c. Clitoris
d. Vestibule
e. Vagina

40-3. Which of the following statements about the labia majora is correct?

a. The labia majora are embryologically homologous with the male scrotum.
b. The uterosacral ligaments terminate at the upper borders of the labia majora.
c. In multiparous women, the labia majora are more prominent than in nulliparous women.
d. In nulliparous women, the labia majora lie in close apposition.
e. Posteriorly, the labia majora merge into the perineum.

40-4. Which types of tissue are prominent in the labia majora?

a. Fat
b. Sebaceous glands
c. Muscle
d. Connective tissue

40-5. Which of the following statements about the labia minora is correct?

a. In nulliparous women, the labia minora usually project beyond the labia majora.
b. The labia minora are covered by stratified squamous epithelium.
c. There are numerous hair follicles in the labia minora.
d. Superiorly, the labia minora form the frenulum of the clitoris and the prepuce.
e. Inferiorly, the labia minora form the fourchet.

40-6. Which of the following statements about the clitoris is correct?

a. It is homologous to the male scrotum.
b. It contains many smooth muscle fibers.
c. The free end of the clitoris points toward the vaginal opening.
d. The glans is very sensitive to touch.
e. The vessels of the clitoris are connected with the vestibular bulbs.

40-7. Which of the following organs is erectile?

a. Clitoris
b. Frenulum
c. Labia majora
d. Labia minora

40-8. Which of the following are boundaries of the vestibule?

    a. Labia majora
    b. Clitoris
    c. Fourchet
    d. Labia minora

40-9. The Bartholin glands

    a. Are also termed the major vestibular glands
    b. Are situated beneath the vestibule on either side of the vaginal opening
    c. Do not possess a duct
    d. Are sometimes partially covered by the vestibular bulbs
    e. Can harbor bacterial pathogens

40-10. Which of the following structures is *not* richly supplied with nerve fibers?

    a. Labia minora
    b. Labia majora
    c. Hymen
    d. Clitoris

40-11. Which of the following statements about the hymen is correct?

    a. Among women, there is a marked similarity in the shape and consistency of the hymen.
    b. The surfaces of the hymen are covered by stratified squamous epithelium.
    c. The hymen is comprised mainly of muscle.
    d. In virgins, the hymen covers the labia minora.

40-12. Presence of an unruptured hymen is a sure indication that the patient is virginal.

    a. True
    b. False

40-13. The cicatrized nodules of various sizes, which are hymenal remnants after childbirth, are called _____ .

Instructions for Items 40-14 to 40-18: Refer to Figure 6. Match the letter with the appropriate description.

40-14. Site of the greatest concentration of genital corpuscles.

40-15. Rich supply of sebaceous glands and hair follicles

40-16. Remnants of the relatively avascular connective tissue covering of the vaginal opening

40-17. Distensible posterior extension of the labia majora and minora

40-18. Distensible anterior extension of the labia majora and minora

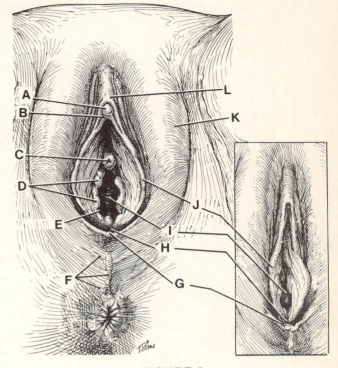

FIGURE 6

40-19. Which of the following is a function of the vagina?

    a. Excretory duct for the uterus
    b. Female organ of copulation
    c. Excretory duct for the bladder
    d. Birth canal

40-20. Which of the following statements about the vagina is correct?

    a. It arises embryologically from the müllerian ducts and the urogenital sinus.
    b. It is in contact with both the rectum and bladder.
    c. A transverse section of a nondistended vagina is H-shaped.
    d. The vagina is distensible only during childbirth.
    e. Vaginal length varies among women.

40-21. The upper one-quarter of the vagina is separated from the rectum by the rectouterine pouch, also called the

_____ .

40-22. The anterior and posterior walls of the vagina are of equal length.

    a. True
    b. False

40-23. In which of the following situations are vaginal rugae *not* prominent.

   a. In nulliparous women
   b. In multiparous women
   c. Before menarche
   d. After menopause

40-24. Which of the following statements about the vagina is correct?

   a. Glycogen begins to appear in the superficial layer of vaginal mucosa after menarche.
   b. There are numerous glands present in the vagina.
   c. Exfoliated vaginal epithelial cells can be used to identify various hormonal events of the ovarian cycle.
   d. Uterine secretions contribute to vaginal moisture in nonpregnant women.
   e. During pregnancy, vaginal secretions decrease.

Instructions for Items 40-25 to 40-27: Match the portion of the vagina with its arterial blood supply.

   a. Inferior vesical arteries
   b. Middle hemorrhoidal artery
   c. Cervicovaginal branches of uterine arteries
   d. Internal pudendal artery

40-25. Upper one-third of vagina
40-26. Middle one-third of vagina
40-27. Lower one-third of vagina

40-28. Which of the following vascular structures contained within the external genital organs are prone to rupture and hematoma formation during vaginal delivery?

   a. Venous plexus of the labia majora
   b. Vestibular bulbs
   c. Venous plexus of the vagina
   d. Venous plexus of the labia minora

40-29. Vessels from the venous plexus around the vagina eventually empty into the _____ veins.

40-30. The lymphatics from the lower third of the vagina and the vulva drain into the

   a. Inguinal nodes
   b. Hypogastric nodes
   c. Iliac nodes

40-31. The vagina contains a rich supply of special nerve endings (genital corpuscles).

   a. True
   b. False

Instructions for Items 40-32 and 40-33: Match the muscles with the appropriate support structures of the perineum.

   a. Deep transverse perineal
   b. Levator ani
   c. Coccygeus
   d. Constrictor of urethra

40-32. Pelvic diaphragm
40-33. Urogenital diaphragm

40-34. The perineal body is formed by which of the following muscles?

   a. External anal sphincter
   b. Bulbocavernosus muscles
   c. Superficial transverse perineal muscles
   d. Deep transverse perineal muscles

40-35. The entire surface of the uterus is covered by serosa or peritoneum.

   a. True
   b. False

Instructions for Items 40-36 to 40-39: Match the portion of the uterus with its correct description.

   a. Cornua
   b. Cervix
   c. Fundus
   d. Corpus

40-36. Upper triangular portion
40-37. Lower, fusiform (cylindrical) portion
40-38. Junction of superior and lateral margins
40-39. Convex segment between the insertion points of the fallopian tubes

40-40. In the nulliparous woman, the ratio of uterine body length to cervix length is approximately

   a. 1:2
   b. 1:1
   c. 2:1

40-41. During pregnancy, which portion of the uterus forms the lower uterine segment?

   a. External cervical os
   b. Isthmus
   c. Fundus
   d. Cornua

40-42. Which of the following statements about the anatomy of the cervix is correct?

   a. The external os approximates the level at which the peritoneum reflects on the bladder.
   b. The posterior surface of the supravaginal segment is covered by peritoneum.
   c. The cervix is attached laterally to the cardinal ligaments.
   d. The portio vaginalis is synonymous with the internal os.

40–43. The appearance of the external cervical os can be sufficiently characteristic to allow an examiner to ascertain whether a woman has borne children by vaginal delivery.

a. True
b. False

40–44. Incompetent cervixes have a greater proportion of muscle fibers than normal cervixes.

a. True
b. False

40–45. Which of the following statements about the structure of the cervix is correct?

a. The cervix is composed mainly of smooth muscle cells.
b. A histologic section taken through the cervical canal resembles a section taken through the endometrium.
c. The endocervical mucosa consists of a single layer of ciliated columnar epithelial cells.
d. Occlusion of the ducts of cervical glands give rise to Nabothian cysts.

40–46. The peritoneum that forms the serosal layer of the uterus is not firmly adherent _____ .

40–47. Which of the following statements about the endometrium is correct?

a. In nonpregnant women, it varies in thickness from 0.5 to 5 mm.
b. The endometrium is attached to the underlying uterine submucosa.
c. The endometrial epithelium consists of a single layer of ciliated, columnar cells.
d. The endometrial glands secrete a thin, acidic fluid.

40–48. The blood supply of the uterus is derived from the

a. Uterine artery
b. Ovarian artery

40–49. Which of the following statements about the blood supply of the endometrium is correct?

a. The coiled arteries (arterioles) supply most of the midportion and the superficial third of the endometrium.
b. The basal arteries usually extend only into the basal layer of the endometrium.
c. The coiled arteries (arterioles) are responsive to hormone action.
d. The basal arteries are responsive to hormone action.

40–50. In pregnancy the myometrium increases mainly through hyperplasia.

a. True
b. False

40–51. Which of the following are portions of the broad ligament?

a. Mesosalpinx
b. Infundibulopelvic ligament
c. Cardinal ligament

Instructions for Items 40–52 to 40–55: Match the ligaments of the uterus with the appropriate statements.

a. Infundibulopelvic ligament
b. Cardinal ligament
c. Round ligament
d. Uterosacral ligament

40–52. Encloses the uterine vessels and the lower portion of the ureter
40–53. Encloses the ovarian vessels
40–54. Corresponds embryologically to the gubernaculum testis in the male
40–55. Forms the lateral boundaries of the pouch of Douglas

Instructions for Items 40–56 to 40–60: Refer to Figure 7. Match the letter with the appropriate structure.

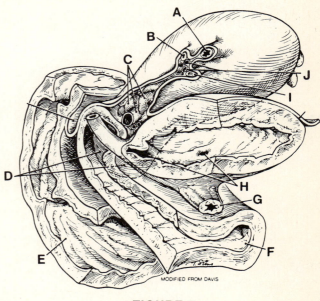

MODIFIED FROM DAVIS

FIGURE 7

40–56. Cervix
40–57. Round ligament
40–58. Ovarian artery and veins
40–59. Urethra
40–60. Utero-ovarian ligament

40-61. In a nonpregnant woman, which of the following statements about the position of the uterus is correct?

 a. The position of the body of the uterus varies with the degree of bladder or rectal distention.
 b. The uterus is free to move in the anteroposterior plane.
 c. Posture and gravity influence the position of the uterus.
 d. The position of the uterus in a woman who is standing and a woman who is supine is the same.

40-62. The uterine artery is a branch of the _____ .

40-63. Which structures are supplied by branches of the uterine artery?

 a. Vagina
 b. Cervix
 c. Body of uterus
 d. Oviduct

40-64. Which of the following statements regarding the position of the ureter in relation to the uterine artery is correct?

 a. About 2 cm lateral to the cervix, the uterine artery crosses under the ureter.
 b. About 3 cm lateral to the cervix, the uterine artery crosses under the ureter.
 c. About 2 cm lateral to the cervix, the uterine artery crosses over the ureter.
 d. About 3 cm lateral to the cervix, the uterine artery crosses over the ureter.

40-65. What is the clinical significance of the anatomical relationship between the uterine vessels and the ureter?

40-66. The ovarian artery

 a. Is a branch of the hypogastric artery
 b. Traverses the infundibulopelvic ligament
 c. Has branches that enter the ovarian hilum
 d. Anastamoses with the ovarian branch of the uterine artery

40-67. Which of the following statements about the venous drainage of the uterus is correct?

 a. The uterine vein empties into the hypogastric (internal iliac) vein.
 b. The pampiniform plexus in the broad ligament terminates in the ovarian vein.
 c. The right ovarian vein empties into the right renal vein.
 d. The left ovarian vein empties into the left renal vein.

Instructions for Items 40-68 and 40-69: Match the segment of the uterus with its lymphatic drainage.

 a. Hypogastric nodes
 b. Periaortic nodes

40-68. Cervix
40-69. Body of uterus

40-70. Which of the following statements regarding the innervation of the genital organs is correct?

 a. The nerve supply of the uterus is derived principally from the sympathetic nervous system.
 b. Sensory fibers from the uterus are carried through the 11th and 12th thoracic nerve roots.
 c. Sensory fibers from the cervix and upper portion of the birth canal pass through the second, third, and fourth sacral nerves.
 d. Sensory fibers from the lower portion of the birth canal pass through the pudendal nerve.

40-71. Which is the correct sequence of oviduct segments through which a sperm travels?

 a. Infundibulum, ampulla, isthmus, interstitium
 b. Interstitium, isthmus, ampulla, infundibulum
 c. Isthmus, interstitium, infundibulum, ampulla
 d. Ampulla, interstitium, infundibulum, isthmus

40-72. Which of the following statements about the structure of the oviducts is correct?

 a. The musculature of the tube is usually arranged in two layers.
 b. The tubal musculature undergoes rhythmic contractions that vary with the ovarian cycle.
 c. The tubal muscular contractions are strongest during pregnancy.
 d. The tubal mucosa undergoes cyclic histologic changes.
 e. Histologic cross-sections taken at various points along the oviduct appear similar.

40-73. Tubal cilia produce a current in the direction of the uterine cavity.

 a. True
 b. False

40-74. Innervation of the oviduct is principally from the _____ system.

 a. Sympathetic
 b. Parasympathetic

40-75. _____ in the wall of the oviduct may contribute to the development of ectopic pregnancy.

40-76. Which of the following statements about the embryologic development of the uterus and oviducts is correct?

  a. The uterus and oviducts arise from the müllerian ducts.
  b. The müllerian ducts initially appear in the coelomic epithelium at the level of the fourth thoracic segment.
  c. The two müllerian ducts approach each other in the midline in the sixth week and begin to fuse a week later.
  d. The uterine lumen is completed in the seventh week.
  e. The vaginal canal is not patent in its entire length until the sixth month.

40-77. Which of the following statements about the anatomy of the ovary is correct?

  a. A normal ovary in the childbearing years may be up to 5 cm long.
  b. The ovary normally lies in the ovarian fossa of Waldeyer.
  c. The ovary is attached to the broad ligament by the mesosalpinx.
  d. The ovary is attached to the uterus by the suspensory ligament of the ovary.
  e. The ovarian vessels are contained within the infundibulopelvic ligament.

Instructions for Items 40-78 to 40-83: Match the histologic finding with the appropriate portion of the ovary.

  a. Cortex
  b. Medulla

40-78. Ova
40-79. Connective tissue
40-80. Tunica albuginea
40-81. Germinal epithelium of Waldeyer
40-82. Arteries and veins
40-83. Smooth muscle fibers

40-84. The ovary is only supplied by sympathetic nerves.

  a. True
  b. False

40-85. When and where does the earliest sign of a developing gonad appear in the embryo?

40-86. The female primordial germ cells originate in the

  a. Mesenchyme of the developing ovary
  b. Yolk sac
  c. Genital ridge
  d. Germinal epithelium

40-87. Which of the following statements about the embryology of the testis is correct?

  a. The testis is recognizable in the seventh week by the presence of well-defined sex cords.
  b. Sex cords develop into seminiferous tubules and tubuli reti.
  c. The mesonephric ducts become the vas deferens.
  d. The rete establishes connection with the mesonephric tubules that develop into the epididymis.

40-88. In the developing ovary

  a. The proliferation of germinal epithelium continues longer than in the testis
  b. The medulla and cortex are not defined until the fifth month
  c. The medulla makes up the bulk of the organ
  d. There are distinct sex cords present from about the third month
  e. Synapsis is first visible in developing oogonia between the third and fourth months

40-89. By 8 months, the ovary is attached to the body wall along the line of hilum by the _____ .

40-90. In the young girl (before puberty), the primordial follicles nearest the central portion of the ovary are at the most advanced stages of development.

  a. True
  b. False

Instructions for Items 40-91 to 40-93: Match the embryologic remnant with its origin.

  a. Wolffian (mesonephric duct)
  b. Mesonephric tubules

40-91. Gartner duct
40-92. Paroophoron
40-93. Parovarium

41. REPRODUCTIVE SUCCESS AND FAILURE: OVULATION AND FERTILIZATION

41-1. In most species the limiting resource with respect to reproduction is the

  a. Female
  b. Male

41-2. Which of the following statements regarding human reproduction is true?

    a. Humans are the only primate in which puberty is delayed until the second decade of life.
    b. Humans are the only primate to undergo full breast development at adolescence rather than with the first pregnancy.
    c. Intercourse in other primates is a far more social function than in the human.
    d. The human female is more attractive to the male during her estrus.

Instructions for Items 41-3 to 41-5: Match the correct percentage with the condition it describes.

    a. Less than 20 percent
    b. Up to 25 percent
    c. Nearly 100 percent

41-3. Mortality rate of acquired immune deficiency syndrome (AIDS)
41-4. Relative infertility rate for couples in the United States
41-5. Success of the better in vitro fertilization programs

41-6. Breast feeding has never been shown to have a contraceptive value.

    a. True
    b. False

41-7. Few spermatozoa are capable of fertilization after _____ hours, and the life span of the ovum may be as short as _____ .
    (1)
    (2)

41-8. The maximum fecundability rate for human menstrual cycles is estimated to be about

    a. 90 percent
    b. 60 percent
    c. 30 percent
    d. less than 10 percent

41-9. Which of the following statements is true?

    a. About 95 percent of menstrual cycles are ovulatory.
    b. The maximum natural fecundability rate appears to be about 28 percent.
    c. Intercourse must occur within 3 days to ensure fertility.
    d. There is predisposing of ovulation for weekends in the United States thought to be secondary to stress-related factors.

41-10. Of early pregnancies what percentage will end in a term pregnancy if not voluntarily terminated?

41-11. What four factors are important in the maintenance of reproductive equilibrium?

41-12. Cyclic, predictable spontaneous menses is strong evidence for _____ , which in turn implies normal sex hormone production.

41-13. Which of the following migration pathways of germ cells in the fetus is correct?

    a. Epithelium of yolk sac, hindgut, gonadal ridge
    b. Epithelium of yolk sac, gonadal ridge, hindgut
    c. Gonadal ridge, epithelium of yolk sac, hindgut
    d. Hindgut, epithelium of yolk sac, gonadal ridge

41-14. The number of germ cells in the ovary increases by

    a. Mitosis
    b. Meiosis

41-15. Ooogonia are formed in the ovaries until puberty.

    a. True
    b. False

Instructions for Items 41-16 to 41-19: Match the number of germ cells in the ovary with the appropriate age.

    a. 400,000
    b. 600,000
    c. 2,000,000
    d. 6,800,000

41-16. 2 months' gestation
41-17. 5 months' gestation
41-18. Birth
41-19. 10 years of age

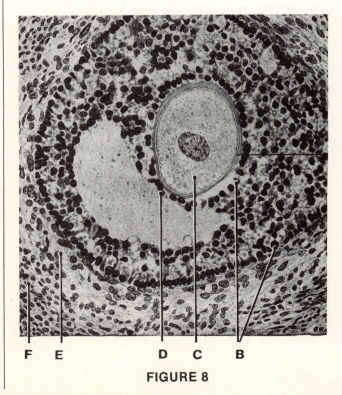

FIGURE 8

Instructions for Items 41–20 to 41–25: Refer to Figure 8. Match the letter with the appropriate part of the maturing graafian follicle.

41–20. Granulosa cell layer
41–21. Theca interna
41–22. Theca externa
41–23. Cumulus oophorus
41–24. Ovum
41–25. Zona pellucida

Instructions for Items 41–26 to 41–28: Match the cell type with the part of the graafian follicle that it forms.

    a. Ovarian stromal cell
    b. Follicular cell

41–26. Theca externa
41–27. Cumulus oophorus
41–28. Membrana granulosa/granulosa cell layer

41–29. Primary oocytes are arrested in which stage of the first meiotic division?

    a. Leptotene
    b. Zygotene
    c. Pachytene
    d. Diplotene
    e. Metaphase

41–30. Oocyte meiosis can be reinitiated by

    a. In vitro culture
    b. Gonadotropin stimulation
    c. Low oxygen levels
    d. Steroids

41–31. Which of the following is an action of FSH?

    a. It increases aromatization of C_{19}-steroids in granulosa cells.
    b. It primes cells to become competent to LH action.
    c. It stimulates the production of LH receptors.
    d. It stimulates the production of prolactin receptors.

41–32. The unique process by which either mature ova or spermatids are produced through reduction and division is called _____ .

41–33. The number of autosomes in mature gametes is

    a. 48
    b. 46
    c. 23
    d. 22
    e. 2
    f. 1

41–34. What is the number of chromosomes in a primitive germ cell (oogonium or spermatogonium)?

    a. 48
    b. 46
    c. 24
    d. 22
    e. 2
    f. 1

41–35. The basic difference between mitosis and meiosis is the prolonged prophase in mitosis, where pairing of homologous chromosomes occurs.

    a. True
    b. False

Instructions for Items 41–36 to 41–39: Match the stage of meiosis with the appropriate events.

    a. Leptotene
    b. Zygotene
    c. Pachytene
    d. Diplotene

41–36. Homologous chromosomes aligned in synapsis
41–37. Chromatids in tetrads, joined at the centromere
41–38. 46 chromosomes appear as single slender threads
41–39. Homologous strands separate

41–40. The acellular glycoprotein layer deposited by follicular cells around the primary oocyte is called the _____ .

41–41. Which of the following events occurs during the maturation phase of oogenesis?

    a. The germ cells divide mitotically.
    b. The cells enter prophase of the first meiotic division.
    c. A ring of granulosa cells surrounds the oogonium.
    d. Definitive oocytes are formed within the primary follicles.

41–42. Which of the following is the correct sequence of events in the development of the human ovum?

    a. Migration, division, maturation
    b. Migration, maturation, division
    c. Division, maturation, migration
    d. Maturation, division, migration
    e. Maturation, migration, division

41–43. As a result of the second meiotic division, each daughter cell contains _____ chromosomes?

    a. 46
    b. 44
    c. 23
    d. 22

41-44. In oogenesis, the haploid number of chromosomes first appears in the

   a. Primitive germ cell
   b. Primary oocyte
   c. Secondary oocyte
   d. Oogonium

41-45. If x is the amount of DNA in a mature oocyte, the amount of DNA present at the end of the first meiotic division is

   a. x
   b. $2x$
   c. $3x$
   d. $4x$

41-46. Oocyte maturation inhibitor, a substance in follicular fluid that inhibits oocyte maturation, is believed to be

   a. Cyclic AMP
   b. A cybernin
   c. LH
   d. FSH

41-47. Approximately what percent of sperm in the ejaculate reaches the site of ovum fertilization?

   a. 100 percent
   b. 10 percent
   c. 1 percent
   d. 0.1 percent
   e. 0.01 percent

41-48. The time from insemination to arrival of sperm at the site of fertilization is compatible with migration by flagellar action.

   a. True
   b. False

41-49. Which of the following statements about fertilization is correct?

   a. At the time of fertilization, the oocyte is usually in the ampulla of the fallopian tube.
   b. The oocyte must complete the second meiotic division before fertilization.
   c. The zona pellucida must disappear for fertilization to occur.
   d. Only one sperm can enter the ovum at the time of fertilization.

41-50. In women, _____ is the most exclusive source of cholesterol for progesterone biosynthesis.

   a. De novo synthesis
   b. High density lipoprotein (HDL)
   c. Low density lipoprotein (LDL)

41-51. At ovulation, the ovum is extruded along with the

   a. Zona pellucida
   b. Corona radiata
   c. Follicular fluid
   d. Theca interna

41-52. The time of ovulation is better determined from the date of onset of the next menstrual period than from the previous menses.

   a. True
   b. False

41-53. A woman's normal menstrual cycle is 22 days in length. If her menstrual bleeding began on March 30, when did she last ovulate?

   a. March 22
   b. March 19
   c. March 16
   d. March 13

41-54. The temperature elevation seen just before or during ovulation is primarily caused by

   a. Intraperitoneal irritation from the released ovum
   b. A thermogenic effect of FSH
   c. A thermogenic effect of progesterone
   d. A thermogenic effect of estrogen
   e. A sympathetic neural response to ovum release

41-55. Which of the following constitutes proof that ovulation has already occurred?

   a. Biphasic basal body temperature chart
   b. Maximal Spinnbarkeit
   c. Ferning of dried mucus
   d. Presence of a secretory endometrium
   e. Elevated levels of plasma progesterone

41-56. Which cells of the corpus luteum are physiologically active?

   a. K cells
   b. Theca interna cells
   c. Granulosa cells
   d. Fibroblasts in the central coagulum

41-57. Which of the following statements about corpus luteum regression is correct?

   a. Complete regression occurs prior to menstruation.
   b. Capillary proliferation continues throughout the menstrual cycle.
   c. There is a loss of lipid-staining material throughout the corpus luteum.
   d. Degenerative changes are postponed if pregnancy occurs.

41-58. A functional corpus luteum is required throughout pregnancy.

    a. True
    b. False

41-59. Surgical ablation of the corpus luteum of early pregnancy

    a. Predisposes the patient to spontaneous abortion
    b. Requires that the patient be treated with exogenous progestin
    c. Removes the sole endogenous source of progesterone
    d. Interferes with implantation of the embryo

41-60. If pregnancy does not occur, the corpus luteum is replaced by a connective tissue structure called the _____ .

41-61. During the process of follicular atresia, the

    a. Ovum undergoes cytolysis
    b. Membrana granulosa degenerates
    c. Theca lutein cells proliferate
    d. Granulosa lutein cells proliferate

41-62. Which of the following are causes of infertility in the human?

    a. Anovulation
    b. Obstruction of the fallopian tubes
    c. Male sterility
    d. Immunological phenomenon
    e. Inadequacy of the corpus luteum
    f. Genetic factors

42. FAMILY PLANNING

42-1. When a fertile couple does not use any contraceptive method, what percent of the women will conceive within 1 year?

    a. 20
    b. 40
    c. 60
    d. 80
    e. 98

42-2. RU 486 is an oral abortificant that may become available to be used once per month.

    a. True
    b. False

42-3. Which of the following statements about fertility in older women is correct?

    a. Women with regular menstrual cycles almost always ovulate normally.
    b. Extremely irregular or absent menstrual cycles usually mean the absence of ovulation.
    c. Pregnancy is rare over the age of 50.
    d. Documented hypergonadotropic, hypoestrogenic amenorrhea eliminates the possibility of pregnancy.

42-4. Supply the actual failure rates of the following common methods of contraception during the first year of their use.

METHOD	PERCENT
Combination birth control pills	___ (1)
Intrauterine devices	___ (2)
Condom	___ (3)
Spermicides	___ (4)
Diaphragm with spermicide	___ (5)
Rhythm	___ (6)

42-5. There is a strong negative correlation between the failure rate for a given method and both the age of the woman and the length of time she has been using the method.

    a. True
    b. False

42-6. Which of the following statements about estrogen–progestin contraceptives is correct?

    a. Ethinyl estradiol, or estrogens that metabolize to it, are used in most estrogen–progestin pills in the United States.
    b. Virtually all pills use norethindrone as the progestational agent.
    c. The main effect of estrogen–progestin pills is the suppression of hypothalamic-releasing factors.
    d. Oral estrogen–progestin contraceptives probably alter the receptiveness of the endometrium to implantation and also make cervical mucus less penetrable to sperm.
    e. Phasic pills offer the basic advantage of a lower total dose with the same efficacy and no more side effects or pregnancy than combination fixed dose pills.

42-7. Which of the following statements about the administration of estrogen–progestin oral contraceptives is correct?

   a. It is generally recommended that oral contraceptive use be initiated on the fifth day of the menstrual cycle.
   b. An additional method of birth control should be used during the first pill cycle by any woman who does not begin oral contraceptive use immediately after a normal menstrual cycle or within 3 weeks of delivery.
   c. Women should be encouraged to establish a regular routine for pill ingestion.
   d. If a woman misses one pill, she should use an additional method of birth control for the remainder of the cycle.
   e. An oral contraceptive should not be restarted immediately after withdrawal bleeding.

42-8. The amount of estrogen in oral contraceptives has been steadily reduced in recent years because of the rising cost of synthetic hormones.

   a. True
   b. False

42-9. Most estrogen–progestin oral contraceptives used in the United States contain _____ μg of either mestranol or ethinyl estradiol.

   a. 10 to 15
   b. 30 to 50
   c. 70 to 90
   d. 110 to 130

42-10. All estrogen–progestin oral contraceptives are formulated to deliver a constant daily dosage of progestin throughout the cycle.

   a. True
   b. False

42-11. When used correctly by appropriately selected patients, effects of estrogen–progestin oral contraceptives include a reduced incidence of

   a. Functional ovarian cysts
   b. Cervical cancer
   c. Endometrial cancer
   d. Ovarian cancer
   e. Rheumatoid arthritis
   f. Pelvic inflammatory disease

42-12. The major adverse reaction to the estrogen–progestin oral contraceptive may be the anxiety generated in the public and medical community by any reported side effects.

   a. True
   b. False

42-13. Which of the following statements about the metabolic effects of estrogen–progestin oral contraceptives is correct?

   a. Some of the metabolic changes are qualitatively similar to those seen in pregnancy.
   b. Plasma thyroxine, thyroid-binding globulin, and triiodothyronine uptake by resin are all elevated.
   c. Plasma cortisol and transcortin levels are lowered.
   d. Serum glucose levels are lowered.
   e. Lower doses of progestin may allow less metabolic changes with the use of triphasic pills.

42-14. Estrogen–progestin oral contraceptives should be withheld from women with a history of viral hepatitis.

   a. True
   b. False

42-15. Which of the following statements about complications from the use of estrogen–progestin oral contraceptives is correct?

   a. Contraceptive steroids may intensify existing diabetes.
   b. Cholestasis and cholestatic jaundice are relatively common complications that do not usually clear when oral contraceptive use is discontinued.
   c. Hepatic focal nodular hyperplasia and tumor formation have been linked to oral contraceptive use.
   d. Oral estrogen–progestin contraceptives may decrease the risk of developing endometrial and ovarian cancers.
   e. Oral estrogen–progestin contraceptives greatly increase a patient's risk for development of breast cancer.

42-16. Use of oral estrogen–progestin contraceptives results in _____ menstrual blood loss and _____ dysmenorrhea.
   (1)   (2)

   a. Increased
   b. Decreased

42-17. Which of the following statements about the cardiovascular effects of oral estrogen–progestin contraceptives is correct?

   a. The risk of deep vein thrombosis and pulmonary embolism may be increased.
   b. The risk of postoperative thromboembolic disease is unchanged.
   c. The risk of stroke in all women taking oral contraceptives is increased about fourfold.
   d. The risk of developing hypertension is increased, especially in older patients.
   e. The frequency and intensity of migraine headache is increased.
   f. The risk of myocardial infarction is increased.
   g. Even in young, healthy women, the risk of death as a consequence of oral contraceptive use is greater than the risk from pregnancy and delivery.

42-18. List the important contraindications to the use of estrogen–progestin oral contraceptives.

42-19. Most women resume regular ovulation within 3 months after discontinuing the use of oral estrogen–progestin contraceptives.

    a. True
    b. False

42-20. Estrogen–progestin oral contraceptives

    a. Are a common cause of cervical mucorrhea
    b. Are associated with *Candida* vulvovaginitis
    c. Can aggravate acne in some cases
    d. May result in the increased growth of uterine myomas
    e. Are a troublesome cause of weight gain in most women
    f. Are a relatively common cause of congenital malformations in the children of women who become pregnant soon after taking them

42-21. Breast feeding should not be combined with the use of estrogen–progestin oral contraceptives because of the large amounts of hormones excreted in the milk.

    a. True
    b. False

42-22. Why have oral progestin-only contraceptives not achieved widespread popularity in the United States?

42-23. Which of the following statements about injectable hormonal contraceptives is correct?

    a. The effectiveness of injected medroxyprogesterone acetate is comparable to that of combined oral contraceptives.
    b. Lactation is not likely to be impaired.
    c. Prolonged amenorrhea or uterine bleeding may occur with the use of LHRH analogues.
    d. There may be prolonged anovulation after their use is discontinued.
    e. Currently the use of progestational implants is being studied in the United States.

42-24. The "morning after pill" is composed of what compound?

42-25. The "ideal" intrauterine device would have what properties?

42-26. What are the two general types of intrauterine devices?

42-27. Which of the following meets the criteria of the "ideal" intrauterine device?

    a. Copper T
    b. Progestasert

42-28. Which type of intrauterine device (IUD) may be effective where use of another type of IUD has caused bleeding or cramping?

    a. Lippes Loop
    b. Copper T
    c. Cu7
    d. Progestasert

42-29. How does the chemically inert type of intrauterine device prevent pregnancy?

42-30. Copper-containing intrauterine devices work through a long-range, systemic action.

    a. True
    b. False

42-31. In general, the serious side effects of intrauterine devices have not been common while the common side effects have not been serious.

    a. True
    b. False

42-32. Which of the following statements about the side effects of intrauterine devices (IUDs) is correct?

    a. Most uterine perforations are due to migration of the IUD through the uterine wall over the period of several years.
    b. Bleeding and cramping are more likely with a larger device.
    c. Blood loss during menstruation may be twice normal when an IUD is in place.
    d. An increased incidence of pelvic infections is associated with the use of an IUD.
    e. Mortality due to the uses of an IUD is higher than either that due to pregnancy or to the use of oral contraceptives.

42-33. The use of an intrauterine device is usually discouraged in women

    a. Of no parity
    b. Of high parity
    c. At increased risk of developing infections of the pelvic viscera
    d. Who smoke

42-34. If actinomyces bodies are identified in Papanicolaou smears from an asymptomatic patient with an intrauterine device, it should be removed immediately and parenteral antibiotics should be administered.

    a. True
    b. False

42-68. What factors appear to increase morbidity in patients undergoing tubal sterilization?

a. Previous abdominal or pelvic surgery
b. Diabetes
c. General anesthesia
d. Obesity
e. History of previous pelvic infection

42-69. The "posttubal ligation syndrome," which includes pain, cyst formation, and abnormal bleeding, can be prevented by utilizing the Pomeroy procedure when performing a tubal sterilization.

a. True
b. False

42-70. The patient who is considering tubal sterilization should be informed that reversal of the procedure is possible and often successful.

a. True
b. False

42-71. Which of the following factors makes hysterectomy for the purpose of sterilization (in the absence of uterine and/or pelvic disease) difficult to justify?

a. Cost
b. Blood loss potentially leading to blood transfusion
c. Potential injury to the urinary tract
d. Risk of death

42-72. Which of the following is the most cost-effective method of female sterilization?

a. Hysterectomy
b. Tubal sterilization
c. Hysteroscopic tubal occlusion

42-73. Which of the following statements about vasectomy is correct?

a. The cost is approximately one-fifth that of tubal sterilization.
b. The failure rate is 1 in 100.
c. Sterility is immediate.
d. Restoration of fertility occurs in over 90 percent of all cases of surgical reversal.

42-74. What factors are important in the restoration of fertility after previous vasectomy?

42-75. Which of the following statements about male contraception is correct?

a. Storage of sperm prior to vasectomy has had excellent results.
b. Antibodies to sperm are rarely found after vasectomy in humans.
c. Vasectomy predisposes to atherosclerosis.
d. A safe and effective reversible male contraceptive is as yet to be developed.

Answers

1-1. b
p 1*
obstetrics, definition

1-2. c
p 2
fertility rate

1-3. a
p 2
birth rate

1-4. c
p 2
live birth

1-5. a
p 2
abortus

1-6. b
p 2
stillbirth

1-7. a, b, c
p 2
live birth criteria

1-8. the number of fetal deaths (stillbirths) plus neonatal deaths per 1,000 total births
p 2
perinatal mortality rate, definition

1-9. c
p 2
stillbirth rate; fetal death rate

1-10. d
p 2
postterm infant, definition

1-11. e
p 2
low-birthweight infant, definition

1-12. b
p 2
preterm infant, definition

1-13. c
p 2
term infant, definition

1-14. b
p 2
maternal death, indirect

1-15. d
p 2
maternal death rate, definition

1-16. deaths resulting from the use of contraceptive techniques plus deaths that are the consequence of pregnancy per 100,000 women
p 2
reproductive mortality, definition

1-17. a, c, d
pp 2–3
maternal mortality

1-18. a, c, d
p 3
maternal mortality

1-19. d
p 4
obstetric care, quality; perinatal mortality rate

1-20. a, c, d
p 4
neonatal death

1-21. a, b, c, d
p 5
birth certificate

2-1. a
p 7
contraception; reproductive function in women

---

*All page numbers refer to Cunningham FG, et al: *Williams Obstetrics*, 18th Edition.

2–2. a, b, c, d
p 7
estrogen; bone density; ovarian function

2–3. a, b, d
p 7
estradiol-17β; ovarian function

2–4. a, b
pp 7–8
progesterone; corpus luteum; endocrinology of menstruation

2–5. a, b
p 8
fallopian tube; uterotropins; decidua; estrogen and ovulation; reproductive function in women

2–6. a, b, c
pp 8–9
communication system; nidation; parturition; blastocyst; paracrine arm

2–7. c
pp 9–10
fetal–placental unit; dynamic role of the fetus in pregnancy

2–8. c
p 9
fertilization; fallopian tube

2–9. c, d
pp 10–11
fetus; fetal nutrition; placental transfer; fetal membranes; endocrinology of pregnancy

2–10. b
p 11
maternal recognition and fetal maintenance of pregnancy; corpus luteum; progesterone

2–11. d
pp 11–12
fetal–placental function; endocrinology of pregnancy

2–12. b
pp 11–12
oxytocin; myoepithelial cells; lactation and milk letdown

2–13. c
p 12
progesterone; lactation

2–14. a
p 12
estrogen; development of the breast

2–15. a, b
p 12
diagnosis of pregnancy

2–16. a, b, c, d
p 12
diagnosis of pregnancy

2–17. c, d, e
p 12
pregnancy, positive evidence; pregnancy, diagnosis; fetal movement; fetal heart tones

2–18. 120 to 160 beats per minute
p 18
fetal heart rate

2–19. c, d
pp 18–19
ultrasonography, real time; fetal heart activity; echocardiography

2–20. a, d, e, f
p 18
fetal heart sounds

2–21. b
pp 18–19
uterine souffle; auscultation of abdomen

2–22. a
pp 18–19
funic souffle; auscultation of abdomen

2–23. d
p 18
auscultation of abdomen; intestinal peristalsis, maternal

2–24. c
p 18
auscultation of abdomen; fetal movement

2–25. a
p 18
funic souffle; auscultation of abdomen

2–26. b
p 19
uterine souffle; auscultation of abdomen

2–27. a
pp 18–19
funic souffle; auscultation of abdomen

2–28. b
pp 18–19
uterine souffle; auscultation of abdomen; leiomyoma uteri

2–29. b, c, d, e
p 19
fetal movement

2–30. a, c, d
p 19
diagnosis of pregnancy; ultrasonography

2–31. a, b, c
p 19
blighted ovum; abortion, spontaneous; ultrasonography

2–32. a, b, c, d, e, f
pp 19–20
ultrasonography

2–33. a
pp 19–20
ultrasonography

2–34. 16
p 20
diagnosis of pregnancy; radiography; ossification, fetal bones

2–35. a, b
pp 13–14
pregnancy, nulliparous; pregnancy, multiparous

2–36. b
p 14
pregnancy, multiparous

2–37. b
p 14
pregnancy, multiparous

2–38. a, b
p 14
pregnancy, nulliparous; pregnancy, multiparous

2–39. a, c, f
p 14
pregnancy, probable evidence; uterus, pregnancy; cervix, pregnancy

2–40. e
p 14
pregnancy, probable evidence; Braxton Hicks contractions

2–41. ballottement
p 14
pregnancy, probable evidence; ballottement

2–42. diagnostic errors may arise from the presence of anatomic abnormalities (such as leiomyomata) or variations in the size of the normal uterus
p 14
pregnancy, probable evidence

2–43. b
pp 14–16
pregnancy tests

2–44. human chorionic gonadotropin (hCG)
pp 15–16
pregnancy tests; hCG

2–45. c, d
p 16
pregnancy tests; hCG; LH; radioimmunoassay

2–46. b
pp 15–16
hCG, levels

2–47. a
pp 17–18
pregnancy, diagnosis; pregnancy tests; hCG; ultrasonography

2–48. b
pp 15–18
pregnancy tests, ELISA, hCG

2–49. c
p 17
pregnancy tests, home kits; pregnancy, diagnosis

2–50. b
p 17
pregnancy tests, progesterone withdrawal; amenorrhea; pregnancy, diagnosis

2–51. a, c
pp 17–18
pregnancy tests; hCG; ectopic pregnancy

2–52. d
p 18
hCG, postabortion monitoring

2–53. a, b, c, d, e, f, g, i, j
p 18
pregnancy, presumptive evidence; pregnancy, diagnosis

2–54. c, e
p 13
pregnancy, presumptive evidence; amenorrhea

2–55. a, b, c, d
pp 13–14
pregnancy, presumptive evidence; breasts

2–56. a
pp 12–13
pregnancy, presumptive evidence; skin pigmentation; oral contraceptives, side effects

2–57. b, c, e
pp 12–13
pregnancy, presumptive evidence

2–58. b
p 20
pregnancy, differential diagnosis; hematometra

2–59. a, b, c, e, f
p 20
pseudocyesis, spurious pregnancy

2–60. a, b
p 20
pregnancy, multiparous; pregnancy, nulliparous; striae gravidarium

2–61. a
p 20
pregnancy, nulliparous; labia majora

2–62. b
p 20
pregnancy, multiparous

2–63. b
p 20
pregnancy, multiparous; myrtiform caruncles

2–64. a
p 20
pregnancy, nulliparous

2–65. b, d
pp 20–21
fetal death; ultrasonography, real time

2–66. a, e
pp 20–21
fetal death

3–1. a, b, c, d
p 24
endometrium; menstrual cycle; menstruation

3–2. c
pp 24–25
decidua

3–3. c
pp 24–25
decidua; parturition

3–4. a, b, c, d
p 25
estrogen, action; estradiol-17β; progesterone, receptors

3–5. a, b, c
p 25
progesterone action; estradiol-17β

3–6. b
pp 25–26
progesterone, receptors; breast, tumors

3–7. c
p 28
menstruation

3–8. a
pp 28, 30
menstrual cycle; ovarian cycle

3–9. b
pp 28, 30
ovarian cycle; follicular phase; endometrial cycle, follicular phase

3–10. a
p 27
ovarian cycle; follicular phase; endometrial cycle, follicular phase

3–11. c
p 27
ovarian cycle; endometrial cycle; luteal phase

3–12. a, c
p 27
menstrual cycle; ovarian cycle; follicular phase; proliferative phase

3–13. a
p 27
endometrial cycle, secretory phase

3–14. a
p 27
endometrial cycle, secretory phase

3–15. b
p 27
endometrial cycle, proliferative phase

3–16. c
pp 27–28
endometrial cycle, premenstrual phase

3–17. d
p 27
endometrium cyclical changes

3–18. a
p 27
endometrium, cyclical changes

3–19. c
p 27
endometrium, cyclical changes

3–20. e
pp 27–28
endometrium, cyclical changes

3–21. b
p 27
endometrium, cyclical changes

3–22. a, b
p 27
menstrual cycle; menstruation

3–23. a, b, c
pp 35–36
decidua

3–24. a, b, c, d
pp 28–30
prostaglandins

3–25. a, b, c
pp 31–34
menstrual cycle

3–26. b
 p 31
 ovulation; menstruation

3–27. a, c
 p 36
 cervical mucus; menstrual cycle

3–28. d
 p 36
 menstrual cycle; cervical mucus

3–29. a
 p 36
 cervical mucus; estrogen, actions

3–30. b
 p 36
 cervical mucus; progesterone, actions

3–31. a
 pp 36–37
 vagina, menstrual cycle

3–32. b
 pp 36–37
 vagina, menstrual cycle

3–33. a
 pp 36–37
 vagina, menstrual cycle

3–34. b
 pp 36–37
 vagina, menstrual cycle

3–35. b, c
 p 32
 menarche; puberty

3–36. c
 p 34
 menopause

3–37. b
 p 32
 puberty

3–38. a
 p 34
 menarche

3–39. d
 p 34
 climacteric

3–40. a, b, c
 pp 34–35
 menstrual cycle

3–41. b
 pp 34–35
 menstrual cycle; fertility

3–42. b, d
 pp 34–35
 menstrual cycle

3–43. b
 pp 34–35
 menstrual cycle

4–1. e, c, b, f, d, a
 p 40
 embryonic development

4–2. a, b, c, d
 pp 40–41
 embryonic development; implantation

4–3. a
 p 43
 inner cell mass; embryonic development

4–4. b, c
 p 40
 syncytiotrophoblast

4–5. g
 pp 45–48
 embryonic period

4–6. e
 pp 45–48
 embryonic period

4–7. c
 pp 45–48
 embryonic period

4–8. h
 pp 45–48
 embryonic period

4–9. i
 pp 45–48
 embryonic period

4–10. d
 pp 45–48
 embryonic period

4–11. a
 pp 45–48
 embryonic period

4–12. f
 pp 45–48
 embryonic period

6–56. d
p 102
hemoglobin, fetus; hemoglobin F

6–57. b
p 102
hemoglobin, fetus; hemoglobin A

6–58. a
p 102
hemoglobin, fetus; hemoglobin A₂

6–59. b
p 102
hemoglobin, fetus; hemoglobin A

6–60. at higher temperatures, the affinity of fetal blood for oxygen decreases
p 102
hypoxia, fetus; hemoglobin, fetus; oxygenation, fetal

6–61. a, b, c, d, f
p 101
hematopoiesis, fetus; erythropoietin

6–62. a
p 101
erythropoietin

6–63. b
p 102
coagulation factors, neonate

6–64. b
p 102
coagulation factors, neonate

6–65. b
p 102
coagulation factors, neonate

6–66. b
p 102
coagulation factors, neonate

6–67. b
p 102
coagulation factors, neonate

6–68. a
p 102
platelets; blood, fetus

6–69. a
p 102
coagulation factors, neonate; thrombin time, neonate

6–70. VIII
p 102
coagulation factors, fetus; hemophilia; Factor VIII

6–71. a, c
p 103
immunoglobulins, fetus

6–72. fetal infection has provoked a fetal immune response
p 103
immunoglobulins, fetus; infection, fetal

6–73. a, b, d
p 102
B lymphocytes; antibodies; immunology; complement

6–74. a, b, c, d
p 102
nervous system; sensory organs

6–75. a, b, c
pp 103–104
digestive system, fetus; fetal swallowing; amnionic fluid

6–76. a, b, c
pp 103–104
digestive system, fetus; meconium; biliverdin; hypoxia, fetal

6–77. a, b, e
p 104
liver, fetus; bilirubin, fetal

6–78. b, c, d
p 105
pancreas, fetus; insulin, fetus

6–79. b
p 105
pancreas, fetus; glucagon, fetus

6–80. a, c, e
p 105
urinary system, fetus; intrauterine growth retardation; urinary tract, anomalies

6–81. b
p 105
urinary system, fetus

6–82. a, b, c, d
pp 105–106
amnionic fluid

6–83. b
pp 105–106
amnionic fluid; hydramnios; postterm pregnancy; prolonged pregnancy

6–84. a, c, d
pp 105–106
amnionic fluid

6–85. urinary, gastrointestinal, respiratory
pp 105–106
amnionic fluid

6–86. b
pp 105–106
hydramnios; esophageal atresia

6–87. a
pp 105–106
oligohydramnios; renal agenesis

6–88. a
p 106
oligohydramnios; rupture of the membranes

6–89. a, b, c, d, e
p 106
respiratory system, fetus; surfactant

6–90. d
pp 106–108 (Fig. 6–19)
surfactant; phosphatidylcholine

6–91. phosphatidylglycerol
p 108
phosphatidylglycerol; surfactant; respiratory distress syndrome

6–92. 1 = lecithin; 2 = sphingomyelin
p 108
surfactant; L/S ratio; lung maturity, fetal

6–93. a, b, c, d
p 108
surfactant; phosphatidylglycerol

6–94. phosphatidate phosphohydrolase (PAPase)
p 108
surfactant

6–95. 1=; a; 2 = c
p 109
surfactant; lung maturation, fetus; phosphatidylglycerol; phosphatidyl-inositol

6–96. 1 = phosphatidylcholine and phosphatidylinositol; 2 = phosphatidylglycerol
p 110
respiratory distress syndrome; diabetes, maternal; surfactant; phosphatidylcholine; phosphatidylglycerol; phosphatidylinositol

6–97. b, d
pp 113–115
surfactant; corticosteriods, actions; prolactin, actions; respiratory distress syndrome

6–98. d
p 114
type II pneumocytes; surfactant; fetal lung maturity

6–99. a, b, c, e
p 116
respiratory system, fetus; fetal breathing

6–100. a, b, c, d, e
p 116
pituitary, fetus

6–101. b
pp 116–117
pituitary, fetus; growth hormone

6–102. a, c, d, f
pp 117–118
thyroid function, fetus

6–103. a
p 118
parathyroid, fetus

6–104. antidiuretic hormone
p 118
antidiuretic hormone, fetus; urine production, fetal

6–105. b
p 118
testosterone, fetus

6–106. b
p 118
sex ratios

6–107. b
pp 118–119
sex differentiation

6–108. a, b, c, d, e
pp 118–119
sexual differentiation

6–109. androgens
pp 118–119
sexual differentiation; ambiguous genitalia

6–110. a, c
pp 120–121
sex differentiation; female pseudohermaphroditism; dysgenetic gonads; true hermaphroditism

6–111. b
p 121
sex differentiation; male pseudohermaphroditism

6–112. a
pp 121–122
sex differentiation; female pseudohermaphroditism

6–113. a, c
pp 121–122
female pseudohermaphroditism; dysgenetic gonads; true hermaphroditism

6–114. b
p 121
sex differentiation; male pseudohermaphroditism

6–115. a
p 121
sex differentiation; female pseudohermaphroditism

6–116. c
p 121
sex differentiation; dysgenetic gonads; true hermaphroditism

6–117. adrenal gland
p 121
female pseudohermaphroditism; sex differentiation

6–118. capacity of trophoblast to convert aromatizable C_{19}–steroids to estrogens
p 121
female pseudohermaphroditism; virilization, fetal

6–119. a
p 121
sex differentiation; female pseudohermaphroditism

6–120. a,b
pp 121–122
sex differentiation

6–121. a, b, c, e
p 122
testicular feminization; sex differentiation

6–122. familial male pseudohermaphroditism; a spectrum of abnormalities affecting genital virilization
p 122
sex differentiation; male pseudohermaphroditism

6–123. c
pp 123–124
Turner syndrome; dysgenetic gonads; sex differentiation

6–124. a, b, d
pp 123–124
sex differentiation

6–125. b
p 124
genital ambiguity; sex differentiation

7–1. a
p 129
uterus, pregnancy; myometrial cell hypertrophy

7–2. a, b, d, e
p 129
uterus, pregnancy; uterus, blood supply; uterus, nerve supply

7–3. b
p 129
uterus, pregnancy; uterine enlargement, pregnancy; uterine hypertrophy; pregnancy, first trimester

7–4. b
p 129
polyamine levels, pregnancy; pregnancy, first trimester

7–5. c
pp 129–130
uterus, pregnancy; uterine enlargement, pregnancy

7–6. a
p 130
uterine enlargement pregnancy; placenta, implantation site

7–7. a, b, d
p 130
uterus, pregnancy

7–8. a, c, d, e
p 130
uterus, pregnancy; uterine contractions; Braxton Hicks contractions

7–9. c
p 131
uteroplacental blood flow; cardiovascular changes, pregnancy

7–10. a
p 131
uteroplacental blood flow; uterus, contractions

7–11. a, b, c, e
pp 131–132
uteroplacental blood flow; estrogen, actions; angiotensin II; fetal hypoxia

7–12. cyanosis and softening
pp 132–133
cervix, pregnancy

7–13. a, b
pp 133–134
cervix, pregnancy; cervical mucus; erosions of the cervix

7–14. b, c
p 134
ovary, pregnancy; corpus luteum, pregnancy

7–15. a, c
p 134
relaxin, pregnancy; corpus luteum, pregnancy

7–16. b, c, d
pp 134–135
luteoma, pregnancy; virilization, maternal; virilization, fetal

7–17. a
p 135
ovary, pregnancy; decidual reaction, ovary

7–18. c
p 135
oviduct, pregnancy

7–19. a, c, d
p 135
vagina, pregnancy

7–20. a, b, c, d
 p 135
 hyperreactio luteinalis; virilization

7–21. a, c, d
 pp 135–136
 vagina, pregnancy; vaginal secretions, pregnancy; vagina, pH; Lactobacillus; cervix, pregnancy; cervical secretions, pregnancy

7–22. b, c
 p 136
 striae gravidarum; cutaneous changes, pregnancy

7–23. diastasis recti
 p 136
 diastasis recii

7–24. a
 p 136
 linea nigra; cutaneous changes, pregnancy

7–25. b
 p 136
 chloasma; cutaneous changes, pregnancy

7–26. b
 p 136
 chloasma; oral contraceptives, side effects

7–27. a, b
 p 136
 vascular spiders; palmar erythema; cutaneous changes, pregnancy

7–28. a, b
 p 136
 vascular spiders; palmar erythema; hyperestrogenemia, pregnancy; cutaneous changes, pregnancy

7–29. a, b
 p 136
 vascular spiders; palmar erythema; cutaneous changes, pregnancy

7–30. a
 p 136
 vascular spiders; nevus; telangiectasis; cutaneous changes, pregnancy

7–31. a, b, c, d, e
 p 136
 breasts, pregnancy; colostrom; striae gravidarum

7–32. glands (follicles) of Montgomery
 p 136
 breasts, pregnancy; glands of Montgomery

7–33. 24 to 28 pounds
 p 137 (Table 7–1)
 pregnancy, weight gain

7–34. a, c, d
 p 137
 water metabolism, pregnancy; pregnancy, weight gain; puerperium, weight loss; puerperium, diuresis, vasopressin

7–35. b
 p 137
 protein metabolism, pregnancy

7–36. a
 p 137
 protein metabolism; nutrition

7–37. b
 p 138
 carbohydrate metabolism, pregnancy; lipid metabolism, pregnancy; fatty acid metabolism, pregnancy

7–38. a, b, c, d
 p 138
 carbohydrate metabolism, pregnancy; hPL; pancreas, pregnancy

7–39. a, b, d
 p 139 (Figs. 7–6 and 7–7)
 lipid metabolism, pregnancy; free fatty acids; cholesterol

7–40. a, d, e
 p 139
 lipid metabolism, pregnancy; breast feeding; progesterone, actions

7–41. a, b, c, d
 p 140
 acid–base equilibrium, pregnancy; 2,3–diphosphoglycerate; respiratory function, pregnancy

7–42. a
 p 140
 minerals, pregnancy; copper

7–43. b
 p 140
 sodium levels, pregnancy

7–44. b
 p 140
 minerals, pregnancy; magnesium

7–45. c
 p 140
 minerals, pregnancy; phosphorus

7–46. b
 p 141
 potassium levels, pregnancy

7–47. b, d
 p 141
 blood volume, pregnancy; hematologic changes, pregnancy

7–48. c
 p 141
 blood volume, pregnancy; hematologic changes, pregnancy; erythrocyte volume, pregnancy

7–49. 33
 p 141
 hematologic changes; pregnancy; erythrocytes, pregnancy

7–50. b, c, d
  p 141
  hematologic changes; pregnancy; erythrocytes, pregnancy

7–51. a, b, c
  p 141
  atrial natriuretic peptide

7–52. b
  pp 141–142
  iron requirements, pregnancy

7–53. a
  p 142
  iron requirements, pregnancy; hematologic changes, pregnancy; erythrocytes, pregnancy

7–54. b, d
  p 142
  iron requirements, pregnancy; iron absorption, pregnancy

7–55. c
  p 142
  blood loss, vaginal delivery

7–56. b
  p 142
  blood loss; vaginal delivery; blood loss, cesarean section; multifetal pregnancy, blood loss

7–57. a, b
  p 142
  blood volume, labor; blood volume, delivery; blood volume, puerperium; erythrocytes, pregnancy

7–58. c
  p 143
  leukocyte count, pregnancy; leukocyte count, labor; puerperium

7–59. a
  p 143
  interferon

7–60. a
  p 143
  blood coagulation, pregnancy

7–61. a (slightly)
  p 143
  blood coagulation, pregnancy

7–62. a
  p 143
  blood coagulation, pregnancy

7–63. a
  p 143
  blood coagulation, pregnancy

7–64. a
  p 143
  blood coagulation, pregnancy

7–65. a
  p 143
  blood coagulation, pregnancy

7–66. b
  p 143
  blood coagulation, pregnancy

7–67. b
  p 143
  blood coagulation, pregnancy

7–68. a
  p 143
  sedimentation rate, pregnancy

7–69. b
  p 143
  blood coagulation, pregnancy; Quick one-stage prothrombin time

7–70. b
  p 143
  blood coagulation, pregnancy; partial thromboplastin time

7–71. c
  p 143
  blood coagulation, pregnancy; clot retraction test

7–72. a, b
  p 143
  blood coagulation, pregnancy; platelets, pregnancy; fibrinogen

7–73. a, b, d, e
  p 143
  blood coagulation, pregnancy; fibrinolysis, pregnancy; fibrin degradation products

7–74. a, b, c, d
  p 144
  cardiovascular system, pregnancy; heart displacement, pregnancy

7–75. b
  p 144
  cardiovascular system, pregnancy; cardiomegaly

7–76. a
  p 144
  cardiovascular system, pregnancy; cardiac volume

7–77. a
  p 144
  cardiovascular system, pregnancy; ventricular wall mass

7–78. a
  p 144
  cardiovascular system, pregnancy; stroke volume

7–79. c
  p 144
  cardiovasculalr system, pregnancy; inotropic state of the myocardium

7–80. a
  p 144
  cardiovascular system, pregnancy; heart rate, pregnancy

7–81. a, c, d, e, f
  p 144
  cardiovascular system, pregnancy; heart sounds; heart murmurs

7–82. a, d
  p 144
  cardiovascular system, pregnancy; angiotensin; fetal acidosis; calcium channel blockers; electrocardiogram changes, pregnancy

7–83. a, c, d
  p 144
  cardiovascular system, pregnancy; cardiac output; labor, cardiovascular function

7–84. c
  p 144
  circulation, pregnancy; blood pressure, pregnancy

7–85. a
  p 144
  blood pressure, pregnancy

7–86. c, d
  pp 144–145
  venous pressure, pregnancy; supine hypotension, pregnancy; blood flow; pregnancy

7–87. b, c, d
  p 145
  venous pressure, pregnancy; hemorrhoids; varicose veins; edema; pregnancy; circulation, pregnancy

7–88. a, b, c, d
  p 145
  circulatory system, pregnancy; supine position, pregnancy; supine hypotension, pregnancy; cardiac output, pregnancy

7–89. b
  p 145
  circulatory system, pregnancy; blood pressure, pregnancy; uteroplacental function

7–90. b, c
  p 145
  circulatory system, pregnancy; supine position, pregnancy; blood pressure; cardiac output, pregnancy; blood flow, pregnancy

7–91. a
  p 147
  circulatory system, pregnancy; cutaneous changes, pregnancy; blood flow, pregnancy

7–92. a, b, c
  p 147
  respiratory function, pregnancy; musculoskeletal system, pregnancy

7–93. b
  p 147
  respiratory tract pregnancy; pulmonary function, pregnancy; maternal arteriovenous oxygen difference

7–94. c
  p 147 (Table 7–3)
  respiratory system, pregnancy; pulmonary function, pregnancy; maximum breathing capacity

7–95. b
  p 147
  respiratory system, pregnancy; pulmonary function, pregnancy; functional residual capacity

7–96. c
  p 147
  respiratory system, pregnancy; pulmonary function, pregnancy; lung compliance

7–97. a
  p 147
  respiratory system, pregnancy; pulmonary function, pregnancy; airway conductance

7–98. a
  p 147
  respiratory system, pregnancy; pulmonary function, pregnancy; tidal volume

7–99. b
  p 147
  respiratory system, pregnancy; pulmonary function, pregnancy; total pulmonary resistance

7–100. the effects of progesterone and to a lesser extent estrogen on the respiratory center
  p 147
  respiratory system, pregnancy; progesterone, actions; estrogen, actions

7–101. a, c, d
  p 147
  urinary system, pregnancy; vitamins, pregnancy; renal function, pregnancy

7–102. c
  pp 148–149
  renal function tests, pregnancy; creatinine clearance

7–103. water accumulated during the day as dependent edema is mobilized and excreted at night (therefore, concentrated urine may not be excreted even after withholding fluids for 18 hours)
  p 149
  renal function tests, pregnancy

7–104. a, b
  p 149
  urinary system, pregnancy; glucosuria, pregnancy

7–105. b
p 149
urinary system, pregnancy; proteinuria, pregnancy; preeclampsia

7–106. a, b, c, d
pp 149–150
urinary system, pregnancy; progesterone, actions; ureters, pregnancy

7–107. b, c
pp 149–150
urinary system, pregnancy; bladder, pregnancy; urinary tract infection, pregnancy

7–108. a, b, c
pp 150–151
gastrointestinal system, pregnancy; gastric-emptying time

7–109. upward and laterally
p 151
gastrointestinal system, pregnancy; appendix, pregnancy

7–110. b
p 151
liver, pregnancy

7–111. a
p 151
liver, pregnancy; alkaline phosphatase activity, serum

7–112. b
p 151
liver, pregnancy; allbumin concentration, plasma

7–113. b
p 151
liver, pregnancy; cholinesterase activity, plasma

7–114. a
p 151
liver, pregnancy; leucine aminopeptidase activity, serum

7–115. a, c, d, e
p 152
gastrointestinal system, pregnancy; gallbladder, pregnancy; hemorrhoids, pregnancy

7–116. b
p 152
pituitary gland, pregnancy

7–117. a, c, d
pp 152–153
pituitary gland, pregnancy; prolactin; microadenomas, pituitary; growth hormone

7–118. b
pp 152–153
pituitary gland, pregnancy; prolactin

7–119. a, b, d
pp 152–153
pituitary gland, pregnancy; β-endorphins

7–120. a, d
p 153
thyroid gland, pregnancy; goiter, maternal; hydatidiform mole; hCG, actions

7–121. a = increased; b = not increased; c = increased; d = increased; e = increased; f = increased; g = increased; h = increased; i = not increased; j = not increased; k = not increased; l = increased; m = not increased; n = not increased; o = increased
p 154 (Table 7–4)
thyroid gland, pregnancy

7–122. 1 = a; 2 = c
pp 153–154
thyroid gland, pregnancy

7–123. c, d
pp 154–155
parathyroid gland, pregnancy; calcitonin; vitamin D

7–124. c, d, e
p 154
adrenal gland, pregnancy; aldosterone, pregnancy; renin; angiotensin

7–125. a, b, c
p 157
musculoskeletal system, pregnancy; lordosis, maternal

7–126. b
p 157
musculoskeletal system, pregnancy

7–127. b
p 157
precocious puberty; menarche

7–128. a
p 157
pregnancy, complications; maternal age, effect on pregnancy

8–1. accommodation
p 163
labor; pelvis; accommodation

8–2. linea terminalis
p 163
pelvis, anatomy; linea terminalis

8–3. c
p 163
pelvis, anatomy; false pelvis

8–4. b
p 163
pelvis, anatomy; false pelvis

8–5. a
p 163
pelvis, anatomy; false pelvis

8-6. d
p 163
pelvis, anatomy; false pelvis

8-7. a = pubic bones, the ascending superior rami of the ischial bones; b = anterior surface of sacrum; c = inner surface of the ischial bones, sacrosciatic notches, and sacrosciatic ligaments; d = promontory and alae of sacrum, linea terminalis, and the upper margins of the pubic bones; e = pelvic outlet
pp 163–164
pelvis, anatomy; true pelvis

8-8. a, c, e, f, g
p 163
pelvis, anatomy; true pelvis

8-9. a, b
p 163
pelvis, anatomy; sacrum; clinical pelvimetry

8-10. b
p 164
clinical pelvimetry; pelvic inlet; obstetric conjugate

8-11. b
p 164
clinical pelvimetry; obstetric conjugate

8-12. subtract 1.5 to 2.0 cm from the measured length of the diagonal conjugate (which is the distance from the lower margin of the symphysis to the promontory of the sacrum)
p 166
clinical pelvimetry; obstetric conjugate

8-13. b
pp 168–169
pelvis, anatomy; clinical pelvimetry

8-14. a = horizontal rami of the pubic bones and symphysis pubis; b = pubic arch; c = linea terminalis; d = sacrosciatic ligaments and the ischial tuberosites; e = promontory and alae of the sacrum; f = tip of sacrum; g = obstetric conjugate; h = lower margin of the symphysis pubis to the top of the sacrum; i = greatest distance between the linea terminalis; j = from the tip of the sacrum to a right angled intersection with a line between the ischial tuberosities
p 169
pelvis, anatomy; planes of the pelvis

8-15. d
p 169 (Fig. 8–13)
pelvis, anatomy; midpelvis

8-16. b
p 169 (Fig. 8–13)
obstetric conjugate; pelvis, anatomy

8-17. a
p 169 (Fig. 8–13)
true conjugate; pelvis, anatomy

8-18. c
p 169 (Fig. 8–13)
diagonal conjugate; pelvis, anatomy

8-19. d
p 169
midpelvis; pelvis, anatomy

8-20. a, e
p 169
pelvis, anatomy

8-21. e
pp 163–164
pelvis, anatomy; pelvic joints

8-22. a
p 170
x-ray pelvimetry

8-23. b, c
pp 170, 172–174
x-ray pelvimetry

8-24. a, b
pp 167–169
pelvic types; Caldwell-Moloy classification

8-25. a
p 167 (Fig. 8–10)
pelvic shape; gynecoid pelvis

8-26. d
p 167–168 (Fig. 8–10)
pelvic shape; platypelloid pelvis

8-27. b
p 167 (Fig. 8–10)
pelvic shape; android pelvis

8-28. c
p 167 (Fig. 8–10)
pelvic shape; anthropoid pelvis

8-29. c
p 167
pelvic shape, frequency; anthropoid pelvis

8-30. a
pp 166–167
pelvic shape, frequency; gynecoid pelvis

8-31. b
p 167
pelvic shape, frequency; android pelvis

8–32. d
  p 167
  pelvic shape, frequency; platypelloid pelvis

8–33. a, c
  p 167
  pelvic shape, frequency; gynecoid pelvis; anthropoid pelvis

8–34. b
  pp 166–167
  pelvic shape; Caldwell-Moloy classification

8–35. b
  p 167
  pelvic shape; android pelvis

8–36. b, c, d
  p 168
  pelvis, anatomy; pelvic size

8–37. a
  p 168
  pelvis, anatomy; diagonal conjugate; clinical pelvimetry

8–38. descent of the biparietal plane of the fetal head to a level below that of the pelvic inlet
  p 169
  engagement

8–39. a, b, c
  p 169
  engagement

8–40. b
  p 169
  engagement

8–41. a, c, d
  p 169
  engagement

8–42. a, b, c
  p 170
  pelvis, anatomy; pelvic outlet

8–43. c
  p 170
  pelvis, anatomy; pelvic outlet

8–44. d
  p 170
  midpelvis; pelvimetry, x-ray; clinical pelvimetry

8–45. a
  pp 170–171
  pelvimetry, x-ray

8–46. a, d, e
  pp 170–171
  pelvis, anatomy; pelvimetry, x-ray

8–47. a, b
  p 171
  pelvimetry, x-ray

9–1. habitus/attitude
  p 177
  fetus, attitude; habitus

9–2. a, c, d, e
  p 177
  fetus, attitude

9–3. b
  p 177
  fetus, posture; accommodation

9–4. relation of the long axis of the fetus to that of the mother
  p 177
  fetus, lie

9–5. b
  p 177
  fetus, lie; oblique lie

9–6. c
  p 177
  fetus, lie

9–7. a, b
  p 177
  fetus, presentation; fetus, lie; longitudinal lie

9–8. A
  p 177
  cephalic presentation, vertex; fetus, presentation

9–9. d
  p 177
  cephalic presentation, face; fetus, presentation

9–10. b
  p 177
  cephalic presentation, sinciput; fetus, presentation

9–11. c
  p 177
  cephalic presentation, brow; fetus, presentation

9–12. b
  p 177
  cephalic presentation, vertex; fetus, presentation

9–13. a
  p 177
  cephalic presentation, face; fetus, presentation

9–14. c
  p 177
  cephalic presentation, brow; fetus, presentation

9–15. d
p 177
cephalic presentation, sinciput; fetus, presentation

9–16. a
p 177
cephalic presentation, sinciput; cephalic presentation, brow; fetus, presentation

9–17. b
p 177
breech presentation, complete; fetus, presentation

9–18. a
p 177
breech presentation, frank; fetus presentation

9–19. c
p 177
breech presentation, incomplete; breech presentation, footling; fetus, presentation

9–20. the right or left side of the maternal birth canal
p 177
fetus, position

9–21. a = 96 percent; b = 3.5 percent; c = 0.3 percent; d = 0.4 percent
p 178
fetus, vertex presentation

9–22. c
p 178
breech presentation; prematurity, presentation

9–23. a, c, d, e
pp 179–180
fetus, presentation; hydrocephalus

9–24. a, b, c, d, e
pp 180–181
fetus presentation, diagnostic methods; fetus position, diagnostic methods; ultrasonography; x-ray

9–25. c
pp 180–181
Leopold maneuvers; fetus presentation, diagnostic methods; fetus position, diagnostic methods

9–26. b
pp 180–181
fetus presentation, diagnostic methods; fetus position, diagnostic methods

9–27. a
pp 180–181
Leopold maneuvers; fetus presentation, diagnostic methods; fetus position, diagnostic methods

9–28. d
p 181
Leopold maneuvers; fetus presentation, diagnostic methods; fetus position, diagnostic methods

9–29. a, b, c, d
p 181
Leopold maneuvers; fetus presentation, diagnostic methods; fetus position, diagnostic methods

9–30. sagittal
pp 181–183
presentation; position; sagittal suture

9–31. b, c
p 184
presentation; position; auscultation

9–32. b
p 185
ultrasonography; x-ray; fetus presentation, diagnostic methods; fetus position, diagnostic methods

10–1. a, b, c
p 187
parturition

10–2. b, c, d
p 187
parturition

10–3. b
p 187
uterotonin

10–4. a
p 187
uterotropin

10–5. b
p 187
uterotonin; prostaglandins; oxytocin

10–6. a
p 187
uterotropin; cervix

10–7. a
p 187
uterotropin; myometrium; oxytocin receptors

10–8. c
p 189
parturition

10–9. a, c
p 189
progesterone; mechanisms of labor

10–10. a, b, d
pp 189, 192
progesterone; corpus luteum; parturition

10–11. b, c, d, e
pp 195–196
oxytocin, pregnancy; labor, third stage; blood loss, postpartum; lactation

10–12. a, b, d
p 190
prostaglandins; parturition

10–13. a, b, d, e
p 190
cortisol, labor; labor, initiation

10–14. a, b, c, d
p 197
prostaglandins, labor; labor, induction

10–15. a, b, c
pp 197–199, 200–202
decidua; interleukin; prostaglandin synthesis

10–16. a, b, c
pp 207–210
preterm labor

10–17. a, b
pp 198–201
organ communication system; fetal membranes; prostaglandins

10–18. a
p 210
uterus, contractions; uterus, smooth muscle; calcium

10–19. b
p 210
uterus, contractions; uterus, smooth muscle; calcium

10–20. it functions to facilitate and integrate transmission of forces generated by the contraction of myometrial cells
p 210
myometrium, extracellular matrix; uterus, contractions; labor

10–21. facilitate intercellular communication by the passage of current (electrical or ionic coupling) or metabolites (metabolic coupling) between cells
p 210
gap junctions; uterus, contractions

10–22. b, e, g
pp 210–211
gap junctions; uterus, contractions; progesterone, actions; estrogen, actions

10–23. a, b, c, e
p 211
smooth muscle contraction; calcium, muscle contraction; myosin

10–24. calmodulin
p 212
cervix, ripening; calmodulin

10–25. a, c, e
p 212
cervix, ripening; collagen, cervix; glycosamoglycans

10–26. a, b
p 212
cervix, ripening; prostaglandins, actions

10–27. a
pp 212–213
prostaglandins, synthesis; estrogen, actions

10–28. a = uterine contractions reach sufficient frequency, intensity, and duration to bring about readily demonstrable effacement and dilation of the cervix; b = the cervix is sufficiently dilated to allow passage of the fetal head; c = dilation of the cervix is complete; d = the fetus is expelled; e = delivery of the infant; f = delivery of the placenta and fetal membranes
p 213
labor, stages

10–29. b
p 213
labor, latent phase

10–30. a
p 213
prelabor

10–31. fourth stage of labor
p 213
labor, fourth stage

10–32. a
p 213
cervix, ripening; labor, prelabor

10–33. a, b, c, d
p 307
lightening, labor; lower uterine segment; fundal height

10–34. b
p 213
labor, false

10–35. a
p 213
labor, true

10–36. b, c
p 213
labor, false

10–37. ''show'' or ''bloody show''
p 213
cervix, mucus; bloody show

10–38. a, b, d
p 214
uterus, contractions; labor; paraplegia; epidural block; pain, labor

10–39. Ferguson reflex
p 214
Ferguson reflex; labor

10–40. a, b, c, d
p 214
labor; uterus, contractions; Ferguson reflex

10–41. a
p 214
labor; uterus, contractions; fetal distress; fetal hypoxia

10–42. 1 = b; 2 = a
pp 214–215
upper uterine segment; lower uterine segment; labor

10–43. b
pp 214–215
lower uterine segment

10–44. a
pp 214–215
upper uterine segment

10–45. a
pp 214–215
upper uterine segment

10–46. b
pp 214–215
lower uterine segment

10–47. a
pp 214–215
upper uterine segment

10–48. b
pp 214–215
lower uterine segment

10–49. a
pp 215–216 (Fig. 10–15)
upper uterine segment; uterus, corpus

10–50. b
p 216 (Fig. 10–15)
lower uterine segment; uterus, isthmus

10–51. pathologic retraction ring (the ring of Bandl)
p 216
pathologic retraction ring; labor, obstructed; Bandl's ring

10–52. a
p 216
labor; upper uterine segment; lower uterine segment; labor, contractions

10–53. 1 = b; 2 = a
p 216
labor; uterus, contractions; uterus, shape

10–54. b, c
p 217
labor stages; "pushing"

10–55. b
p 217
labor

10–56. cervical effacement
p 217
labor; cervix; effacement; lower uterine segment

10–57. a, d
pp 217–218
cervix, dilation; labor

10–58. cervical dilation and fetal descent
pp 218–219
labor; Friedman's curve; fetal descent; cervical dilation

10–59. a
p 219
labor, latent phase

10–60. b
p 219
labor, active phase

10–61. a
p 220
labor, latent phase

10–62. b
p 220
labor, active phase

10–63. 1 = b; 2 = c; 3 = a
p 220
labor, acceleration phase; labor, maximum slope; labor, deceleration phase; cervix, dilation; Friedman's curve

10–64. b
p 219
labor; engagement

10–65. a
p 217
labor, preparatory phase; cervix, ripening

10–66. b
p 218
labor, dilational phase; cervix, dilation

10–67. a
p 217
labor, preparatory phase

10–68. c
pp 219, 220–221
labor, pelvic phase

10–69. c
p 221
labor, pelvic phase; labor, cardinal movements

10–70. caul
p 220
fetal membranes; caul

10–71. f, e, a, d, h, g, b, c
p 221
pelvic floor, anatomy

10–72. b, c, e
p 221
pelvic floor, anatomy

10–73. a, b, e, f
pp 221–222
urogenital diaphragm; perineum, anatomy

10–74. stretching of fibers of the levator ani muscles and the thinning of the central portion of the perineum
pp 221–223
perineum, anatomy; labor

10–75. a disproportion between the relatively unchanged size of the placenta and the reduced size of the uterus
p 223
labor, third stage

10–76. c, d
p 223
labor, third stage

10–77. a
p 224
placenta, extrusion; mechanism of Schultze

10–78. b
p 224
placenta, extrusion; mechanism of Duncan

10–79. a
p 224
placenta, extrusion; mechanism of Schultze

10–80. a
p 225
placenta, extrusion; mechanism of Schultze

11–1. 95
p 227
occiput (vertex) presentation

11–2. a, c, d
p 227
occiput (vertex) presentation; labor

11–3. a
p 227
occiput (vertex) presentation; labor

11–4. b, c, d
p 227
occiput posterior presentation; labor

11–5. e, d, c, b, a, f, g
pp 227–228
labor, cardinal movements

11–6. a, d, e, f
pp 227–228
labor, cardinal movements

11–7. b
pp 227–228
labor, engagement; labor, cardinal movements

11–8. asynclitism
p 229
asynclitism; labor; sagittal suture

11–9. a
p 229
asynclitism; labor; sagittal suture

11–10. a
p 229
asynclitism; labor

11–11. a, b, c, d
p 229
labor, cardinal movements

11–12. occipitofrontal
p 229
labor, flexion; labor, cardinal movements; accommodation

11–13. ischial spines
pp 229–230
labor, internal rotation; labor, cardinal movements; engagement

11–14. a, b, c, d
p 230
labor, extension; labor, external rotation; labor, cardinal movements

11–15. a
p 232
persistent occiput posterior presentation; labor, transverse arrest

11–16. a, b, c, d
pp 232–233
caput succedaneum; fetal head, molding

12–1. b
p 235
respiration, newborn; respiration, fetal; fetal breathing movements

12–2. a, c, d, e
p 235
respiration, newborn; transcient tachypnea of the newborn

12–3. fifth
  p 235
  respiration, newborn

12–4. a
  p 235
  ductus arteriosus; circulation, fetal

12–5. respiratory distress syndrome (hyaline membrane disease)
  p 235
  respiratory distress syndrome; surfactant; hyaline membrane disease

12–6. a, b, c, d
  pp 235–236
  respiration, newborn

12–7. a
  p 236
  respiration, newborn; cesarean section

12–8. a, b, c
  p 236
  neonate, immediate care; umbilical cord, management

12–9. a, b, c, d, e, f, g
  p 236
  neonate, immediate care; fetal well-being

12–10. auscultation over the chest; palpation of the base of the umbilical cord
  p 237
  neonate, heart rate; newborn, initial evaluation

12–11. c
  p 237
  neonate, heart rate

12–12. a
  p 237
  neonate, heart rate; neonate, respiration; neonate, resuscitation; suctioning, newborn nasopharynx

12–13. c, d
  pp 236–237
  neonate, respiration; neonate, resuscitation

12–14. a, b, c, d, e, f, g, h
  p 237
  respiration, initiation

12–15. heart rate; respiratory effort; muscle tone; reflex irritability; color
  p 237
  Apgar score; fetal well-being

12–16. a
  p 237
  Apgar score; perinatal asphyxia; neonatal resuscitation

12–17. 7
  p 237
  Apgar score

12–18. 4–7
  p 237
  Apgar score

12–19. failure to check equipment; use of a cold resuscitation table; unsuccessful intubation; inadequate ventilation; failure to manage bradycardia or poor chest movement; failure to manage hypovolemia; failure to perform cardiac massage
  p 241
  resuscitation, neonate

12–20. skilled personnel immediately available; large, well-heated and lighted work area; equipment to deliver oxygen, positive pressure and suction; drugs and appropriate accompanying equipment
  p 239
  resuscitation, neonate

12–21. b
  p 239
  resuscitation, neonate

12–22. a, d
  p 238
  hypoxia; acidemia; umbilical blood sampling

12–23. a, c, d
  p 240
  resuscitation, neonate; endotracheal intubation

12–24. intermittent positive pressure ventilation with oxygen delivered from a bag; resuscitator puffing oxygen-rich air into the endotracheal tube
  p 240
  resuscitation, neonate; endotracheal intubation

12–25. a
  p 240
  endotracheal intubation, complications; pneumothorax

12–26. b
  p 240
  endotracheal intubation, complications

12–27. a
  p 240
  endotracheal intubation, complications; pneumomediastinum

12–28. a, b, c, d, e
  p 240
  resuscitation, neonate; acidosis; sodium bicarbonate

12–29. naloxone (Narcane)
  p 240
  resuscitation, neonate; respiratory depression; naloxone (Narcan); narcotics, respiratory depression

12–30. a, b, c, d, e
  p 240
  resuscitation, neonate; hypovolemia, newborn; sepsis, neonatal; twin-to-twin transfusion; hemorrhage; fetal to maternal

12–31. a
  pp 240–241
  cardiac massage; resuscitation, neonate

12–32. a, b, e
  pp 240–241
  cardiac massage; resuscitation, neonate

12–33. b
  p 241
  resuscitation, neonate; epinephrine; intracardiac injection

12–34. a
  p 241
  gestational age, determination

12–35. c, d
  p 241
  gonorrheal ophthalmia; silver nitrate; penicillin; tetracycline

12–36. a, d
  p 242
  newborn, identification

12–37. a, b
  p 242
  newborn, temperature

12–38. a
  p 242
  vitamin K administration; coagulation defects

12–39. a, b, d, e
  p 242
  umbilical cord, management

12–40. a
  p 242
  skin care, neonate; vernix caseosa

12–41. a, b, c, d
  pp 242–243
  meconium

12–42. a, c
  pp 242–243
  stool production, neonate

12–43. a, d, e
  p 243
  hyperbilirubinemia; icterus neonatorum; physiologic jaundice of the newborn

12–44. a, b, c, d
  p 243
  physiologic jaundice of the newborn; prematurity, effects; bilirubin; hemolysis, newborn

12–45. a, b, c, d
  p 243
  weight loss, newborn

12–46. a, c, d
  p 243
  weight loss, newborn; weight gain, infant; prematurity, effects

12–47. a, d
  p 243
  feeding, newborn; breast feeding

12–48. b
  p 243
  circumcision

12–49. a, b, d
  p 243
  circumcision, contraindications

13–1. b
  p 245
  puerperium, definition

13–2. a
  p 245
  uterus, involution; puerperium

13–3. f
  p 245
  uterus, involution; puerperium

13–4. h
  p 245
  uterus, involution; puerperium

13–5. a
  p 245
  uterus, involution; puerperium

13–6. e
  p 245
  uterus, involution; puerperium

13–7. f
  p 245
  uterus, involution; puerperium

13–8. c, d
  p 245
  uterus, involution; puerperium

13–9. 1 = b; 2 = c
  p 245
  myometrium, involution

13–10. c
  p 245
  endometrium, postpartum regeneration

13–11. late puerperal hemorrhage
p 245
placental site, involution; hemorrhage, postpartum

13–12. a, b
p 245
placental site, involution

13–13. a
p 245
puerperium; regeneration of endometrium

13–14. b
p 246
cervix, puerperium; lower uterine segment, puerperium; vagina, puerperium; hymen, puerperium

13–15. a, d
p 247
abdominal wall, puerperium; striae gravidarum; diastasis recti

13–16. a, b
p 247
urinary system, puerperium; bladder, pregnancy

13–17. a, b, e
p 247
breast development; lactation

13–18. a, d
p 248
colostrum; lactation

13–19. b, d
p 248
colostrum; breast feeding, immunology

13–20. a, b, c, e, f
pp 248–250
lactation, vitamins, breast milk; minerals, breast milk; breast milk; iodine

13–21. a, b, c, d, e, f
p 250
lactation, hormonal control

13–22. progesterone and estrogen
p 250
lactation, hormonal control; estrogen, actions; progesterone, actions

13–23. a, b, c, d, e
p 250
lactation; oxytocin, actions; prolactin, actions; suckling; milk letdown

13–24. a, b, c
p 250
breast feeding, immunology; breast milk, IgA; colostrum

13–25. a, b
pp 250–251
breast feeding

13–26. b, c, e
p 251
afterpains; puerperium

13–27. a, b, c, d
p 251
lochia

13–28. a, d, e
p 251
lochia; oxytocics, puerperium; methylergonovine maleate

13–29. a, b
pp 251–252
preeclampsia; puerperal diuresis

13–30. b, c, d
p 252
puerperium; puerperal diuresis; urinary tract infection, puerperium; afterpains; leukocytosis, postpartum

13–31. a, b, d
p 252
puerperium; leukocytosis; lymphopenia; sedimentation rate (ESR)

13–32. a
p 252
puerperium, weight loss

13–33. b, c, d, e
p 252
puerperium; postpartum hemorrhage; episiotomy

13–34. a, c, d
pp 252–253
postpartum depression

13–35. a, b, c
p 253
puerperium, early ambulation; puerperium, constipation; thromboembolism

13–36. a, c
p 253
puerperium, abdominal wall

13–37. d
p 253
puerperium, diet; lactation

13–38. a, b, c, d
p 253
puerperium, bladder function; puerperium, oxytocics

13–39. a
p 253
puerperium, bladder

13–40. a, b
p 253
puerperium, breast care; puerperium, constipation

13–41. c
p 254
puerperium

13–42. a, d, e
p 254
puerperium; postpartum, menstruation; postpartum, ovulation

13–43. none of these
p 255
puerperium

14–1. a, b, c
p 257
prenatal care

14–2. b; ideally, prenatal care should be a continuation of a regimen of physician-supervised health care already established for the woman
p 257
prenatal care

14–3. d
p 258
primipara

14–4. b
p 258
gravida

14–5. c
p 258
nullipara

14–6. g
p 258
puerpera

14–7. f
p 258
parturient

14–8. e
p 258
multipara

14–9. a
p 257
nulligravida

14–10. primipara
p 258
primipara

14–11. d
p 258
obstetric history

14–12. d
p 258
pregnancy, duration

14–13. March 10
p 258
Naegele's rule; gestational age, determination; EDC (estimated date of confinement)

14–14. b
p 258
gestational age; menstrual age

14–15. c
p 258
gestational age

14–16. a, b, c, d
pp 258–259
prenatal care, initial comprehensive obstetrical evaluation; gestational age, determination

14–17. a, b, c
p 259
gestational age; prenatal care, initial comprehensive obstetrical evaluation; oral contraceptives, effects

14–18. a, d
pp 259–260
prenatal care, initial comprehensive obstetrical evaluation; cervical cytology; gonorrhea, culture

14–19. c
p 259
vaginal secretions, pregnancy; prenatal care, initial comprehensive obstetrical evaluation

14–20. b
p 259
prenatal care, initial comprehensive obstetrical evaluation; clinical pelvimetry

14–21. the height of the fundus in cm equals the gestational age in weeks in most normal singleton pregnancies
p 260
gestational age; prenatal care; fundal height

14–22. b
p 260
dental care, pregnancy; caries, pregnancy

14–23. (1) vaginal bleeding; (2) swelling of the face or fingers; (3) severe or continuous headache; (4) dimness or blurring of vision; (5) abdominal pain; (6) persistent vomiting; (7) chills or fever; (8) dysuria; (9) escape of fluid from the vagina; (10) marked change in frequency or intensity of fetal movements
p 260
pregnancy, danger signals; prenatal care

14–24. a, b, c, d
p 260
high-risk pregnancy

14–25. c
  p 260
  prenatal care, return visits

14–26. b
  p 260
  prenatal care, return visits

14–27. a
  p 260
  prenatal care, return visits

14–28. a, b, e
  pp 260–261
  prenatal care, return visits; fundal height; fetal heart sounds; gestational age, determination

14–29. a, b, c, d, e
  p 261
  prenatal care, routine monitoring; fetal heart rate; fetal movement

14–30. a, b, c
  p 261
  prenatal care, routine monitoring; fundal height

14–31. none of the tests *must* be repeated at *every* prenatal visit
  p 261
  prenatal care, routine monitoring; prenatal care, laboratory testing

14–32. a, b, c
  p 261
  neural tube defect; gestational diabetes; human immunodeficiency syndrome; Chlamydia trachomatis

14–33. seven
  p 262
  low birthweight; neonatal mortality rate; weight gain, pregnancy

14–34. a, b, c, d, e, f
  p 263
  nutrition, pregnancy; high-risk pregnancy; weight gain, pregnancy

14–35. a, b, c, d
  pp 262–263
  weight gain, pregnancy; birthweight; low birthweight; diet, pregnancy

14–36. 300
  p 263 (Table 14–1)
  nutrition, pregnancy; caloric requirements, pregnancy

14–37. a, b
  pp 263–264
  nutrition, pregnancy; protein requirements, pregnancy; caloric requirements, pregnancy

14–38. iron; iodized salt should be utilized
  p 264
  nutrition, pregnancy; minerals, pregnancy; iron, pregnancy; iodine, pregnancy

14–39. a, d, e
  pp 264–265
  iron, pregnancy; nutrition, pregnancy

14–40. a, c, d
  pp 264–265
  iron, pregnancy; nutrition, pregnancy; nausea, pregnancy

14–41. b, c
  p 265
  calcium, pregnancy; nutrition, pregnancy

14–42. a, b, d
  p 265
  zinc, pregnancy; nutrition, pregnancy; wound healing; acrodermatitis enteropathica

14–43. b, c, e
  p 265
  minerals, pregnancy; nutrition, pregnancy; cretinism; goiter, fetal; potassium, pregnancy

14–44. b
  pp 265–266
  sodium, pregnancy; nutrition, pregnancy; preeclampsia, etiology

14–45. c
  p 266
  fluoride, pregnancy

14–46. b
  pp 266–267
  vitamins, pregnancy

14–47. a, c
  p 266
  folic acid, pregnancy; vitamins, pregnancy

14–48. a, b, c, d
  p 266
  vitamin B_{12}, pregnancy; vitamins, pregnancy; breast milk, composition

14–49. a, c
  pp 266–267
  vitamin B_6, pregnancy; vitamins, pregnancy

14–50. b
  p 266
  vitamin C, pregnancy; vitamins, pregnancy

14–51. b
  p 265
  iodine, pregnancy; minerals, pregnancy; cretinism, fetal

14–52. d
  p 266
  folic acid, pregnancy; vitamins, pregnancy

14–53. e
  p 265
  zinc, pregnancy; minerals, pregnancy; acrodermatitis enteropathica

14–54. c
p 265
iodine, pregnancy; vitamins, pregnancy; goiter, fetal

14–55. a
p 267
vitamin C, pregnancy; vitamins, pregnancy; scurvy

14–56. d
p 266
folic acid, pregnancy; vitamins, pregnancy; megaloblastic anemia

14–57. h
pp 266–267
vitamin B₆, pregnancy; vitamins, pregnancy; progressive sensory ataxia

14–58. b, c
p 262
nutrition, pregnancy; weight gain, pregnancy; iron, pregnancy

14–59. a
p 267
exercise, pregnancy

14–60. a, b, c
p 267
exercise, pregnancy; multifetal pregnancy; hypertension, pregnancy; intrauterine growth retardation

14–61. a, b, c, d
p 267
prenatal care; high-risk pregnancy, activity

14–62. b, c
p 268
prenatal care; travel, pregnancy

14–63. b
p 268
prenatal care

14–64. b
p 268
prenatal care; gastrointestinal system, pregnancy; laxatives, pregnancy

14–65. a
pp 268–269
prenatal care; coitus, pregnancy

14–66. b, c
p 269
prenatal care; douching, pregnancy; air embolism, pregnancy

14–67. b
p 269
striae gravidarum

14–68. a, c
p 269
smoking, pregnancy; perinatal death; low birthweight

14–69. a, b, c, d
pp 269–270
smoking, pregnancy

14–70. a, b, c, d, e, f
p 270
fetal alcohol syndrome; alcohol, pregnancy; birth defects; intrauterine growth retardation

14–71. b, c, d
p 270
drug abuse, pregnancy; low birthweight

14–72. b, c, e
p 269 (Table 14–3)
prenatal care; immunization, pregnancy

14–73. b
p 270
medications, pregnancy; placental function

14–74. b, e
pp 270–271
pregnancy, common complaints; nausea, pregnancy

14–75. a, c
p 271
pregnancy, common complaints; back pain, pregnancy; musculoskeletal system, pregnancy

14–76. b
p 271
pregnancy, common complaints; varicosities, pregnancy

14–77. a, b, c, d
pp 271–272
pregnancy, common complaints; hemorrhoids, pregnancy

14–78. b
p 272
pregnancy, common complaints; gastrointestinal system, pregnancy

14–79. b
p 272
nutrition, pregnancy; pica

14–80. b, d
pp 272–273
pregnancy, common complaints

14–81. a, b, c, d
p 273
vagina, pregnancy; vaginitis, pregnancy; Trichomonas; Candida

15–1. a, b, c, d, e, f, g, h
pp 277–278
antepartum care; fetal well-being; perinatal death rate

15–2. a, b, c, d, e, f
p 278
amniocentesis, risks; abortion; premature labor; Rh isoimmunization; umbilical cord trauma; intrauterine infection

15–3. a, b, c, d, e, f
pp 278–279
amniocentesis; amnionic fluid; congenital abnormalities; birth defects

15–4. a, b, c, d
p 278
amniocentesis; Rh isoimmunization; ultrasonography

15–5. a, b, c, d, e
pp 278–279
amniocentesis, risks; postterm pregnancy; oligohydramnios

15–6. when the fetus is mature enough to have a reasonable chance of survival if delivery becomes necessary. This is especially the case after a suspected traumatic tap.
p 279
amniocentesis, risks; electronic fetal monitoring

15–7. e
p 279
amniocentesis; prenatal diagnosis

15–8. a, c
pp 279–280
amniocentesis, bloody tap; L/S ratio

15–9. type II pneumocytes
p 279
surfactant; fetal lung maturity

15–10. d
p 279
respiratory distress syndrome; L/S ratio; fetal lung maturity

15–11. a, b
p 280
L/S ratio; respiratory distress syndrome

15–12. 14
p 280
L/S ratio; respiratory distress syndrome; perinatal mortality; neonatal mortality

15–13. a, b, d
p 280
respiratory distress syndrome; L/S ratio; diabetes; erythroblastosis fetalis

15–14. a
p 280
respiratory distress syndrome; phosphatidylglycerol, amnionic fluid

15–15. a, b, c, d, e, f
p 280
surfactant; L/S ratio; foam stability test; phosphatidylglycerol

15–16. b
pp 280–281
surfactant; foam stability test

15–17. a, c
p 281
bilirubin, amnionic fluid

15–18. a, b, c
p 281
bilirubin, amnionic fluid; sickle cell anemia

15–19. a, b, c, d, e
pp 281–282
amniocentesis, cytogenetic studies; spontaneous abortion; Down syndrome; neural tube defects; birth defects

15–20. c, d
p 278
amniocentesis

15–21. d
p 278
amniocentesis

15–22. e
pp 278–279
amniocentesis; bloody tap

15–23. c
pp 277–278
amniocentesis; techniques; risks

15–24. c
p 278
amniocentesis; techniques; risks

15–25. f
pp 278–279
amniocentesis; techniques; risks

15–26. a, b, c
p 282
fetal blood sampling

15–27. b
p 280
amnionic fluid surfactant (fetal lung maturity); lecithin-to-sphingomyelin (L/S) ratio

15–28. b
p 280
amnionic fluid surfactant; foam stability (shake) test

15–29. b, c
p 280
amnionic fluid surfactant; phosphatidylglycerol

15–30. b
p 280
amnionic fluid surfactant; foam stability test

15–31. a
p 280
amnionic fluid surfactant; lecithin-to-sphingomyelin ratio

15–32. a
p 282
fetal blood sampling

15–33. a, b, c, d
pp 253–254
fetal blood sampling

15–34. b
p 284
sonography

15–35. a, b
pp 279, 284
amniocentesis, fetal blood sampling

15–36. a
p 280
amniocentesis, supernatant fraction; fetal lung maturity

15–37. a, b
pp 280, 284
amniocentesis, supernatant fraction; bilirubin; hemolytic disease of the newborn

15–38. a
p 280
amniocentesis, supernatant fraction

15–39. a
p 284
ultrasound, clinical application

15–40. b
pp 285–286
Doppler ultrasound, wave form analysis

15–41. a, b, c, d, e, f
p 284
ultrasonography; multifetal pregnancy; oligohydramnios; hydramnios; placentation; gestational age, determination

15–42. a, b, c, d
pp 284–285
ultrasonography; fetal movement; fetal heart activity

15–43. a, b, c, d
p 285
ultrasonography; radiography; hydatidiform mole; gestational age

15–44. b
p 282
fetoscopy

15–45. a
pp 281–282
amnioscopy

15–46. d
p 289
fetography

15–47. a, b, c
p 282
fetal blood sampling

15–48. a, b, c, d
pp 281–282
amnioscopy

15–49. a, c
p 285
Doppler ultrasound

15–50. c, e
p 290
fetal movement; fetal well-being

15–51. b, e
p 290
fetal well-being; contraction stress test

15–52. a, b, c, e, f, g, h, i
pp 290–291
contraction stress test; oxytocin

15–53. b
pp 290–291
contraction stress test

15–54. b
pp 290–291
contraction stress test, interpretation; contraction stress test, negative

15–55. d
pp 290–291
contraction stress test, interpretation

15–56. c
p 291
contraction stress test, interpretation; contraction stress test, suspicious

15–57. e
p 291
contraction stress test, interpretation; contraction stress test, unsatisfactory

15–58. a
p 291
contraction stress test, interpretation; contraction stress test, positive

15–59. c
p 291
contraction stress test; fetal well-being; contraction stress test, negative

15–60. a
p 291
contraction stress test; fetal well-being; contraction stress test, negative

15–61. 1 percent or less
p 291
contraction stress test; contraction stress test, false negative

15–62. b
p 291
contraction stress test; fetal well-being; contraction stress test, positive

15–63. a
pp 291–292
fetal heart rate, acceleration; nonstress test; electronic fetal monitoring

15–64. three or more fetal movements are accompanied by acceleration of the fetal heart rate of 15 beats/minute or more
pp 291–292
nonstress test

15–65. a
p 295
fetal well-being

15–66. a, c, e, f, i
p 293
biophysical profile

15–67. b, c, d
pp 293–294
biophysical profile

15–68. a, c, d
p 296
fetal monitoring, internal; spiral electrode

15–69. b
p 296
fetal monitoring; fetal heart rate; spiral electrode

15–70. b, c, d
pp 296–298
fetal monitoring, internal; fetal monitoring, external

15–71. a
p 300
fetal monitoring

15–72. c
p 298
fetal heart rate, baseline

15–73. a
p 299
fetal heart rate, baseline; bradycardia, fetal

15–74. d
p 299
fetal heart rate, baseline; tachycardia, fetal

15–75. deviations from baseline that are related to uterine contractions
p 300
fetal heart rate, periodic

15–76. c
p 298
fetal heart rate, deceleration; variable deceleration; cord compression

15–77. b
p 298
fetal heart rate, deceleration; type II deceleration; uteroplacental insufficiency

15–78. a
p 298
fetal heart rate, deceleration; type I deceleration; fetal head compression

15–79. a
p 298
fetal heart rate, deceleration; type I deceleration; vagus nerve, effect of stimulation

15–80. a
p 298
fetal heart rate, deceleration; type I deceleration; atropine, maternal stimulation

15–81. a, b, c
p 298
fetal heart rate, deceleration; type I deceleration; type II deceleration; variable deceleration; maternal position, labor

15–82. a, b, c
p 298
fetal heart rate, deceleration; type I deceleration; type II deceleration; variable deceleration; fetal distress

15–83. a
p 298
fetal heart rate, deceleration; type I deceleration

15–84. b
p 298
fetal heart rate, deceleration; type II deceleration

15–85. a, b, c, d, e
p 299
fetal heart rate; beat-to-beat variability

15–86. a, c, d, e
p 299
fetal heart rate; sinusoidal pattern; tachycardia, persistent; bradycardia, persistent; hypoxia, fetal; hypothermia, maternal

15–87. a
p 299
fetal heart rate; sinusoidal pattern; anemia, fetal

15–88. d
p 299
persistent fetal bradycardia, severe; heart block, fetal

15–89. b
p 299
persistent fetal tachycardia; fever, maternal

15–90. a, b, c, d
p 300
fetal well-being; fetal blood sampling

15–91. c
p 300
fetal blood sampling; fetal distress; fetal blood, pH; cesarean delivery, indications

15–92. b
p 300
fetal blood sampling; fetal distress; fetal blood, pH

15–93. a
p 300
fetal blood sampling; fetal distress; fetal blood, pH

15–94. b, c
p 300
fetal blood sampling; fetal blood, pH

15–95. b, c, d
p 300
amniotomy; fetal monitoring, internal; umbilical cord, prolapse

15–96. a, b, c, d
p 301
fetal monitoring, internal

15–97. b
pp 301–302
fetal monitoring, external

15–98. c, d, e
p 301
fetal blood sampling; vacuum extraction; hemophilia; coagulation defect, fetal

15–99. b
p 302
fetal monitoring; fetal well–being

16–1. a, c, d
p 307
labor, antepartum care; psychoprophylaxis

16–2. b
pp 307–308
labor, false

16–3. a
p 307
labor, true

16–4. a
p 307
labor, true

16–5. b
p 307
labor, false

16–6. b
p 307
labor, false

16–7. b
p 307
labor, initial presentation; antepartum care

16–8. a, b, c, d, e, f
p 308
labor; bloody show; admissions procedures; membranes, rupture

16–9. b
p 308
admissions procedures; bloody show; third trimester bleeding; labor

16–10. c, d, f
p 308
labor; vaginal examination; clinical pelvimetry

16–11. c
p 308
labor; vaginal examination; cervical effacement

16–12. c
p 308
labor; vaginal examination; cervical dilation

16–13. c
p 308
cervix, position; premature labor

16–14. a, b, c
p 308
labor, station; vaginal examination; cervix; engagement

16–15. c
p 308
labor, station

16–16. a, b, c
pp 308–309
labor, membranes, rupture; labor, infection; umbilical cord prolapse

16–17. 1 = 4.5 to 5.5; 2 = 7.0 to 7.5
p 309
amnionic fluid; membranes, rupture; vagina, pH

16–18. a, c, d
pp 308–309
membranes, rupture; bloody show; rupture of membranes, detection; amnionic fluid, pH

16–19. d
p 309
vaginal examination; labor, management

16–20. b
pp 309–310
labor, first stage

16–21. c, d
pp 310–311
labor, management; fetal monitoring; fetal heart rate; fetal distress, diagnosis

16–22. a, b, e
p 312
labor, management; uterus, contractions; fetal monitoring

16–23. a, b, c, d
p 313
labor, management; analgesia

16–24. c, d
p 313
labor, management; amniotomy; umbilical cord prolapse

16–25. d
pp 313–314
labor, management

16–26. a, d
p 314
labor, management; bladder function; urinary tract infection

16–27. b
pp 313–314
active management of labor

16–28. b
p 314
labor, second stage

16–29. a, c, d, e
p 314
labor, second stage; fetal heart rate; placental abruption; fetal distress; nuchal cord; electronic fetal monitoring

16–30. a, d
p 314
labor, second stage; maternal expulsive efforts (pushing)

16–31. dorsal lithotomy position
pp 314–315
delivery, dorsal lithotomy position

16–32. b
p 315
labor, second stage; leg cramps, labor

16–33. none of these absolutely assures a noninfected outcome, especially since the advent of human immunodeficiency virus infections
p 315
labor, infection; perineal preparation, labor

16–34. crowning
pp 315–316
labor, second stage; crowning

16–35. a, b, c
p 315
delivery, head; episiotomy; pelvic relaxation

16–36. Ritgen maneuver (modified)
pp 316–317
Ritgen maneuver; labor, second stage

16–37. a, b, c, d
p 317
delivery, head; umbilical cord; nuchal cord

16–38. a, b
p 317
delivery, shoulders; second stage, management

16–39. a, b
p 317
fetus, injury; delivery, shoulders; second stage, management

16–40. b, d, f
pp 318–319
umbilical cord; labor, second stage; hyperbilirubinemia; nuchal cord; infant transfusion syndrome

16–41. a, b, d, e
p 319
labor, third stage; placenta, separation; third stage management

16–42. a, b, c, e
p 319
labor, third stage; postpartum hemorrhage; placental separation

16–43. inversion of the uterus
p 320
uterine inversion; placenta, delivery

16–44. a
pp 320–321
placenta, manual removal; postpartum hemorrhage

16–45. a, c, d, e
p 321
placenta, manual removal; third stage, management

16–46. a, b, c, d
p 321
labor, fourth stage; hemorrhage, obstetric; uterus, atony

16–47. vasoconstriction produced by a well-contracted myometrium
p 321
postpartum hemorrhage

16–48. a, b, d
p 321
oxytocic agents; labor, third stage; labor, fourth stage; oxytocin; ergonovine maleate; methylergonovine maleate

16–49. b, e, f
p 321
oxytocin

16–50. a, b, c, d, e
p 322
ergonovine; methylergonovine

16–51. entrapment of a second, undiagnosed twin
p 322
oxytocics; multifetal pregnancy

16–52. b
pp 322–323
birth canal, lacerations

16–53. c
pp 322–323
birth canal, lacerations

16–54. a
pp 322–323
birth canal, lacerations

16–55. d
p 323
birth canal, lacerations

16–56. a, b, c, d, e
p 323
episiotomy; birth canal, lacerations

16–57. a
p 323
episiotomy, midline

16–58. b
pp 323–324
episiotomy, mediolateral

16–59. b
pp 323–324
episiotomy, mediolateral

16–60. a
pp 323–325
episiotomy, midline

16–61. a
pp 323–325
episiotomy, midline

16–62. b
pp 323–325
episiotomy, mediolateral

16–63. a
pp 323–325
episiotomy, midline

16–64. hemostasis; anatomic restoration without excessive suturing
p 325
episiotomy, repair

16–65. d, e, f
p 325
episiotomy

16–66. vulvar, paravaginal, or ischiorectal hematoma or abscess
p 325
episiotomy

17–1. a, b, c, d
p 327
anesthesia, surgical; anesthesia, obstetrical

17–2. a, b, c, d, e
pp 327–328
anesthesia, obstetric; analgesia, obstetrical; labor, management

17–3. a, b, c
p 328
analgesia; pain control in labor

17–4. none; all narcotics and tranquilizers used for analgesia during labor can reach the fetus
p 328
analgesia, obstetric; analgesia, fetal effects; placental transfer

17–5. a
p 329
narcotic antagonists; fetal respiratory depression; naloxone (Narcan)

17–6. a, d, e
p 329
narcotic antagonists; fetal respiratory depression; naloxone (Narcan)

17–7. c, d
p 329
anesthesia, obstetric; anesthesia, general; placental barrier

17–8. a, c, d, e
p 329
anesthesia, obstetric; nitrous oxide; anesthetics, volatile

17–9. none; all are capable of crossing the placenta and producing fetal narcosis
pp 329–330
anesthesia, obstetric; anesthetics, volatile; placental barrier; ether; halothane (Fluothane); methoxyflurane (Penthrane); enflurane (Ethrane)

17–10. a, b, c, d
pp 329–330
anesthesia, obstetric; anesthetics, volatile; ether; halothane (Fluothane); methoxyflurane (Penthrane); enflurane (Ethrane)

17–11. c
pp 329–330
anesthesia, obstetric; anesthetics, volatile, methoxyflurane (Penthrane)

17–12. b
p 329
anesthesia, obstetric; anesthetics, volatile; halothane

17–13. a, b, c, d, e
p 330
anesthesia, obstetric; anesthetics, intravenous; thiopental

17–14. c, d
p 330
anesthesia, obstetric; anesthetics, intravenous, thiopental

17–15. b
p 330
anesthesia, obstetric; anesthetics, intravenous, fetal respiratory depression

17–16. a, b, c, d
pp 330–331
anesthesia, obstetric; anesthetics, intravenous; ketamine; hypertension, maternal; respiratory depression of the newborn

17–17. aspiration and consequent chemical pneumonitis from the inhalation of acidic gastric contents
p 331
anesthesia, obstetric; aspiration, pneumonia; maternal death, causes

17–18. b, d, e
p 331
anesthesia, obstetric; aspiration, prevention

17–19. a
p 331
anesthesia, obstetric; aspiration

17–20. a, b, e
pp 331–332
anesthesia, obstetric; aspiration; aspiration pneumonitis

17–21. a, d
p 332
anesthesia, obstetric; aspiration, treatment; aspiration pneumonitis

17–22. a
p 330
anesthesia, obstetric; anesthesia, risks of exposure

17–23. a, b, c, d
p 332
uterus, innervation; Frankenhaüser's ganglion; analgesia, labor

17–24. a, b, c
p 332
genital tract, innervation; pudendal nerve

17–25. second, third, and fourth sacral
p 332
genital tract, innervation; pudendal nerve

17–26. b, c, d, e, f
p 334
anesthesia, obstetric; anesthesia, CNS toxicity; regional anesthesia; ephedrine; succinylcholine; thiopental; diazepam; convulsions, maternal

17–27. b, c, e
p 334
anesthesia, obstetric; anesthesia, local

17–28. a, b, c, d, e, f
p 334
anesthesia, obstetric; pudendal block; local infiltration; cardiovascular toxicity

17–29. d
p 334
anesthesia, obstetric; pudendal block; vaginal delivery

17–30. a, b, c
p 334
anesthesia, obstetric; pudental block; convulsions, maternal

17–31. a, b, d
p 335
anesthesia, obstetric; paracervical block; bradycardia, fetal; postparacervical bradycardia

17–32. a, c, d
p 335
anesthesia, obstetric; spinal block

17–33. a, b, c, d, e, f
pp 335–336
anesthesia, obstetric; spinal block, complications; spinal headache

17–34. a, b, c
pp 335–336
anesthesia, obstetric; spinal block, complications, ephedrine; maternal hypotension

17–35. too large a dose of anesthetic
p 336
anesthesia, obstetric; spinal block, complications; total spinal block

17–36. a, b, c, d
p 336
anesthesia, obstetric; spinal block, complications; nitrous oxide; morphine; meperidine; fentanyl

17–37. leakage of cerebrospinal fluid from the site where the meninges have been punctured
p 336
anesthesia, obstetric; spinal block, complications; spinal headache

17–38. a, b, e, f, g
p 336
anesthesia, obstetric; spinal block, complications; spinal headache

17–39. a
p 337
anesthesia, obstetric; spinal block, complications; epidural block; hypertension, regional anesthesia; ergotamine

17–40. maternal hypovolemia; maternal hypotension or hypertension; maternal coagulation disorders; skin infection at the possible puncture site; maternal neurologic disorders
pp 336–337
anesthesia, obstetric; spinal block, contraindications

17–41. a, b, c
p 337
anesthesia, obstetric; epidural/peridural block; analgesia, obstetric

17–42. a, b, c, d, e
p 337
anesthesia, obstetric; epidural block, complications; hypotension, maternal; labor, inhibition; spinal block

17–43. a
p 337
anesthesia, obstetric; epidural block; delivery, midforceps

17–44. maternal hemorrhage; overt hypertension; skin infection at or near the possible puncture site; neurologic disease
p 338–339
anesthesia, obstetric; epidural block, contraindications

17–45. a, c
p 339
anesthesia; analgesia

18–1. insufficiently strong or coordinated uterine forces that cannot efface and dilate the cervix; abnormalities of presentation, position, or fetal development; abnormalities of the maternal bony pelvis; abnormalities of the birth canal other than those of the bony pelvis
p 341
dystocia, causes

18–2. pelvis contraction accompanied by uterine dysfunction
p 341
dystocia; pelvic contraction; uterine dysfunction

18–3. a
p 341
uterine dysfunction; fetopelvic disproportion

18–4. a
p 341
cervical effacement; labor, latent phase

18–5. b
pp 341–342
cervical dilation; labor, active phase

18–6. 1 = mild; 2 = strong; 3 = short; 4 = long; 5 = irregular; 6 = regular
p 342
labor, Friedman curve; labor, latent phase; labor, active phase; uterine contractions

18–7. c, d
pp 341–342
uterine dysfunction; cervical dilation rates; protracted labor, active phase

18–8. b
p 343
uterine dysfunction, hypertonic

18–9. a
p 343
uterine dysfunction, hypotonic

18–10. a
p 343
uterine dysfunction, hypotonic

18–11. b
p 343
uterine dysfunction, hypertonic

18–12. a
p 343
uterine dysfunction, hypotonic

18–13. b
p 343
uterine dysfunction, hypertonic

18–14. a
p 343
uterine dysfunction, hypotonic

18–15. 1 = >14 hr; 2 = <1.2 cm per hr; 3 = <2.0 cm per hr; 4 = >3 hr; 5 = >2 hr; 6 = >1 hr; 7 = no descent in the deceleration phase or in the second stage of labor
p 342 (Table 18–1)
abnormal labor; prolongation disorders, labor; protraction disorders, labor; arrest disorders, labor

18–16. 1 = therapeutic rest; 2 = oxytocin or cesarean delivery for urgent problems; 3 = expectant management and support; 4 = cesarean delivery for cephalopelvic disproportion
p 342 (Table 18–1)
prolongation disorder, labor; protraction disorder, labor

18–17. b
p 343
uterine dysfunction; dystocia

18–18. a, b, c, d
pp 343–344
uterine dysfunction

18–19. the patient must be in active labor; there must be no cephalopelvic disproportion
pp 344–345
uterine dysfunction, hypotonic; cephalopelvic disproportion; oxytocin stimulation; augmentation of labor

18–20. Usually, spontaneous activity does not persist and the normal forces of labor are replaced by hypotonic uterine dysfunction.
p 344
uterine dysfunction, hypotonic; cephalopelvic disproportion; uterine rupture

18–21. a, b, c, d, e
pp 344–345
uterine dysfunction, hypotonic

18–22. b
p 344
dysfunctional labor; uterine dysfunction

18–23. b
pp 344–345
uterine dysfunction, hypotonic; oxytocin, uterine dysfunction

18–24. Oxytocin has a potent antidiuretic action. Fluids may precipitate water intoxication that may lead to convulsions, coma, or death.
p 344
oxytocin, actions; water intoxication

18–25. a, c, e
p 345
oxytocin, uterine dysfunction; uterine dysfunction

18–26. a, c, e
pp 344–345
uterine dysfunction, hypotonic; oxytocin, uterine dysfunction; labor, stimulation

18–27. a
p 345
oxytocin, uterine dysfunction; cesarean delivery

18–28. b
p 346
labor, latent phase; uterine dysfunction, hypotonic; labor, false

18–29. c
pp 345–346
prostaglandins; cervical ripening; induction of labor; augmentation of labor

18–30. a, c
p 346
uterine dysfunction, hypertonic

18–31. a, b, c, d
p 347
pushing; labor, second stage; voluntary expulsive forces

18–32. a, b, c, f
pp 347–348
precipitate labor; postpartum hemorrhage; amnionic fluid embolism

18–33. a, b, c, d
p 347
contraction ring; protracted labor; pathologic retraction ring, Bandl

18–34. Uterine contractions begin at or near term but then disappear without the birth of a fetus. The fetus then dies and is retained in utero.
p 347
missed labor

19–1. 1 = 33; 2 = 3 to 4 (6 to 7)
pp 349–350 (Table 19–1)
breech presentation, incidence

19–2. a, b, c, e, g, h, i, j, k, l, m
p 349
breech presentation, incidence; grand multiparity; multifetal pregnancy; hydramnios; hydrocephalus; anencephaly; uterine anomaly; placenta previa; breech presentation, recurrent

19–3. increased perinatal morbidity and mortality; low birth weight; umbilical cord prolapse; placenta previa; fetal anomalies and perinatal developmental abnormalities; multiple fetuses; need for operative intervention, especially cesarean delivery
p 349
breech presentation, associated complications; perinatal mortality; umbilical cord prolapse; intrauterine growth retardation; multifetal pregnancy, cesarean delivery; fetal growth retardation

19–4. b
p 349
breech, complete

19–5. a
p 349
breech, frank

19–6. c
p 349
breech, incomplete

19–7. a
p 349
breech, frank

19–8. b
pp 349–350
abdominal examination, breech presentation; Leopold maneuvers

19–9. 1 = slightly above the umbilicus; 2 = below the umbilicus
p 350
fetal heart sounds, cephalic presentation; fetal heart sounds, breech presentation

19–10. a, b, d
p 350
vaginal examination, breech presentation

19–11. b
p 350
ultrasonography, breech presentation; x-ray, breech presentation

19–12. a
p 350
breech presentation, maternal mortality; maternal morbidity, maternal mortality

19–13. prematurity; congenital anomalies; birth trauma
p 350
breech presentation, perinatal mortality; breech presentation, perinatal morbidity; prematurity; birth trauma; congenital anomalies; perinatal mortality

19–14. e
pp 350–351
brain injury, breech presentation

19–15. b
p 352
breech presentation, perinatal mortality; cesarean delivery

19–16. b, c
pp 352–353
breech presentation, perinatal mortality; umbilical cord prolapse

19–17. a
pp 353–354
breech presentation, perinatal mortality

19–18. a
pp 353–354
breech presentation, perinatal mortality; prematurity

19–19. a, c, d
p 354
external version; antepartum hemorrhage; premature labor

19–20. a, c
p 354
breech presentation, vaginal delivery; asphyxia, fetal; accommodation, fetal head

19–21. large fetus (>3,500 g); contracted or unfavorably shaped pelvis; hyperextended head; maternal or fetal indications for delivery when the mother is not in labor; uterine dysfunction; footling breech; premature fetus (>26 weeks) with the mother in labor or in need of delivery; severe fetal growth retardation; history of previous perinatal death or children with birth trauma; firm request for sterilization by the mother
p 355
breech presentation, cesarean delivery; cesarean delivery, breech presentation

19–22. b, d
pp 355–356
pelvic shape, breech presentation

19–23. injury to the cervical spinal cord
p 356
hyperextended fetal head; spinal cord injury, fetal

19–24. b, c, d
p 356
vaginal delivery, breech presentation; breech presentation, delivery

19–25. b
p 357
face presentation

19–26. a, c, d
p 357
face presentation; pelvic contraction; anencephaly; macrosomia

19–27. a, b, d
pp 357–358
face presentation; cesarean delivery, face presentation

19–28. a, b, c, d
pp 358–359
brow presentation; caput succedaneum

19–29. b
p 359
brow presentation; vaginal examination, brow presentation

19–30. a
p 359
face presentation; vaginal examination, face presentation

19–31. b
p 359
transverse lie

19–32. a
p 360
transverse lie

19–33. a, b, c, d
pp 360–361
transverse lie

19–34. b, d, f, h
p 360
prematurity; placenta previa; contracted pelvis; fetopelvic disproportion; transverse lie

19–35. spontaneous rupture of the uterus or traumatic rupture consequent upon late and ill–advised version and extraction
p 362
transverse lie; uterus, rupture; maternal mortality

19–36. a, b, c, d
p 362
transverse lie; maternal mortality; maternal morbidity

19–37. a, d
pp 361–363
transverse lie, postpartum infection; conduplicato corpore; cesarean delivery

19–38. b
pp 360–362
cesarean delivery; transverse lie

19–39. a, b, c
p 362
compound presentation; perinatal mortality

19–40. d
pp 362–363
occiput posterior position, persistent; forceps delivery; episiotomy; midforceps rotation; Scanzoni maneuver

19-41. a, d
pp 362–363
occiput posterior position, persistent; episiotomy; perinatal mortality

19-42. a, b, c, d
p 363
occiput transverse position, persistent; hypotonic uterine dysfunction; deep transverse arrest; cesarean delivery, deep transverse arrest

19-43. With platypelloid and android pelves, there may not be adequate room for rotation of the occiput to either the anterior or posterior positions.
p 364
deep transverse arrest; android pelvis; platypelloid pelvis

19-44. >4000 g
p 365
fetal macrosomia

19-45. a, c, e, f, g, h
p 365
fetal macrosomia; prolonged gestation; diabetes, maternal; multiparity

19-46. a, c, d
p 365
fetal weight measurement; perinatal mortality; fetal macrosomia

19-47. a
pp 365–366
shoulder dystocia; fetal macrosomia

19-48. The head is delivered causing the umbilical cord to be drawn into the pelvis and then compressed when the shoulders cannot be delivered.
p 365
shoulder dystocia; umbilical cord compression

19-49. a, b
pp 366–367
shoulder dystocia; ultrasonography

19-50. Fundal pressure, "corkscrewing" the fetus, the "McRoberts maneuver," delivery of the posterior shoulder, fundal pressure, rocking of the fetal shoulders, "shoulder horn," pressure of the head and jaw, cephalic replacement, fracture of the clavicle, cleidotomy
p 369
shoulder dystocia; fetal macrosomia

19-51. a
p 366
shoulder dystocia; ultrasound

19-52. b, c, d
p 371
hydrocephalus, internal; uterus, rupture

19-53. a, c
pp 371–372
hydrocephalus, internal; x-ray

19-54. a, b, c, d
p 374
fetal abdomen, enlargement; ascites, fetal; kidney, fetal

19-55. b
p 374
fetal abdomen, enlargement; ascites, fetal

20-1. a, b, c
p 377
pelvic contraction; dystocia

20-2. a, b, c
p 377
pelvic inlet contraction; diagonal conjugate

20-3. c
p 377
pelvic inlet contraction

20-4. 1 = a; 2 = a
p 377
pelvic contraction

20-5. d
pp 377–378
contracted pelvic inlet; presentation and position of the fetus

20-6. c
p 377
contracted pelvic inlet; sonographic measurements

20-7. a, c, d
p 378
face presentation; shoulder presentation; pelvic inlet contraction; umbilical cord prolapse

20-8. b, c, d, e, f
p 378
pelvic inlet contraction; cervix, dilation; intrapartum infection; rupture of the membranes, spontaneous; dystocia, complications; uterine rupture

20-9. a
p 378
pelvic inlet contraction; pathologic contraction ring; cesarean delivery, indications; uterine rupture

20-10. a, b
p 379
pelvic contraction; intracranial hemorrhage, fetal; molding; caput succedaneum; station, clinical determination

20-11. a
pp 379–380
vaginal delivery, pelvic inlet contraction; occiput presentation; pelvic inlet contraction

20-12. b
p 380
vaginal delivery, pelvic inlet contraction; breech presentation; pelvic inlet contraction

20-13. b
p 380
vaginal delivery, pelvic inlet contraction; fetal macrosomia; pelvic inlet contraction

20-14. b
p 380
vaginal delivery, pelvic inlet contraction; android pelvis; pelvic inlet contraction

20-15. a
p 380
vaginal delivery, pelvic inlet contraction; cervix, dilation; pelvic inlet contraction

20-16. b
p 380
vaginal delivery, pelvic inlet contraction; uterine dysfunction; pelvic inlet contraction

20-17. b
p 380
vaginal delivery, pelvic inlet contraction; pelvic inlet contraction

20-18. b
p 380
vaginal delivery; pelvic inlet contraction; asynclitism; pelvic inlet contraction

20-19. c
p 380
pelvic inlet contraction; oxytocin; uterine rupture

20-20. The plane extends from the inferior margin of the symphysis pubis, through the ischial spines, and touches the sacrum near the junction of the fourth and fifth vertebrae.
p 381
midpelvis

20-21. ischial spines
p 381
midpelvis; interspinous diameter

20-22. 1 = 10.5; 2 = 11.5; 3 = 5.0
p 381
midpelvis, measurements

20-23. d
p 381
pelvic contraction, midpelvis; midpelvis, measurements

20-24. c
p 381
pelvic contraction, midpelvis; interspinous diameter, midpelvis, measurements

20-25. b
p 381
pelvic contraction, midpelvis; pelvimetry, x-ray; ultrasonography

20-26. a
p 381
pelvic contraction, midpelvis; pelvic inlet contraction

20-27. b, c, d, e
p 381
pelvic contraction, midpelvis; forceps delivery; midforceps delivery; labor

20-28. an interischial tuberous diameter of 8 cm or less
p 381
pelvic outlet contraction; interischial tuberous diameter

20-29. 1 and 2 = interischial tuberous diameter; 3 = pubic rami; 4 = pelvic soft tissue, no bony margins; 5 = inferior posterior surface of the symphysis pubis; 6 = tip of the last sacral vertebra
p 381
pelvic outlet; interischial tuberous diameter

20-30. b
pp 380–381
contracted midpelvis

20-31. perineal tears secondary to distension caused by the fetal head
pp 381–382
contracted pelvic outlet

20-32. b
p 382
generally contracted pelvis

20-33. 1 = cardiorespiratory compromise; 2 = midpelvic contraction; 3 = cardiorespiratory compromise and midpelvic contraction
p 383
rare pelvic contractions

20-34. a
p 383
rare pelvic contractures

21-1. a, b, c
p 385
vulva, atresia; Condylomata acuminata; dystocia, vulva

21-2. d, e, f
pp 385–386
vaginal septa; vagina, atresia; Gartner duct, cyst; levator ani, tetanic contraction, vagina, annular stricture

21-3. a, b, c, d, e
p 386
cervix, stenosis; conization

21-4. a, b
p 386
cervix, stenosis; cervix, conglutination

21-5. a
p 386
cervical carcinoma, invasive

21-6. a
p 386
uterus, anteflexion; diastasis recti; uterine displacement

21-7. b
p 386
uterus, retroflexion; abortion, spontaneous; uterine displacement

21-8. b
p 386
uterus, retroflexion; sacculation; uterus, rupture; uterine displacement

21-9. a, b
p 386
uterus, anteflexion; uterus, retroflexion; cervical dilation, impeded

21-10. a, b, c, d
p 386
uterine displacement, management; uterine displacement, effects on pregnancy

21-11. c
p 387
uterus, myoma; myoma, intramural

21-12. b
p 387
uterus, myoma; myoma, subserous

21-13. a
p 387
uterus, myoma; myoma, submucous

21-14. d
p 387
uterus, myoma; myoma, pedunculated

21-15. b, d
p 387
uterus, myoma; hemorrhagic infarction; myoma, submucous

21-16. a, b, d, e
p 387
hemorrhagic infarction; placental abruption; appendicitis; ureteral stone; pyelonephritis

21-17. d
p 389
myomectomy, pregnancy; uterus, myoma; dystocia, myomas, uterine

21-18. a, d
p 391
ovarian tumors, pregnancy; torsion, ovarian tumors; teratoma, cystic; cystadenoma, mucinous

21-19. a, b
p 391
ovarian tumors, pregnancy; laparotomy, pregnancy

21-20. d, e
p 392
cystocele; enterocele; bladder distension, labor; rectum, tumors

22-1. a, b, d
p 393
breech presentation, labor; breech presentation, vaginal delivery

22-2. a, b, c, d, e
p 393
breech delivery

22-3. a
p 393
breech extraction, partial; breech presentation, vaginal delivery

22-4. a
p 393
breech delivery, spontaneous; breech presentation, vaginal delivery

22-5. c
p 393
breech extraction, total; breech presentation, vaginal delivery

22-6. an obstetrician skilled in breech deliveries; a gowned associate to aid in the delivery; an anesthesiologist; an individual able to perform infant resuscitation; someone available to render general assistance
p 394
vaginal delivery, breech presentation; breech presentation, vaginal delivery

22-7. a
p 394
perinatal mortality; perinatal morbidity; breech presentation, vaginal delivery

22-8. cesarean delivery; total breech extraction
p 394
cesarean delivery, breech presentation; breech extraction, total; fetal distress; breech presentation, cesarean delivery

22-9. a, d, e, f
p 394
breech extraction; breech presentation, complete; breech presentation, incomplete; episiotomy, breech presentation

22-10. a
pp 394–395
breech presentation, vaginal delivery; breech extraction; breech presentation, complete; breech presentation, incomplete

22-11. (1) Rotate the trunk until the anterior arm and shoulder appear at the vulva; deliver the anterior shoulder and arm; rotate the body in the reverse direction to deliver the other shoulder and arm; (2) deliver the posterior shoulder first by drawing the fetus over the maternal groin; then depress the fetal body to deliver the anterior shoulder and arm
pp 394–395
breech extraction, delivery of shoulders; breech presentation, vaginal delivery

22-12. a
p 397
breech extraction; breech presentation, vaginal delivery

22–13. a, c
p 397
breech extraction, delivery of arm; breech presentation, vaginal delivery

22–14. a, c, e
p 397
breech extraction; nuchal arm; breech presentation, vaginal delivery

22–15. a
p 397
Mauriceau maneuver, breech extraction; breech presentation, vaginal delivery

22–16. a, b, c, d, e, f
p 397
Mauriceau maneuver, breech extraction; delivery of the head; breech presentation, vaginal delivery

22–17. a, b, c
p 397
breech extraction, frank breech; Pinard maneuver; breech decomposition

22–18. a
p 397
breech extraction, forceps; Piper forceps; breech presentation, forceps delivery; breech presentation, vaginal delivery

22–19. Suspending the fetus keeps the arms out of the way and prevents excessive abduction of the trunk
p 397
breech extraction, forceps; Piper forceps; breech presentation, forceps delivery; breech presentation, vaginal delivery

22–20. a
p 397
breech presentation

22–21. a, c, d
pp 398–400
breech presentation, vaginal delivery; anesthesia, breech delivery

22–22. risks due to manipulation: infection, rupture of the uterus, laceration of the cervix, perineal tears, extension of the episiotomy; risks due to anesthesia: uterine atony, postpartum hemorrhage
p 400
breech extraction, maternal risks

22–23. 1 = a; 2 = b
p 400
breech extraction, maternal risks; breech extraction, fetal risks

22–24. a, b, c, d, e, f
pp 400–401
breech extraction, fetal risks

22–25. In a version operation, the presentation of the fetus is altered artificially.
p 401
breech presentation; version operation

22–26. b
p 403
podalic version

22–27. a
pp 401–402
cephalic version

22–28. c
p 401
external version

22–29. d
pp 401–403
internal version

22–30. c, d
p 401
breech presentation; external cephalic version

22–31. b, d
p 401
breech presentation; external cephalic version

22–32. a, b, c
pp 401–402
breech presentation; external cephalic version

22–33. b, c, d
p 403
breech presentation; internal podalic version

23–1. a, b, c, d
p 405
obstetric lacerations, perineum; rectocele; cystocele; uterine prolapse; vaginal relaxation

23–2. b, d, e
p 405
obstetric lacerations, vagina; pelvic relaxation; urinary incontinence; periurethral laceration

23–3. a, b, c
p 405
genital tract, lacerations; retained placental fragments

23–4. a, d, e
p 405–406
cervix, lacerations; obstetric hemorrhage; annular cervical detachment; leukorrhea

23–5. c, d, e
p 405–406
obstetric laceration, cervical; leukorrhea; vaginal packing; cautery, cervical; cryotherapy

23–6. a
p 406
uterine rupture

23–7. 1 = cesarean section or hysterotomy; repaired previous uterine rupture; myomectomy incision to endometrium; deep cornual resection; excision of uterine septum; 2 = instrumented abortion; sharp or blunt trauma; silent rupture during previous pregnancy
p 407 (Table 23–1)
uterine rupture, etiology; cesarean delivery; myomectomy; hysterotomy; abortion, induced; cornual resection

23–8. 1 = persistent, intense, spontaneous contractions; oxytocin/prostaglandin administration; intraamnionic injection of hypertonic solution; perforation by monitor catheter; external trauma, blunt or sharp; marked uterine overdistention; 2 = internal podalic version; difficult forceps delivery; breech extraction; fetal anomaly that overdistends the lower uterine segment; vigorous fundal pressure; difficult manual removal of placenta
p 407 (Table 23–1)
uterine rupture, etiology

23–9. d
pp 407–408
uterine rupture, etiology; placenta accreta

23–10. b
p 408
uterine rupture, complete

23–11. a
pp 407–408
uterine rupture, incomplete

23–12. b
p 408
uterine rupture, complete; uterine rupture, incomplete

23–13. d
p 408
uterine rupture; cesarean section scar, rupture; cesarean section scar, dehiscence

23–14. through the body of the pregnant uterus
p 407
cesarean section scar, classical; classical cesarean section

23–15. b, e
p 408
cesarean section, classical; cesarean section, lower segment; uterine rupture, cesarean delivery

23–16. b
p 408
cesarean section scar, healing

23–17. b, c, e
p 408
uterine rupture, complete; uterine rupture, incomplete; oxytocin; uteroabdominal pregnancy

23–18. a, b, c, d
p 409
uterine rupture, labor

23–19. a, b
p 409
uterine rupture, labor; hemoperitoneum

23–20. 50 and 75 percent
p 411
perinatal mortality, uterine rupture; uterine rupture, perinatal mortality

23–21. a, b
pp 411–413
uterine rupture, management; hysterectomy; obstetric hemorrhage; oxytocin

23–22. vesicovaginal
p 413
vesicovaginal fistula

24–1. 500 ml
p 415
postpartum hemorrhage; obstetric hemorrhage; labor, third stage

24–2. hemorrhage after the first 24 hours following birth
p 415
postpartum hemorrhage, late obstetric hemorrhage

24–3. b
p 415
postpartum hemorrhage; obstetric hemorrhage

24–4. a, b, c, d, e, f, g
p 415
postpartum hemorrhage; obstetric hemorrhage; hypotonic myometrium; uterine atony

24–5. c, d
p 415
postpartum hemorrhage, immediate; obstetric hemorrhage; uterine atony; hypotonic myometrium; cervix, lacerations; vagina, lacerations; retained placenta

24–6. a, b
pp 415–416
postpartum hemorrhage; postpartum hemorrhage, delayed; retained placenta; obstetric hemorrhage

24–7. b, c, d
pp 415–416
postpartum hemorrhage

24–8. b
pp 415–416
placental separation; labor, third stage

24–9. the condition (degree of contraction) of the uterus
p 416
postpartum hemorrhage; uterine atony; genital tract, laceration

24–10. a, b, c
pp 415–416
postpartum hemorrhage; labor, third stage; breech extraction

24–11. a, b
p 416
postpartum hemorrhage; labor, third stage; vaginal delivery

24–12. a, b, c
p 416
postpartum hemorrhage; labor, third stage; internal podalic version

24–13. a, b, c
p 416
postpartum hemorrhage; labor, third stage; previous cesarean section, vaginal delivery

24–14. failure in lactation, atrophy of the breasts, loss of pubic and axillary hair, superinvolution of the uterus, hypothyroidism, and adrenal cortical insufficiency, though pituitary symptoms may be delayed for years beyond the initial failure to lactate
p 417
Sheehan's syndrome; pituitary, anterior; obstetric hemorrhage

24–15. d
p 416
human immunodeficiency virus; transfusion; Sheehan's syndrome

24–16. a
p 417
mechanism of Duncan; labor, third stage

24–17. b
p 417
mechanism of Schultze; labor, third stage

24–18. a, b, c, d, e
p 417
third stage, management; placenta, separation; manual removal, placenta; postpartum hemorrhage

24–19. b, c, e
pp 417–418
postpartum hemorrhage; oxytocin; uterine massage; prostaglandins; uterine packing; bimanual compression, uterus

24–20. The posterior aspect of the uterus is massaged with the abdominal hand. The vaginal hand, which is formed into a fist with the knuckles in contact with the uterine wall, massages the anterior uterine surface.
p 418
bimanual compression, uterus; postpartum hemorrhage, management

24–21. perform bimanual uterine compression; obtain help; transfuse with whole blood; inspect the birth canal for lacerations; explore the uterine cavity for retained placental fragments and/or lacerations; add a second intravenous line so that oxytocin administration may be maintained along with blood transfusion; constantly monitor maternal cardiovascular status
pp 417–418
postpartum hemorrhage, management

24–22. a
pp 418–419
cervix, lacerations; vagina, lacerations; postpartum hemorrhage, management

24–23. Vigorous transfusion therapy should be begun before surgery to combat the often profound hypovolemia.
p 419
hysterectomy; postpartum hemorrhage, management; transfusion, indications

24–24. b
p 419
placenta percreta

24–25. a
p 419
placenta increta

24–26. d
p 419
placenta accreta, partial

24–27. partial or total absence of the decidua basalis; imperfect development of the fibrinoid layer (Nitabuch's layer)
p 419
placentation, abnormal; Nitabuch's layer; decidua basalis; fibrinoid layer; placenta accreta

24–28. b
p 419
abnormally adherent placenta; placenta accreta

24–29. a, b, c, d
pp 419–420
placenta accreta; placenta previa, multiparity, grand

24–30. a, b, d
p 420
placenta accreta; placenta previa; postpartum hemorrhage; obstetric hemorrhage

24–31. a
pp 420–421
placenta accreta; placenta increta; ultrasonography, hysterectomy

24–32. a, c, e
p 422
uterine inversion; obstetric hemorrhage; postpartum hemorrhage

24–33. obtain anesthesia consultation; if the inversion is fresh, attempt to manually reposition the uterus; institute two intravenous systems (lactated Ringer's and whole blood); remove the placenta only after the uterus is repositioned and transfusion has been initiated; manually compress the uterus; administer intravenous oxytocin (only after uterine reposition and placental removal)
p 422
uterine inversion; obstetric hemorrhage; postpartum hemorrhage; transfusion

24–34. a
p 423
uterine inversion; laparotomy

25–1. extraction of the fetus
p 425
forceps delivery

25–2. blade; shank; lock; handle
p 425
forceps

25–3. 1 = b; 2 = a
p 425
forceps, cephalic curve; forceps, pelvic curve

25–4. a
p 425
forceps, fenestrated

25–5. b
p 425
Kielland forceps

25–6. a
p 426 (Fig. 25–1)
Simpson forceps

25–7. b
p 425
Barton forceps

25–8. a
p 425 (Fig. 25–2)
Tucker-McLane forceps

25–9. none of the above
pp 437–438
vacuum extractor

25–10. 1 = perineal floor; 2 = anterior-posterior diameter or right or left occiput anterior position, not more than 45 degrees from the midline; 3 = vaginal introitus
pp 427–428
forceps delivery; outlet forceps delivery

25–11. a, b, d
pp 432–433
forceps delivery; midforceps delivery; midforceps delivery; engagement, fetal head

25–12. a
pp 432–433
forceps delivery; midforceps delivery

25–13. None, high forceps delivery has no place in modern obstetrics
p 426
forceps delivery; high forceps delivery

25–14. b
pp 435–437
midforceps delivery; perinatal morbidity, midforceps delivery; perinatal mortality, midforceps delivery; maternal morbidity, midforceps delivery

25–15. a, b, c, d
p 427
forceps delivery; low forceps delivery

25–16. traction; rotation
pp 426–427
forceps delivery

25–17. a, b, c
pp 426, 433
deep transverse arrest; midforceps delivery, deep transverse arrest; cesarean delivery; oxytocin stimulation; augmentation

25–18. a, b, c, d, e, f, g
p 427
forceps delivery, indications

25–19. a, b, c, d
pp 428–429
forceps delivery; outlet forceps delivery, elective

25–20. Prophylactic forceps have not proven to be of benefit to the fetus.
p 427
forceps delivery; forceps delivery, prophylactic; low forceps delivery, elective

25–21. b
p 427
forceps delivery; forceps delivery, prophylactic; low forceps delivery, elective; low-birthweight infant, forceps delivery

25–22. head engaged (preferably deeply engaged); vertex or chin anterior presentation; position of the head precisely known; cervix completely dilated; membranes ruptured; no disproportion between the size of the head and the pelvic inlet, midpelvis, or outlet
pp 427–428
forceps delivery

25–23. b, c
p 430
forceps delivery; low forceps delivery

25–24. a, b, c, d, e, f
pp 428–430
forceps delivery; fetus, position

25–25. 1 = a; 2 = b
pp 428–430
forceps delivery; pelvic application, forceps delivery

25–26. a
pp 428–430
forceps delivery; pelvic application, forceps delivery

25–27. insufficient expulsive forces; resistance of the perineum
pp 430–431
forceps delivery; low forceps delivery

25–28. a, b, e
p 431
forceps delivery; low forceps delivery

25–29. occiput anterior—blades should be equidistant from the sagittal suture; occiput posterior—blades should be equidistant from the midline of the face and brow
pp 430–432
forceps delivery; low forceps delivery

25–30. b
p 430
forceps delivery; low forceps delivery

25–31. a, b, d
pp 430–431
forceps delivery; low forceps delivery; Ritgen maneuver, episiotomy

25–32. a, b, c
pp 432–433
forceps delivery; midforceps delivery

25–33. a
p 433
forceps delivery; midforceps delivery; occiput posterior position

25–34. b
pp 433–434
fetal head, manual rotation; occiput posterior position, manual rotation

25–35. b
p 434
fetal head, manual rotation; occiput posterior position, manual rotation; forceps delivery

25–36. a
pp 433, 434
forceps delivery; midforceps delivery, occiput posterior position; Kielland forceps

25–37. a, b, d
pp 434–435
forceps delivery; midforceps rotation; Scanzoni maneuver

25–38. b, c, e
p 435
forceps delivery; midforceps rotation; Kielland forceps

25–39. a
p 435
rotation with Kielland forceps; special forceps maneuvers

25–40. a, b, c, d
pp 433–437
forceps delivery; midforceps delivery, indications; fetal distress, forceps delivery; umbilical cord prolapse, forceps delivery

25–41. 1 = a; 2 = b
pp 436–437
forceps delivery; maternal morbidity, midforceps delivery; perinatal morbidity, midforceps delivery

25–42. b
pp 436–437
forceps delivery; perinatal morbidity, midforceps delivery; cerebral palsy, midforceps delivery

25–43. hollow of the sacrum (also called the mentum posterior)
p 437
forceps delivery; face presentation

25–44. a
p 437
forceps delivery; trial forceps

25–45. b
p 437
forceps delivery; failed forceps

25–46. a
p 437
forceps delivery; trial forceps

25–47. malposition of the fetal head; incomplete dilation of the cervix; disproportion; inexperience of the operator
p 437
forceps delivery; failed forceps

25–48. a, b, c
p 437
vacuum extraction

25–49. scalp abrasion; scalp laceration; cephalohematoma; intracranial hemorrhage; death
pp 437–438
vacuum extraction; cephalohematoma; intracranial hemorrhage, neonatal

25–50. None of these procedures is commonly used in the United States
p 438
Dührssen incision

26–1. incisions in the abdominal and uterine walls
p 441
cesarean delivery

26–2. b
p 441
cesarean delivery

26–3. Cesarean delivery is used when it is believed that further delay would compromise the fetus and/or the mother, yet vaginal delivery is unlikely to be accomplished rapidly and safely.
p 441
cesarean delivery, indications

26–4. a, b, c, d
  p 441
  cesarean delivery, indications; breech presentation; fetal distress; dystocia; cesarean delivery, repeat

26–5. b
  p 441
  cesarean delivery; perinatal mortality

26–6. b
  p 442
  cesarean delivery; neonatal mortality; neonatal morbidity

26–7. b
  p 443
  breech presentation, vaginal delivery

26–8. e
  pp 442–443
  cesarean delivery, maternal mortality; cesarean delivery, maternal morbidity; cesarean delivery, neonatal morbidity; breech presentation; transverse lie

26–9. a, b
  pp 443–444
  cesarean delivery, repeat; repeat cesarean delivery, timing

26–10. the date of onset of the last menstrual period (LMP); results of serial fundal heights initiated in the first half of pregnancy; the time that the fetal heart was first heard with a fetoscope; the estimated size of the fetus
  p 444
  repeat cesarean delivery, timing; gestational age, determination

26–11. None of these is an *absolute* contraindication to cesarean delivery.
  p 445
  cesarean delivery, contraindications

26–12. b, d
  p 445
  vaginal delivery subsequent to cesarean delivery

26–13. The classical cesarean section incision is a vertical incision into the body of the uterus above the lower uterine segment and reaching the uterine fundus.
  p 445
  cesarean delivery; classical cesarean section, incision

26–14. a
  p 447
  technique of cesarean section; type of uterine incision

26–15. Neither of the above; Both should be low segment incisions and be equally strong.
  p 447
  technique of cesarean section; type of uterine incision

26–16. a
  p 447
  cesarean delivery, contraindications

26–17. b
  p 447
  cesarean delivery, contraindications

26–18. c
  p 447
  cesarean delivery, contraindications

26–19. a
  p 447
  cesarean delivery, contraindications

26–20. a
  p 447
  cesarean delivery, contraindications

26–21. c
  p 447
  cesarean delivery, contraindications

26–22. a
  pp 445, 447
  cesarean delivery, lower segment transverse incision

26–23. a, b, c, d
  p 447
  cesarean delivery, preparation

26–24. a, c
  p 447
  cesarean delivery, anesthesia; cesarean delivery, preparation; anesthesia, obstetrical

26–25. a
  p 447
  cesarean delivery, vertical abdominal incision

26–26. a
  p 447
  cesarean delivery, abdominal incision; Pfannenstiel incision

26–27. a, b, c, f
  p 447
  cesarean delivery, abdominal incision; Pfannenstiel incision

26–28. size and presenting part of the fetus; the degree and direction of uterine rotation
  p 447
  cesarean delivery

26–29. b
  p 447
  cesarean delivery, bowel laceration

26–30. The loose reflection of peritoneum above the bladder margin is grasped with forceps in the midline and sharply incised; scissors then develop the incision laterally, aiming cephalad at the lateral ends; the lower peritoneal flap is then bluntly dissected away from the myometrium; the separation of the bladder should not exceed 5 cm in depth.
  p 448
  cesarean delivery

26-31. a, b
p 448
cesarean delivery, uterine incision

26-32. The placenta must be either incised or detached. Especiallly if the placenta is incised, the cord should be clamped as soon as possible to minimize fetal hemorrhage.
pp 450–451
cesarean delivery, management of placenta; cesarean delivery, fetal hemorrhage

26-33. After the retractors are removed, a hand is slipped into the uterine cavity between the symphysis and the fetal head; the head is gently lifted while gentle transabdominal fundal pressure is exerted; the shoulders are then delivered using gentle traction and fundal pressure; the body follows readily.
p 450
cesarean delivery, delivery of infant

26-34. An assistant can apply upward pressure through the vagina with a sterile gloved hand.
p 450
cesarean delivery, cephalopelvic disproportion

26-35. c, d, e, f
p 450
cesarean delivery

26-36. b
pp 450–451
cesarean delivery, delivery of the placenta

26-37. a, c
p 450
cesarean delivery, uterine incision; multifetal pregnancy, cesarean delivery

26-38. advantages: ease of fundal massage; ease of visualization; exposure of adnexa; disadvantages: discomfort; possibility of vomiting with epidural or spinal anesthesia; displacement of a tubal ligation ligature
p 451
cesarean delivery, uterine repair

26-39. b
p 451
cesarean delivery, uterine repair

26-40. a, b, c
p 451
cesarean delivery, uterine repair

26-41. A running–lock suture is begun just beyond one angle of the incision; each stitch penetrates the entire thickness of the myometrium without withdrawing the needle after it has entered; one or two layers of suture can be utilized; the running–lock suture is continued just beyond the opposite angle of the incision.
p 451
cesarean delivery, uterine repair

26-42. b
pp 451–452
cesarean delivery, uterine repair

26-43. a
p 452
cesarean delivery, tubal sterilization

26-44. The entire fallopian tube is visualized; the mesosalpinx is perforated with a hemostat; the tube is ligated proximally and distally with 0 chromic suture to remove a segment at least 2 cm in length; tissue is sent for histologic examination; the site of the section is observed for bleeding.
p 452
cesarean delivery, tubal sterilization; tubal ligation

26-45. b, c, d
pp 452–453
cesarean delivery, abdominal closure

26-46. b
pp 452–453
cesarean delivery, abdominal closure

26-47. a
pp 452–453
cesarean delivery, abdominal closure

26-48. d
p 453
cesarean delivery, abdominal closure

26-49. c
p 453
cesarean delivery, abdominal closure

26-50. a, b, c, d, e
p 453
cesarean delivery; transverse lie; placenta previa; cervical carcinoma, invasive; uterine myoma; cesarean delivery, classical

26-51. e
p 453
cesarean delivery; cesarean delivery, classical

26-52. b
p 453
cesarean delivery, extraperitoneal

26-53. a, b, c, d, e, f
p 453
cesarean delivery, postmortem

26-54. a, b, c, d, g
pp 453–454
cesarean hysterectomy, indications; uterine atony; placenta increta; intrauterine infection

26-55. damage to the urinary tract; increased blood loss
pp 453–454
cesarean hysterectomy

26–56. b
p 454
cesarean delivery, blood loss

26–57. c
p 454
cesarean hysterectomy, blood loss

26–58. b, e
p 454
cesarean hysterectomy

26–59. b
p 454
cesarean hysterectomy; uterine artery, anatomic relationships; ureteral injury, cesarean hysterectomy

26–60. the uterine arteries and veins
p 454
cesarean hysterectomy, supracervical

26–61. a, b, c, d
p 454
cesarean hysterectomy, total

26–62. An "open" vagina may promote drainage and thereby, possibly, avoid hematoma or abscess formation.
p 454
cesarean hysterectomy; vaginal cuff

26–63. c
p 455
cesarean hysterectomy; reperitonealization

26–64. a, c, d
p 455
cesarean delivery, preoperative care

26–65. c, d
p 455
cesarean delivery, fluid management

26–66. blood loss through the vagina or bleeding concealed in the uterus
p 455
cesarean delivery, blood loss; concealed hemorrhage, cesarean delivery; external hemorrhage, cesarean delivery

26–67. d
p 455
cesarean delivery, recovery room care

26–68. a, b, c, d
p 455
cesarean delivery, postoperative care

26–69. meperidine 50 to 100 mg (depending on the size of the patient) every 3 hours as needed; morphine 10 mg every 3 hours as needed
p 455
cesarean delivery, postoperative care; analgesia, cesarean delivery

26–70. hourly for 4 hours, then every 4 hours
p 455
cesarean delivery, postoperative care

26–71. a, b, c, e, f, g
p 456
cesarean delivery, postoperative care

26–72. b
pp 455–456
cesarean delivery, postoperative care; cesarean delivery, management of fluids

26–73. b
p 456
cesarean delivery, postoperative care; oliguria, cesarean delivery

26–74. a
p 456
cesarean delivery, postoperative care

26–75. b
p 456
cesarean delivery, postoperative care

26–76. a
p 456
cesarean delivery, postoperative care

26–77. c
p 456
cesarean delivery, postoperative care

26–78. b, c
p 456
cesarean delivery, postoperative care

26–79. a
p 456
cesarean delivery, postoperative care

26–80. c
p 456
cesarean delivery, postoperative care

26–81. d
p 456
cesarean delivery, postoperative care

26–82. d
p 456
cesarean delivery, postoperative care; anemia; transfusion, cesarean delivery; transfusion, postoperative

26–83. b, c, d
p 456
cesarean delivery, postoperative care; breast feeding; bromocriptine

26–84. fourth or fifth
p 456
cesarean delivery, postoperative care

26-85. For the first week, activities should be limited to self-care and care of the infant with assistance; the return visit for postpartum evaluation should be during the third postpartum week.
p 456
cesarean delivery, postpartum care

26-86. b, c
p 456
cesarean delivery, prophylactic antibiotics; infection, cesarean delivery; febrile morbidity, cesarean delivery

27-1. the infection of the genital tract after delivery
p 461
puerperal infection

27-2. a, b
p 461
puerperal infection; puerperal morbidity

27-3. a, b, c, d
p 461
puerperal morbidity; puerperium, fever; breast engorgement

27-4. a, c, d, e
pp 461-462
postpartum infection; puerperal infection; vaginal examination, intrapartum; obstetrical lacerations; rupture of membranes

27-5. None of the mentioned antepartum factors has been clearly shown to predispose to puerperal infection.
p 462
puerperal infection; transferrin; anemia; nutrition, pregnancy; coitus, pregnancy

27-6. a, b, c
p 462
puerperal infection; vaginal examination, intrapartum; obstetrical trauma

27-7. The postpartum genital tract has several areas that are essentially open wounds, and are consequently susceptible to the entry of infectious organisms. These are the site of placental attachment and the cervix or the birth canal which may have lacerations and/or an episiotomy incision.
pp 462-463
puerperal infection; obstetrical lacerations; implantation site, placenta; episiotomy

27-8. a, b
pp 464-465
puerperal infection; obstetrical lacerations; vagina, lacerations; cervix, lacerations

27-9. a, f
pp 462-463, 465
metritis; postpartum fever; puerperal infection; breast feeding

27-10. b
pp 470-471
thrombophlebitis; ovarian veins

27-11. a
p 471
thrombophlebitis; ovarian veins

27-12. c
p 471
thrombophlebitis; ovarian veins

27-13. a, c
p 471
thrombophlebitis; puerperal infection; pulmonary embolism

27-14. a
pp 472-473
thromboembolism; sudden death, maternal; cor pulmonale; septic thromboembolism

27-15. a, b, c, d
pp 472-473
metritis; pulmonary embolism; sepsis; puerperal infection; pneumonia; thrombus

27-16. a, b
pp 472-473
puerperal infection; blood culture; bacteriology, puerperal infection

27-17. b
p 463
puerperal infection; bacteriology, puerperal infection

27-18. c
p 463
puerperal infections; bacteriology; common pathogens

27-19. a
p 463
puerperal infections; bacteriology; common pathogens

27-20. b
p 463
puerperal infections; bacteriology; common pathogens

27-21. a, b, c, d, e
pp 463-464
cephalosporins; clindamycin; gentamicin; chloramphenicol; vibramycin; pseudomembranous colitis

27-22. a
p 467
pelvic cellulitis, parametritis

27-23. a, b, c
pp 464-465
infections of the perineum; vagina and cervix; necrotizing fascitis

27-24. a, b, c, d, f
pp 468-469
pelvic cellulitis; parametritis; puerperal infection; puerperium, morbidity; puerperium, fever

27–25. a, b, c, d
pp 467–468
puerperal infection; pelvic cellulitis; parametritis; pelvic abscess; space of Retzius; cul-de-sac of Douglas, abscess

27–26. b, c
p 468
toxic shock syndrome; Staphylococcus *sp.*

27–27. a, b, c
pp 468–469
parametrial phlegmon; pelvic cellulitis; metritis

27–28. a
p 469
parametrial phlegmon

27–29. a, b, c
pp 470–472
septic pelvic thrombophlebitis

27–30. a, b, c, d, e, f
pp 472–473
septic shock

27–31. a
p 475
postpartum fever; puerperal infection

28–1. b
p 477
thromboembolism; venous thrombosis

28–2. stasis
p 477
thromboembolic disease; stasis, vascular; venous thrombosis

28–3. b
p 477
thromboembolic disease

28–4. a
p 477
ambulation, puerperium; thromboembolic disease

28–5. a
p 477
thrombophlebitis; venous thrombosis

28–6. b
p 477
phlebothrombosis; venous thrombosis

28–7. b
p 477
venous thrombosis, superficial; venous thrombosis, deep; pulmonary embolism

28–8. d
p 477
deep vein thrombosis

28–9. a, d, e
p 477
venous thrombosis, deep; venous thrombosis, puerperium; venous thrombosis, antepartum; anticoagulation; milk leg

28–10. b
p 478
warfarin (coumadin); coagulation factors

28–11. b
p 478
warfarin (coumadin); congenital malformations

28–12. a
p 478
heparin; thrombocytopenia

28–13. b
p 478
warfarin (coumadin); placental transfer

28–14. a
p 480
heparin; placental transfer

28–15. c
p 479
warfarin (coumadin); venous thrombosis, deep

28–16. b, c
pp 478–479
pelvic vein thrombosis; ovarian vein thrombophlebitis, heparin

28–17. a, e, f
p 479
heparin; warfarin (coumadin); protamine sulfate; coagulation factors; fetus, intrapartum hemorrhage

28–18. dose, route, and time of administration of heparin relative to delivery; magnitude of incisions and obstetric lacerations; intensity of myometrial contraction upon completion of delivery of fetus and placenta (presence or absence of uterine atony); presence of other coagulation defects
p 480
anticoagulation, intrapartum; heparin

28–19. a
p 481
pulmonary embolism; inferior vena cava, ligation

28–20. 1 in 2700 to 1 in 7000
p 479
thromboembolic disease; disorder of the puerperium

28–21. a, b, d, e
p 479
pulmonary embolism

28–22. b
p 479
pulmonary embolism

28–23. a, c, e
pp 479–480
heparin; warfarin (coumadin); pulmonary embolism

28–24. Ligation of the inferior vena cava below the level of the renal veins but above the entry of the right ovarian vein plus ligation of the left ovarian vein below its entry into the left renal vein is usually indicated
p 481
pulmonary embolism, recurrent; inferior vena cava, ligation

28–25. b, c, d
p 481
subinvolution; metritis; ergonovine; methylergonovine

28–26. b
pp 481–482
cervical erosions, puerperium

28–27. abnormal involution of the placental site; a retained portion of the placenta forms a placental polyp, which detaches from the myometrium and results in bleeding
p 483
postpartum hemorrhage, delayed; placental polyp; involution of the placental site, abnormal

28–28. b
p 483
oxytocin; postpartum hemorrhage, delayed

28–29. a, b, c
p 482
hematomas, puerperium; vagina, hematoma; vulva, hematoma

28–30. a, b, c, d, e
p 483
bladder function, puerperium; urinary tract infection, puerperium

28–31. a, d
pp 483–484
breast engorgement; breast fever; breast binders

28–32. a, c, d
p 484
lactation, suppression; bromocriptine

28–33. b, c, e
p 485
mastitis; Staphylococcus aureus; puerperal fever; breast engorgement

28–34. a
p 485
mastitis

28–35. a, c, d
p 485
mastitis, suppurative; bacterial interference; staphylococcal infection; epidemic, nursery

28–36. b
p 485
puerperal infection; mastitis

28–37. a, b, c, e
p 485
mastitis; staphylococcal infection; penicillin G; mastitis, suppurative; breast abscess; nursing, mastitis

28–38. the clogging of a duct and the consequent accumulation of milk in one or more breast lobules
pp 485–486
galactocele

28–39. b, c, d
p 486
polymastia; nipples; nipples, depressed; nipples, fissures; supernumary breasts

28–40. a
p 486
Chiari-Frommel syndrome; pituitary adenoma; amenorrhea; estrogen; galactorrhea

28–41. a, b, d
p 487
footdrop; obstetrical paralysis

28–42. b
p 487
symphysis pubis, separation in labor; sacroiliac synchondroses, separation in labor

29–1. b
p 489
abortion, definition

29–2. b
p 501
abortion; elective abortion

29–3. b
p 499
abortion; therapeutic abortion

29–4. c
p 501
abortion; elective abortion

29–5. a
p 489
abortion

29–6. Viability may be defined as a reasonable potential for subsequent survival if the fetus is removed from the uterus
p 489
viability, definition; abortion, viability

29–7. termination of pregnancy before 38 weeks of gestation but after the fetus has achieved some potential for survival
p 489
prematurity; preterm

29-8. 1 = 20 completed weeks; 2 = 500 g
p 489
abortion, definition

29-9. c
p 489
immaturity; prematurity; gestational age

29-10. failure to include (or recognize) early spontaneous abortions; inclusion of actual induced abortions as early spontaneous abortions; 40 percent may be more accurate
p 489
abortion, incidence; spontaneous abortion

29-11. a, b, c, d
p 491
abortion, spontaneous

29-12. a, b, c, e
p 491
abortion, spontaneous; chromosomal anomalies, abortion; fetal development, abnormal

29-13. 1 = b; 2 = a
p 491
abortion, spontaneous; chromosomal anomalies, abortion; trisomy; monosomy

29-14. a
p 492
abortion, spontaneous; maternal factors

29-15. a, b, c, d
pp 492–493
abortion, spontaneous; uterine environment, abortion

29-16. b; c is still not certain but possible; **e**
p 493
abortion, spontaneous; infection, abortion; toxoplasmosis; Listeria monocytogenes

29-17. b
p 493
abortion, spontaneous

29-18. a, c
p 493
abortion, spontaneous; fetal well-being; hormone levels, spontaneous abortion

29-19. a, b, c
p 493
abortion, spontaneous; alcohol, abortion; smoking, abortion; nutrition, pregnancy

29-20. a
pp 493–494
abortion, spontaneous; immunologic factors, abortion

29-21. b, c, d
p 495
abortion, spontaneous; laparotomy, spontaneous abortion; peritonitis, abortion; myomas, abortion

29-22. a, b
p 494
abortion; immunological factors

29-23. a, c, d
p 495
abortion; DES

29-24. a, b, c, d
pp 489–490
abortion, pathology; blighted ovum; fetus papyraceus; fetus compressus; multifetal pregnancy, fetal demise; twin pregnancy, fetal demise

29-25. a
pp 496–497
abortion, threatened

29-26. c
p 497
abortion, incomplete

29-27. b
p 497
abortion, inevitable

29-28. e
p 498
abortion; recurrent spontaneous abortion

29-29. d
pp 497–498
abortion, missed

29-30. a, c, d
pp 496–497
abortion, threatened; antepartum bleeding

29-31. b, c, d
p 497
abortion, threatened; prematurity; low birth weight; perinatal death, abortion

29-32. b
p 497
abortion, inevitable; rupture of the membranes, preterm

29-33. a, b
p 497
abortion, incomplete

29-34. c
pp 497–498
abortion, missed; fetal death

29-35. a
p 497
abortion, threatened; antepartum bleeding

29-36. 1 = a; 2 = b
p 497
abortion, threatened

29-37. a, b, c
p 497
abortion, threatened; pain, threatened abortion

29-38. b, c, e, f
pp 496–497
abortion, threatened; threatened abortion, management; hCG, serial determinations; progesterone

29-39. a
pp 496–497
abortion, threatened; ultrasonography, abortion

29-40. b
p 497
abortion, threatened; antepartum bleeding; pain, threatened abortion

29-41. a, b, d
p 497
abortion, inevitable; rupture of the membranes; abortion, septic

29-42. a, d
p 497
abortion, incomplete; hemorrhage, abortion; suction curettage

29-43. b
p 497
abortion, missed

29-44. three or more consecutive spontaneous abortions
p 498
abortion, recurrent spontaneous abortion

29-45. a
pp 492–493
cytogenetic abnormalities, spontaneous abortion; abortion, spontaneous

29-46. b
p 493
maternal factors, spontaneous abortion; abortion, spontaneous

29-47. a, c
p 498
abortion; recurrent spontaneous abortion

29-48. a, b, c, d
p 498
incompetent cervix; abortion, habitual

29-49. a
pp 498–499
incompetent cervix; abortion, habitual

29-50. a, b
pp 498–499
incompetent cervix; abortion, habitual; stilbestrol, in utero exposure; cervix, trauma

29-51. b
pp 498–499
incompetent cervix; abortion, habitual

29-52. bleeding; uterine contractions
p 499
cerclage, contraindications; incompetent cervix; abortion, habitual

29-53. a, b, c, e
p 499
incompetent cervix; cerclage; Shirodkar procedure; McDonald procedure; abortion, habitual

29-54. rupture of the uterus or cervix
p 499
incompetent cervix; uterus, rupture; cerclage, complications; abortion, habitual

29-55. b
p 499
incompetent cervix; cerclage; Shirodkar procedure; McDonald procedure; abortion, habitual

29-56. when the pregnancy may threaten the life of the woman or seriously impair her health; when the pregnancy has resulted from rape or incest; when continuation of the pregnancy is likely to result in the birth of a child with severe physical deformities or mental retardation
pp 499, 501
abortion, therapeutic

29-57. b
pp 499, 501
abortion, elective

29-58. a, b, c, d, e
p 502
curettage, complications; suction curettage; abortion, transvaginal

29-59. a
pp 502–503
suction curettage; dilation and curettage

29-60. b
pp 502–503
suction curettage; dilation and curettage

29-61. a, b, c, d
p 503
abortion, transcervical; laminaria, cervical dilation; prostaglandins, cervical softening; paracervical block anesthesia

29-62. Any instrument introduced into the uterine cavity may cause perforation
pp 503–504
uterine perforation; abortion, transvaginal

29-63. adequate dilation of the cervix; uterine evacuation without perforation; removal of all the products of conception but not the decidua basalis
p 504
abortion, transvaginal; morbidity, abortion

29-64. a, b, c
p 504
abortion, transcervical; uterine perforation

29-65. a, d
p 504
abortion, transcervical; uterine perforation

29-66. a, b, c
p 504
abortion, transcervical; uterine synechiae; incompetent cervix; comsump-
tive coagulopathy

29-67. a, b, c, d, e
p 504
menstrual aspiration

29-68. performing the procedure on a woman who is not pregnant; missing the implanted zygote with the small Karman curet; failure to recognize an ectopic pregnancy; uterine perforation
p 504
menstrual aspiration; uterine perforation; incomplete abortion

29-69. a
p 505
Rh isoimmunization, abortion; Rho (D) immune globulin, prophylaxis

29-70. b
p 505
menstrual aspiration

29-71. a, b, c, d
p 505
hysterotomy; hysterectomy; second trimester abortion

29-72. b, c, e
p 505
oxytocin; abortion, induction

29-73. b, d, e
p 506
prostaglandins; abortion, induction

29-74. b, c, d
p 506
hyperosmotic solutions, abortion; abortion, induction

29-75. a, b, c, d, e, f, g, h, i, j, k
p 506
hyperosmotic solutions, abortion; hypertonic saline, side effects; abor-
tion, induction

29-76. b, c, d
pp 506–507
abortion, sequelae; maternal mortality, abortion; Asherman's syndrome;
incompetent cervix

29-77. a, b, c
p 501
elective termination of pregnancy

29-78. uterine evacuation; administration of antibiotics
p 507
septic abortion

29-79. a, b, c, d, e
p 507
septic shock

29-80. a, b, d
p 501
septic shock

29-81. perfusion of vital organs
p 507
septic shock

29-82. b, c, d
p 501
septic shock; renal failure

30-1. b
p 511
ectopic pregnancy

30-2. a, b, c, d, e
p 511
ectopic pregnancy; etiology; pelvic inflammatory disease; endometriosis;
infertility

30-3. a
p 511
ectopic pregnancy; hysterectomy

30-4. c
p 511
ectopic pregnancy, incidence

30-5. increased prevalence of sexually transmitted diseases; popularity of intrauterine devices; unsuccessful previous tubal sterilization; induced abortion followed by infection; fertility induced by ovulatory agents; previous pelvic surgery, specifically tubal surgery; in utero exposure to stilbestrol; better and earlier diagnostic techniques for ectopic pregnancy
p 511–512
ectopic pregnancy, etiology

30-6. b
pp 523–526
ectopic pregnancy, management

30-7. a, b, c, d
p 513
ectopic pregnancy, locations; tubal pregnancy

30-8. b, c, d
pp 513–514
ectopic pregnancy; tubal pregnancy, implantation

30-9. a, b, c
p 514
ectopic pregnancy, uterine changes

30–10. a, c, d
p 514
ectopic pregnancy, endometrial changes; Arias-Stella reaction

30–11. a
p 514
ectopic pregnancy, endometrial changes; Arias-Stella reaction

30–12. a, b, c, d
p 514
ectopic pregnancy, endometrial changes

30–13. separation of the products of conception from the implantation site and extrusion of the abortus through the fimbriated end of the oviduct
pp 514–515
tubal abortion; tubal pregnancy

30–14. a, b, d, e
pp 514–515
tubal abortion; ectopic pregnancy

30–15. a, e
p 515
ectopic pregnancy; tubal rupture; lithopedion; abdominal pregnancy

30–16. a, b, c
p 515
ectopic pregnancy; broad ligament pregnancy; intraligamentous pregnancy

30–17. implants within the segment of the tube that penetrates the uterine wall
p 515
ectopic pregnancy; interstitial pregnancy

30–18. a, c, d, e
p 515
interstitial pregnancy; ectopic pregnancy; cornual; pregnancy

30–19. a
p 515
ectopic pregnancy; cornual pregnancy; interstitial pregnancy; hysterectomy

30–20. a combined pregnancy
p 516
ectopic pregnancy; multifetal pregnancy; combined pregnancy

30–21. a, d
p 516
combined pregnancy; ectopic pregnancy; multifetal pregnancy

30–22. b
p 516
tuboabdominal pregnancy; ectopic pregnancy

30–23. a
p 516
tubouterine pregnancy; ectopic pregnancy

30–24. c
p 516
tuboovarian pregnancy; ectopic pregnancy

30–25. a, b, c, d, e, f
p 517
ruptured tubal pregnancy, signs; ruptured tubal pregnancy, symptoms; tubal pregnancy

30–26. blood irritating the cervical sensory nerves on the inferior surface of the diaphragm
p 517
tubal pregnancy; ruptured tubal pregnancy, symptoms; hemoperitoneum; shoulder pain

30–27. b
pp 517–518
ruptured tubal pregnancy, symptoms; pain, tubal pregnancy; hemoperitoneum

30–28. *None* of these rules out the presence of a ruptured tubal pregnancy.
p 518
ruptured tubal pregnancy, diagnosis; amenorrhea; vaginal bleeding; pregnancy test

30–29. a, b, c
p 518
hypovolemia, detection; ruptured tubal pregnancy; hemorrhage

30–30. normocytic
p 519
ruptured tubal pregnancy; anemia

30–31. a, b, c, d, e
p 519
pregnancy tests; ectopic pregnancy

30–32. acute or chronic salpingitis; threatened or incomplete abortion of an intrauterine pregnancy; torsion of an ovarian cyst; appendicitis; gastroenteritis; pain from an intrauterine device; rupture of a corpus luteum or other ovarian cyst with intraperitoneal bleeding
p 522
ruptured tubal pregnancy, differential diagnosis; abortion; appendicitis; ovarian cyst; corpus luteum cyst; intrauterine device

30–33. b, d
p 522
ruptured tubal pregnancy, differential diagnosis; salpingitis

30–34. c, e
p 522
ruptured tubal pregnancy, differential diagnosis; abortion, intrauterine pregnancy; decidual cast; decidual reaction, ectopic pregnancy

30–35. b
p 522
ectopic pregnancy, diagnosis; multifetal pregnancy, ectopic

30–36. a, b, d
p 520
ectopic pregnancy; ultrasound; serial hCG determinations

30–37. c
p 523
ruptured tubal pregnancy, differential diagnosis; twisted ovarian cyst

30–38. a
pp 522–523
ruptured tubal pregnancy, differential diagnosis

30–39. b
p 523
ruptured tubal pregnancy, differential diagnosis; appendicitis

30–40. a, b, c
pp 523–526
ruptured tubal pregnancy, management

30–41. a
p 523
ruptured tubal pregnancy, differential diagnosis; follicular cyst; corpus luteum cyst

30–42. a, c
p 523
ruptured tubal pregnancy, differential diagnosis; intrauterine device, tubal sterilization

30–43. b
p 520
ectopic pregnancy; other diagnostic aids

30–44. d
p 521
tubal pregnancy, diagnosis; culdocentesis

30–45. b
p 521
tubal pregnancy, diagnosis; curettage

30–46. a
p 521
tubal pregnancy, diagnosis; curettage

30–47. a
p 521
tubal pregnancy, diagnosis; curettage

30–48. b
p 521
tubal pregnancy, diagnosis; colpotomy

30–49. a, b, d
p 522
tubal pregnancy, diagnosis; laparoscopy

30–50. b
pp 521–522
tubal pregnancy, diagnosis; colpotomy; laparoscopy

30–51. d
p 521
tubal pregnancy, diagnosis; laparotomy

30–52. d
p 513
tubal pregnancy, mortality

30–53. b
p 513
tubal pregnancy, sterilization

30–54. b, c, d
pp 523–526
tubal pregnancy, management; salpingectomy; cornual resection; infertility rate; oophorectomy

30–55. b
p 526
tubal pregnancy, management; methotrexate

30–56. a
p 526
autotransfusion; ruptured tubal pregnancy, management

30–57. b
p 526
autotransfusion; ruptured tubal pregnancy, management

30–58. b
p 526
autotransfusion; ruptured tubal pregnancy, management

30–59. b, c, d
p 526
Rh isoimmunization; ruptured tubal pregnancy, management

30–60. b
pp 526–527
abdominal pregnancy

30–61. b, c, d, e
p 528
abdominal pregnancy; lithopedion; adipocere; congenital malformations, abdominal pregnancy

30–62. a, b, c, d, e
p 528
abdominal pregnancy, diagnosis; abdominal pregnancy, symptoms

30–63. a, c, d, e
pp 528–529
abdominal pregnancy, diagnosis; abdominal pregnancy, physical findings

30–64. b
p 529
abdominal pregnancy, diagnosis

30–65. b
p 529
abdominal pregnancy, diagnosis; oxytocin

30–66. a
p 529
abdominal pregnancy, diagnosis; ultrasonography; isotope localization; x-ray

30–67. a, b, c
pp 529–530
abdominal pregnancy, management; hemorrhage

30–68. infection; abscess; intestinal obstruction; adhesions; wound dehiscence
pp 529–530
abdominal pregnancy, complications of management

30–69. detect and manage ectopic pregnancy in the first trimester
p 530
abdominal pregnancy, management; tubal pregnancy, management

30–70. the fallopian tube on the affected side is intact; the fetal sac occupies the position of the ovary; the ovary is connected to the uterus by the ovarian ligament; definite ovarian tissue is found in the wall of the sac
p 530
ovarian pregnancy, Spiegelberg criteria

30–71. a, b
p 530
ovarian pregnancy

30–72. within the cervix below the internal os
p 530
cervical pregnancy

30–73. a, c, d
pp 530–531
cervical pregnancy, symptoms; cervical pregnancy, management

31–1. d
p 533
placenta succenturiata; placental abnormalities

31–2. a
p 533
placenta bipartita; placental abnormalities

31–3. b
p 533
placenta duplex; placental abnormalities

31–4. succenturiate lobe (accessory lobe)
p 533
succenturiate lobe; placenta succenturiata

31–5. b
p 533
succenturiate lobe; placenta succenturiata

31–6. c
p 533
succenturiate lobe; postpartum hemorrhage

31–7. a, c, d
p 533
ring-shaped placenta; fetal growth retardation; antepartum bleeding; postpartum bleeding

31–8. a, b, e
p 533
membranaceous placenta; placenta diffusa, retained placenta

31–9. a placenta in which the central portion is missing
p 533
fenestrated placenta

31–10. a
p 533
extrachorial placenta

31–11. a
pp 533–534
circumvallate placenta

31–12. b
pp 533–534
circummarginate placenta, marginate

31–13. a
pp 533–534
circumvallate placenta

31–14. b
p 533
marginate placenta

31–15. a
pp 533–534
circumvallate placenta; fetal malformations; antepartum hemorrhage

31–16. b
p 534
placenta, weight

31–17. a, d
p 534
placental enlargement; syphilis; Rh sensitization; erythroblastosis fetalis

31–18. parts of a normal placenta or a succenturiate lobe that is retained after delivery
p 534
placental polyp; succenturiate lobe; retained placenta

31–19. Changes associated with trophoblastic aging; impairment of the uteroplacental circulation causing infarction
p 535
placental infarcts; placenta, degeneration

31–20. a, b, c
p 535
placental infarcts; placenta, degeneration

31–21. a, e
p 535
placental infarcts; placenta, degeneration

31–22. c
 pp 535–536
 placental calcification; ultrasonography

31–23. a
 p 536
 villous arterial thrombosis

31–24. a, b, d
 p 536
 chorionic villi, hypertrophy; diabetes, placental effect; erythroblastosis (hydropic type); fetal congestive heart failure

31–25. a, b
 pp 536–537
 syncytial knot; placental abnormalities

31–26. b
 p 537
 umbilical cord, abnormalities; long cord; knot, umbilical cord

31–27. b
 p 537
 umbilical cord, abnormalities; long cord; umbilical cord prolapse

31–28. a
 p 537
 umbilical cord, abnormalities; short cord; placental abruption

31–29. a
 p 537
 umbilical cord, abnormalities; short cord; intrafunicular hemorrhage

31–30. a, b, c, d, f
 p 538
 umbilical cord, abnormalities; velamentous insertion; vasa previa; battledore placenta

31–31. c, d
 p 539
 umbilical cord, abnormalities

31–32. abnormalities of chorionic villi consisting of varying degrees of trophoblast proliferation and edema of the villous stroma
 p 445
 hydatidiform mole; neoplastic trophoblast

31–33. a, b
 p 540
 invasive mole; neoplastic trophoblast

31–34. b
 p 540
 choriocarcinoma; neoplastic trophoblast

31–35. A neoplastic trophoblast without stroma spreads locally or disseminates beyond the original site of zygote implantation and proliferates rapidly.
 p 540
 choriocarcinoma

31–36. a
 pp 540–541
 invasive mole; chorioadenoma destruens

31–37. b
 p 540
 choriocarcinoma; chorionepithelioma

31–38. a, b, c
 p 541
 hydatidiform mole

31–39. Chorionic villi are converted to a mass of clear vesicles that often hang in clusters from thin pedicles. The mass may grow to the size of an advanced pregnancy.
 p 541
 hydatidiform mole, complete; mole

31–40. a
 pp 541–542
 hydatidiform mole, complete

31–41. b
 p 542
 hydatidiform mole, partial

31–42. a
 pp 541–542
 hydatidiform mole, complete

31–43. b
 p 542
 hydatidiform mole, partial

31–44. a
 pp 541–542
 hydatidiform mole, complete

31–45. b
 pp 541–542
 hydatidiform mole, partial

31–46. a, b
 pp 541–542
 hydatidiform mole, complete; hydatidiform mole, partial

31–47. moderate hydropic swelling of some villi without significant trophoblastic proliferation
 p 542
 molar degeneration

31–48. b
 p 542
 hydatidiform mole; choriocarcinoma

31–49. b, c, e
 p 542
 theca lutein cysts; hydatidiform mole

31–50. 1 per 1,500 to 2,000 pregnancies
 p 542
 hydatidiform mole

31–51. c
 p 542
 hydatidiform mole

31–52. a
 p 543
 hydatidiform mole

31–53. a, b, c, d, e
 pp 543–544
 hydatidiform mole, diagnosis

31–54. uterine bleeding
 pp 543–544
 hydatidiform mole; uterine bleeding

31–55. c, d
 pp 543–544
 hydatidiform mole; uterine bleeding; concealed hemorrhage

31–56. a
 p 544
 hydatidiform mole; gestational age

31–57. multiple lutein cysts
 p 542
 hydatidiform mole; theca lutein cysts

31–58. b
 p 544
 hydatidiform mole; hypertension

31–59. b, c
 p 544
 hydatidiform mole; hyperthyroidism, hydatidiform mole; TSH, hydatidiform mole

31–60. b
 p 545
 hydatidiform mole; spontaneous expulsion

31–61. a, b, c, d
 p 545
 hydatidiform mole; myomata; multifetal pregnancy; hydramnios; gestational age, determination

31–62. b
 p 545
 hydatidiform mole; ultrasonography

31–63. a, d
 p 545
 hydatidiform mole; hCG, hydatidiform mole

31–64. a, b, c, d, e, f
 pp 543–545
 hydatidiform mole, complete; hCG, hydatidiform mole; fetal heart sounds; vaginal bleeding, pregnancy; hydatidiform mole, ultrasonography; preeclampsia, hydatidiform mole

31–65. 0 percent
 p 545
 hydatidiform mole

31–66. a
 p 545
 hydatidiform mole; choriocarcinoma

31–67. c, d
 pp 545–546
 hydatidiform mole, treatment

31–68. It allows a better assessment of malignant predisposition and prediction of subsequent biologic behavior of tissue that is left in the uterus.
 p 547
 hydatidiform mole

31–69. laparotomy
 pp 547, 548
 hydatidiform mole; obstetrical hemorrhage, hydatidiform mole

31–70. a, b
 p 547
 hydatidiform mole; oxytocin

31–71. a, b
 p 547
 hydatidiform mole; prostaglandin

31–72. a
 p 548
 hydatidiform mole; hysterectomy

31–73. detection of any change suggestive of trophoblastic malignancy
 p 548
 hydatidiform mole; hydatidiform mole, follow-up

31–74. hCG levels
 pp 548–549
 hydatidiform mole, follow-up; hCG, hydatidiform mole

31–75. a, b, c, d
 p 549
 hydatidiform mole; actinomycin D; methotrexate; trophoblastic disease, treatment; hydatidiform mole, follow-up; persistent trophoblastic disease

31–76. b, c
 p 549
 persistent trophoblastic disease; curettage

31–77. a
 p 549
 persistent trophoblastic disease; hysterectomy

31–78. c
 p 549
 persistent trophoblastic disease; chemotherapy

31–79. a, d, e
p 549
persistent trophoblastic disease; hCG

31–80. b
p 550
hydatidiform mole; choriocarcinoma

31–81. d
p 550
choriocarcinoma

31–82. b
p 550
choriocarcinoma; theca lutein cysts

31–83. a, b, c, d
pp 550–551
choriocarcinoma

31–84. b
p 551
choriocarcinoma

31–85. a, c, d
p 551
choriocarcinoma; hydatidiform mole; hCG, hydatidiform mole

31–86. e
p 552
persistent trophoblastic disease

31–87. a, b, c, d
p 552
choriocarcinoma; methotrexate; radiation therapy; actinomycin D

31–88. 24-hour urine hCG level less than 100,000 IU; duration of disease less than 4 months; no brain or liver metastases
p 550
choriocarcinoma, low risk

31–89. b
pp 551–552
choriocarcinoma, treatment

31–90. b, c, d
p 552
invasive mole; methotrexate; choriocarcinoma

31–91. a, b, e
p 552
hemangioma, placenta; chorioangioma, placenta

31–92. malignant melanoma
p 553
placenta, metastatic tumors; melanoma

31–93. b, c, d
pp 553–554
amnion; amnionic caruncles; amnion nodosum

31–94. excess amnionic fluid (>2,000 mL)
p 554
hydramnios

31–95. a, b, c, d
pp 554–555
hydramnios

31–96. a, b, c, d, e, i
p 555
hydramnios; esophageal atresia; multifetal pregnancy; anencephaly; diabetes, maternal; erythroblastosis fetalis, hydropic; spina bifida

31–97. a, b, c, d, e
p 555
hydramnios

31–98. dyspnea; difficulty in palpating fetal small parts; difficulty in hearing fetal heart tones; pain with rapidly increasing uterine size; edema of the lower extremities, the vulva, and the abdominal wall
p 555
hydramnios

31–99. a, b, c, d
p 557
hydramnios

31–100. d
p 557
hydramnios; amniocentesis, therapeutic

31–101. b
p 557
hydramnios; amniocentesis; infection, fetal; intrauterine infection

31–102. a
p 557
hydramnios; amniocentesis; umbilical cord prolapse

31–103. a
p 557
hydramnios; amniocentesis; placental abruption

31–104. b
p 557
hydramnios; amniocentesis; hemorrhage, fetal

31–105. a, b, d, e
pp 557–558
oligohydramnios; pulmonary hypoplasia, fetal; amnionic band amputation; postmaturity

31–106. a
pp 557–558
oligohydramnios; fetal malformations

32–1. b
p 561
congenital malformations

32–2. e
p 561
genetics and environment

32–3. d
p 562
teratology

32–4. a
p 562
fetal infections; congenital malformations

32–5. b
p 562
maternal diseases; congenital malformations

32–6. c
p 562
maternal diseases; congenital malformations

32–7. c, d, e
p 561
genetics and environment; congenital anomalies

32–8. a, b, d
p 562
teratology

32–9. i
p 562
drugs and medication; Food and Drug Administration

32–10. c
p 563
drugs and medication; Food and Drug Administration

32–11. b
p 563
drugs and medication; Food and Drug Administration

32–12. d
p 563
drugs and medication; Food and Drug Administration

32–13. a
p 563
drugs and medication; Food and Drug Administration

32–14. This one is up to you

32–15. a
p 562
teratology

32–16. a
p 564
diabetes in pregnancy; congenital malformation

32–17. b
p 565
herpes in pregnancy; acyclovir; antiviral drugs

32–18. b, c
p 565
teratology; cardiovascular disease; atenolol; methyl dopa

32–19. b, c, d
p 565
teratology; hypertension in pregnancy

32–20. e
p 566
seizure disorder; congenital malformations; valproic acid

32–21. a
pp 565–566
thromboembolism; teratology; heparin

32–22. a
pp 565–566
thromboembolism; teratology; heparin

32–23. c
p 566
asthma; teratology; terbutaline

32–24. d
p 566
seizure disorder

32–25. a, b, c
p 566
teratology; antiemetics

32–26. a, b, c, d
p 567
teratology; alcoholism; fetal alcohol syndrome

32–27. b, c, d
pp 567–568
illicit drug use

32–28. a, b
p 568
psychotropic drugs

32–29. a, b, d
p 568
aspirin, platelet

32–30. a
p 569
antineoplastic drugs; cancer

32–31. a, d
p 569
oral contraception; teratology

32–32. d
p 569
teratology; radiation in pregnancy

32–33. e
p 569
teratology; radiation in pregnancy

32–34. c
p 569
teratology; agent orange; chemicals

32–35. a
p 569
lead; teratology

32–36. b
p 569
teratology; methyl mercury

32–37. none of these
p 569
Yusho; polychlorinated biphenyl

32–38. c
p 570
inherited disorders; chromosomal abnormalities

32–39. b
pp 570–571
inherited disorders; mosaicism

32–40. a
p 570
inherited disorders; nondisjunction

32–41. a
p 570
inherited disorders; nondisjunction

32–42. b
p 570
inherited disorders; mosaicism

32–43. a
p 570
inherited disorders; nondisjunction, chromosomal abnormalities

32–44. b, c
pp 570–571
Down syndrome

32–45. a
pp 570–571
paternal age; Down syndrome

32–46. a
p 572
Turner syndrome; fragile X syndrome; Klinefelter syndrome

32–47. a, d
pp 572–573
dominant inheritance

32–48. c
p 574
phenylketonuria

32–49. a, c, d
p 574
multifactorial inheritance

32–50. a
p 574
congenital anomalies

32–51. None of these are correct.
pp 574–575
neural tube defects

32–52. d
p 579
omphalocele

32–53. a
p 579
umbilical hernia

32–54. d
p 580
genetic counseling

32–55. a, b, c
pp 580–581
evaluation of malformed infants; genetic counselling

32–56. b, c, d
p 581
Tay Sachs disease; sickle cell anemia; genetic screening

32–57. a, b, c
p 582
prenatal diagnosis; congenital malformations; sonography

32–58. b, c, d
p 582
prenatal diagnosis; amniocentesis; prenatal screening

32–59. c
pp 582–583
α-fetoprotein; neural tube defect

32–60. a, b
p 585
α-fetoprotein; prenatal diagnosis; amnionic fluid; acetylocholinesterase

32–61. c, e
p 585
Down syndrome; α-fetoprotein

32–62. a, b, d
p 586
chorionic villus sampling

32–63. e
p 587
mutation; molecular genetics

32–64. a, f
p 587
gene; purine; pyrimidine

32–65. c
p 587
transcription

32–66. b
p 587
messenger RNA

32–67. i
pp 587–588
restriction fragment length polymorphisms

32–68. b
p 587
messenger RNA

32–69. d
p 587
translation

32–70. g
pp 587–588
probe; complementary DNA

32–71. h
pp 587–588
restriction endonuclease

33–1. Surfactant serves to stabilize the newly-expanded fetal lung alveoli by preventing their collapse during expiration.
p 593
surfactant; hyaline membrane disease; type II pneumocytes; respiratory distress syndrome

33–2. a, b, c
p 593
hyaline membrane disease; surfactant; respiratory distress syndrome

33–3. None of the statements about hyaline membrane disease is correct
p 593
hyaline membrane disease; respiratory distress syndrome; neonatal death rate

33–4. a, b, c, d, e
p 593
hyaline membrane disease; grunting tachypnea; atelectasis, neonatal

33–5. a, b, c, d, e, f, g, h
pp 593–594
hyaline membrane disease; pneumonia, neonatal; sepsis, neonatal; aspiration, neonatal; pneumothorax; diaphragmatic hernia, neonatal; patent ductus arteriosus; myocardiopathy, neonatal; respiratory distress syndrome

33–6. a, b, c, d
p 593–594
hyaline membrane disease; oxygen therapy, neonatal; retrolental fibroplasia

33–7. a
p 594
hyaline membrane disease; neonatal mortality, hyaline membrane disease; respiratory distress syndrome

33–8. c
p 594
pulmonary hypertension, neonatal; oxygen therapy, neonatal; hyaline membrane disease

33–9. a
pp 594–595
retrolental fibroplasia; hyaline membrane disease; hyperoxia, neonatal

33–10. b
p 594
tracheal abrasion, neonatal; hyaline membrane disease; endotracheal intubation

33–11. c
p 594
bronchopulmonary dysplasia; hyaline membrane disease; oxygen therapy, neonatal

33–12. a, b, c
p 594
surfactant; hyaline membrane disease

33–13. b, c, d
p 595
meconium, aspiration; pneumonitis, neonatal; fetal distress; atelectasis, neonatal; pneumothorax, neonatal

33–14. a
p 595
meconium, aspiration

33–15. The mouth and nares should be suctioned thoroughly just after delivery of the head and before delivery of the thorax (whether the delivery is vaginal or cesarean); as soon as possible after delivery, the vocal cords should be visualized and all meconium aspirated from the area; the stomach should be emptied to avoid the possibility of further meconium aspiration; ventilation of the lungs must not be unduly delayed while the above procedures are being accomplished.
p 595
meconium, aspiration; resuscitation, neonatal

33–16. b
p 594
retrolental fibroplasia; blindness, neonatal

33–17. b
p 594
retrolental fibroplasia; hyperoxia, neonatal

33–18. a, b
pp 596, 598
anemia, neonatal; hematocrit, neonatal

33–19. a, b, d
p 596
cerebral trauma; perinatal asphyxia; intraventricular hemorrhage

33–20. a
p 596
intraventricular hemorrhage

33–21. b
p 596
birth injury; intracranial hemorrhage, neonatal

33–22. a
p 596
intraventricular hemorrhage

33–23. b
p 597
cerebral palsy; birth injury; asphyxia, birth; fetal distress

33–24. a, f
pp 599–600
ABO incompatibility; stillbirth

33–25. c
pp 599–600
isoimmunization; ABO incompatibility

33–26. Mother is group O with anti-A and anti-B in her serum, and the fetus is group A, B, or AB; there is the onset of neonatal jaundice within 24 hours of birth; there are varying degrees of anemia, reticulocytosis, and erythroblastosis; there has been the careful exclusion of all other causes of hemolysis.
p 599
ABO incompatibility; hemolysis, ABO incompatibility; isoimmune disease, newborn

33–27. a, d
pp 599–600
ABO incompatibility; Coombs test; exchange transfusion

33–28. a
p 599
Rho(D) isoimmune disease; ABO incompatibility; hemolytic disease, newborn

33–29. a, b, d
p 599
hemorrhage, fetal-maternal; anemia, neonatal

33–30. varying rate of occurrence of antigens; variable antigenicity; insufficient placental transfer of antigen from fetus to mother; insufficient placental transfer of antibody from mother to fetus
p 600
hemolytic disease; Rh isoimmunization; placental transfer, antigenicity

33–31. a, c
p 600
Rh antigen; immunogenicity, Rh antigen

33–32. a
p 600
Rho(D) antigen; antepartum care, routine; Rho(D) isoimmunization

33–33. a, b, d
p 600
Rho(D) isoimmunization; perinatal death, Rho(D) disease; Rho(D) immune globulin

33–34. a, b, c, d, e
pp 600, 603
Rho(D) isoimmunization; Rho(D) immune globulin

33–35. b
pp 603–604
Rho(D) isoimmunization, prophylaxis; Rho(D) immune globulin; transfusion, maternal

33–36. a
pp 603–604
Rho(D) isoimmunization; Rho(D) immune globulin

33–37. A single 300 μg dose should be given at between 28 and 32 weeks of gestation and again within 72 hours of the birth of a Rho(D)-positive infant; a single 300 μg dose should be given at the time of amniocentesis or whenever there is uterine bleeding (unless the routine dose at 28 to 32 weeks had just been given); if a massive fetal to maternal hemorrhage is recognized, immune globulin is administered according to the formula that a 300 μg dose will protect against a bleed of up to 15 ml of Rho(D)-positive fetal red cells.
p 604
Rho(D) isoimmunization; Rho(D) immune globulin, prophylaxis; fetal-maternal hemorrhage

33–38. b
p 604
Rho(D) isoimmunization; Rho(D)immune globulin, prophylaxis; Coombs test, direct

33–39. a, c
pp 604–605
Rho(D) isoimmunization; maternal-fetal bleed, isoimmunization; fetal-maternal bleed, isoimmunization; Rho(D) immune globulin

33–40. 1 = a; 2 = b
pp 599–600 (Fig. 33–3)
acid-elution test; fetal-maternal bleed; fetal hemoglobin

33–41. a
p 605
fetal-maternal bleed; Rho(D) isoimmunization; Rho(D) immune globulin; Rho(D) antibody, maternal serum

33–42. b
p 605
Rho(D) isoimmunization; perinatal mortality, Rho(D) isoimmunization

33–43. past obstetric history; accurate determination of gestational age; determination of paternal Rho(D) zygosity; measurements of maternal antibody levels; spectrophotometric analysis of amnionic fluid samples; identification of other pregnancy complications
p 605
Rho(D) isoimmunization

33–44. a
p 605
Rho(D) isoimmunization; antibody measurement, Rho(D) isoimmunization; hemolytic disease of the newborn

33–45. b
p 605
Rho(D) isoimmunization; amniocentesis, Rho(D) isoimmunization; Rho(D) antibody, maternal

33–46. a
p 606
amnionic fluid, bilirubin; bilirubin, absorption at 450 nm; Rho(D) isoimmunization

33–47. a
p 606 Figs. (33–6 and 33–7)
Liley zone; amniocentesis, Rho(D) isoimmunization; hemolytic disease; Rho(D) isoimmunization

33–48. c
p 606 (Figs. 33–6 and 33–7)
Liley zone; amniocentesis, Rho(D) isoimmunization; hemolytic disease; Rho(D) isoimmunization

33–49. b
p 606
Liley zone; amniocentesis, Rho(D) isoimmunization; hemolytic disease; Rho(D) isoimmunization

33–50. a, b, e
p 606
Rho(D) isoimmunization; hemolytic disease, newborn; Coombs test, direct; Coombs test, indirect; Rho(D) antibodies

33–51. a
pp 606–607
fetal anemia; erythroblastosis

33–52. a, d, f
p 602
immune hydrops; Rho(D) isoimmunization; hematopoiesis, extramedullary; ultrasonography

33–53. a, c
p 606
intrauterine transfusion; respiratory distress syndrome; Rho(D) isoimmunization

33–54. None of these methods has proved to be both safe and effective.
p 606
Rho(D) isoimmunization

33–55. a
pp 607–608
anemia, neonatal; Rho(D) isoimmunization; sinusoidal fetal heart rate

33–56. b
p 608
cesarean delivery; Rho(D) isoimmunization

33–57. a, b
p 608
Rho(D) isoimmunization; exchange transfusion

33–58. lethargy; stiffness of the extremities; retraction of the head; squinting; high-pitched cry; poor feeding; convulsions
p 608
kernicterus; hyperbilirubinemia; Rho(D) isoimmunization; convulsions, neonatal

33–59. a, b, e
p 608
kernicterus; hyperbilirubinemia

33–60. a, b, c, d, e, f
p 608
kernicterus; hyperbilirubinemia; sulfonamides; salicylate; furosemide; gentamicin; vitamin K, analogues; diazepam

33–61. a, b, c
pp 608–609
breast feeding; breast milk jaundice; kernicterus

33–62. a, b, c
p 609
jaundice, physiologic; hyperbilirubinemia; phototherapy, newborn

33–63. a, b, c, d
p 609
jaundice, physiologic; kernicterus; hyperbilirubinemia; icterus

33–64. a, c, d
p 609
hyperbilirubinemia; phototherapy; exchange transfusion; phenobarbital

33–65. a
p 609
nonimmune hydrops fetalis; hydrops fetalis

33–66. a, b, c, d
p 609
nonimmune fetal hydrops

33–67. **a, b, c, e**
p 611
hemorrhagic disease of the newborn; coagulation factors, vitamin K

33–68. consumptive coagulopathy (DIC); hemophilia; congenital syphilis; sepsis; thrombocytopenia purpura; erythroblastosis; traumatic intracranial injury
p 611
hemorrhagic disease of the newborn; consumptive coagulopathy; hemophilia; syphilis, congenital; thrombocytopenia purpura; birth trauma; erythroblastosis

33–69. **a**
p 611
hemorrhagic disease of the newborn; hypoprothrombinemia, neonatal; vitamin K$_1$

33–70. **a, b**
p 611
hemorrhagic disease of the newborn; vitamin K; breast feeding; placental transfer, vitamin K

33–71. **a**
p 612
autoimmune thrombocytopenia purpura

33–72. **b**
p 612
isoimmune thrombocytopenia purpura

33–73. **b**
p 612
isoimmune thrombocytopenia

33–74. **a**
p 612
autoimmune thrombocytopenia purpura

33–75. **b**
p 612
isoimmune thrombocytopenia

33–76. **b**
p 612
isoimmune thrombocytopenia

33–77. **b, c, d, e**
p 612
polycythemia, neonatal; hyperviscosity, neonatal; hypoxia, neonatal

33–78. **a, b, c, e**
pp 612–613
diarrhea, newborn; Escherichia coli; infection, neonatal

33–79. **a, b**
pp 612–613
necrotizing enterocolitis; bowel perforation, neonatal; pneumotosis intestinalis

33–80. **a, b, c, d**
p 613
drug addiction in pregnancy

33–81. **a, c, d, e**
p 613
infection, neonatal; immunologic capacity, neonatal

33–82. **a**
p 614
infection, neonatal; group A β-hemolytic streptococci

33–83. **c**
p 614
infection, neonatal; staphylococci

33–84. **b**
p 614
infection, group B β-hemolytic streptococci, neonatal

33–85. **a**
p 615
rubella; rubella vaccine

33–86. **a, c, d, f**
p 615
rubella; rubella antibody, IgM, rubella

33–87. 1 = 50; 2 = 25; 3 = 15
p 615
rubella; congenital abnormalities

33–88. eye lesions; heart defects; auditory defects; central nervous system defects; fetal growth retardation; hematologic abnormalities; hepatosplenomegaly and jaundice; chronic diffuse interstitial pneumonitis; osseus changes; chromosomal abnormalities
pp 615–616
congenital rubella syndrome; rubella, congenital; cataracts, neonatal; glaucoma; patent ductus arteriosus; thrombocytopenia, neonatal; anemia, neonatal; hepatosplenomegaly, neonatal

33–89. **a**
p 616
diabetes, juvenile; rubella, congenital

33–90. **a**
p 616
placental transfer; rubella; rubella vaccine

33–91. **a, c, e**
p 616
cytomegalovirus; IgM, cytomegalovirus; infection, neonatal

33–92. **a, b, c, d, e, f, g, h, i, j, k**
p 616
infection, neonatal; cytomegalovirus; microcephaly; hydrocephalus; mental retardation; cerebral palsy; epilepsy; deafness; chorioretinitis; blindness; hemolytic disease; thrombocytopenia; hepatosplenomegaly

33–93. TO = toxoplasmosis; R = rubella; C = cytomegalovirus; H = herpes
p 620
TORCH

33–94. b
p 620
TORCH; antenatal testing

33–95. a, b
p 619
Chlamydia trachomatis; pneumonia, neonatal; conjunctivitis, neonatal; infection, neonatal; abortion; premature labor

33–96. eating raw or undercooked meat; contact with infected cat feces; placental transfer from infected mother to fetus
p 619
Toxoplasma gonadii; toxoplasmosis

33–97. a, e
p 619
toxoplasmosis; chorioretinitis; Sabin-Feldman dye test; IgM, toxoplasmosis; infection, neonatal

33–98. elimination of difficult forceps operations; correct management of breech presentations; virtual eradication of internal podalic version operations; liberalized use of cesarean delivery for the treatment of cephalopelvic disproportion
p 793
birth injury; forceps delivery; internal podalic version; cesarean delivery; cephalopelvic disproportion

33–99. b, d
pp 620–621
birth injury; intracranial hemorrhage, neonatal; molding; fetal skull, compression

33–100. b
p 620
birth injury; intracranial hemorrhage, neonatal

33–101. a, b, c, d, e, f
p 620
intracranial hemorrhage, neonatal

33–102. atelectasis; birth asphyxia; meconium aspiration; diaphragmatic hernia; congenital heart disease; idiopathic respiratory distress syndrome; pneumonia
p 620
intracranial hemorrhage, neonatal; atelectasis; meconium aspiration; respiratory distress syndrome; diaphragmatic hernia; asphyxia, birth; congenital heart disease; pneumonia

33–103. periventricular; intraventricular
p 620
intracranial hemorrhage, neonatal; prematurity, neonatal complications

33–104. a, b, e
p 620
intracranial hemorrhage, neonatal

33–105. b
p 621 (Fig. 33–12)
cephalohematoma

33–106. a
p 621 (Fig. 33–14)
caput succedaneum

33–107. b
p 621 (Fig. 33–14)
cephalohematoma

33–108. a
p 621
caput succedaneum

33–109. b
p 621
cephalohematoma

33–110. a
pp 620–621
intracranial hemorrhage, neonatal; birth injury; cephalohematoma; coagulation defects, newborn; thrombocytopenia, newborn

33–111. a
p 621
brachial plexus, injury; Duchenne's paralysis; Erb's paralysis; birth injury

33–112. b
p 621
brachial plexus, injury; Klumpke's paralysis; birth injury

33–113. a
p 621
brachial plexus, injury; Duchenne's paralysis; Erb's paralysis; birth injury

33–114. b
p 621
brachial plexus, injury; Klumpke's paralysis; birth injury

33–115. a
p 621
brachial plexus, injury; Duchenne's paralysis; Erb's paralysis; birth injury

33–116. a
p 621
Duchenne's paralysis; Erb's palsy

33–117. b, c, d
p 621
brachial plexus, injury; birth injury; breech presentation, brachial plexus injury; macrosomia, brachial plexus injury

33–118. b
p 623
facial paralysis, birth injury; forceps delivery

33–119. a, c, d, e
p 623
birth injury; skeletal injury, newborn; shoulder dystocia

33–120. torticollis
p 623
torticollis; birth injury; sternocleidomastoid muscle, birth injury

33–121. b, c, d
p 623
congenital amputations; amnion, premature rupture; constriction bands

33–122. a, b, c, d, f
p 624
oligohydrammnios; talipes; hip dislocation, congenital; limb reduction, congenital; body wall deficiency, congenital

33–123. the shielding provided by the uterus and the amnionic fluid in which the fetus floats
pp 624–625
coincidental injury, fetus; trauma, in pregnancy

33–124. a
pp 624–625
coincidental injury, fetus; trauma, in pregnancy

34–1. abortion; increased perinatal mortality; low birthweight; fetal malformation; fetal–fetal hemorrhage; pregnancy-induced or aggravated hypertension; maternal anemia; placental accidents; maternal hemorrhage; cord accidents; hydramnios; complicated labor
p 629
multifetal pregnancy, complications

34–2. a
p 629
twins, monozygotic

34–3. b
p 629
twins, monozygotic

34–4. c
p 629
twins, monozygotic; monoamnionic, monochorionic twins

34–5. a
pp 629–630
twins, monozygotic; diamnionic, dichorionic twins

34–6. b
pp 629–630
twins, monozygotic; diamnionic, monochorionic twins

34–7. d
pp 629–630
twins, monozygotic; conjoined twins

34–8. c
pp 629–630
twins, monozygotic; monoamnionic, monochorionic twins

34–9. a
pp 629–630
twins, monozygotic; monoamnionic, monochorionic twins

34–10. b
pp 629–630
twins, monozygotic; diamnionic, monochorionic twins

34–11. a
pp 629–630
twins, monozygotic; diamnionic, dichorionic twins

34–12. 1 set/250 births
p 630
twins, monozygotic

34–13. None of the factors seems to influence the incidence of monozygotic twins
p 630
twins, monozygotic

34–14. a, b, c, d, e
p 630
twins, dizygotic

34–15. d, e
pp 630–631
multifetal pregnancy; ovulation induction, multifetal pregnancy

34–16. a
p 630
twins, monozygotic

34–17. b
pp 629, 632
twins, dizygotic; twins, monozygotic

34–18. b, c
pp 632–633
zygosity

34–19. a
pp 633–634
twins, conjoined; thoracopagus

34–20. d
pp 633–634
twins, conjoined; ischiopagus

34–21. c
pp 633–634
twins, conjoined; craniopagus

34–22. b
pp 633–634
twins, conjoined; pyopagus

34–23. thoracopagus
pp 633–634
twins, conjoined; thoracopagus

34–24. a
pp 633–634
twins, conjoined

34–25. a
p 635
twins, monozygotic; arteriovenous anastomoses, twins; twin-to-twin transfusion

34–26. b
p 635
twins, monozygotic; arteriovenous anastomoses, twins; twin-to-twin transfusion

34–27. b
pp 635–636
twins, monozygotic; arteriovenous anastomoses, twins; twin-to-twin transfusion; cardiac hypertrophy, neonatal

34–28. a
pp 635–636
twins, monozygotic; arteriovenous anastomoses, twins; twin-to-twin transfusion; microcardia, neonatal

34–29. b
pp 635–636
twins, monozygotic; arteriovenous anastomoses, twins; twin-to-twin transfusion

34–30. b
pp 635–636
twins, monozygotic; arteriovenous anastomoses, twins; twin-to-twin transfusion; polycythemia, neonatal

34–31. a
pp 635–636
twins, monozygotic; arteriovenous anastomoses, twins; twin-to-twin transfusion; anemia, neonatal

34–32. a, b, c, d
p 636
twins, monozygotic; arteriovenous anastomoses, twins; twin-to-twin transfusion; hyperbilirubinemia

34–33. 1 = b; 2 = a
p 636
mosaicism; chimerism

34–34. b
p 636
chimerism; twin-to-twin transfusion; twins, monozygotic

34–35. multifetal pregnancy; bladder distention; inaccurate menstrual history; hydramnios; hydatidiform mole; uterine myomas or adenomyosis; closely attached adnexal mass; fetal macrosomia
p 636
multifetal pregnancy, diagnosis; uterine enlargement, differential diagnosis

34–36. a, b, c, f
pp 636–637
multifetal pregnancy, diagnosis; ultrasonography; x-ray

34–37. None of these biochemical tests clearly differentiates a multifetal pregnancy from a singleton pregnancy or from other possibilities such as hydatidiform mole.
pp 636–637
multifetal pregnancy, diagnosis; hCG; α-fetoprotein; estriol, urinary

34–38. a, d
pp 638–639
perinatal mortality rate, multifetal pregnancy; intrauterine fetal demise

34–39. 1 = 39; 2 = 35; 3 = 33; 4 = 29
p 640
multifetal pregnancy, duration

34–40. a
p 640
multifetal pregnancy, growth retardation; fetal growth retardation; intrauterine growth retardation

34–41. a
p 640
multifetal pregnancy, growth retardation; fetal growth retardation; intrauterine growth retardation

34–42. b
p 640
multifetal pregnancy, growth retardation

34–43. a
p 641
superfetation

34–44. b
p 641
superfecundation

34–45. a, b, c, d, e
p 642
multifetal pregnancy, maternal adaptation; hypervolemia, pregnancy; anemia, pregnancy; blood loss, vaginal delivery, hydramnios

34–46. a, b, d
p 643
multifetal gestation; preeclampsia; growth retardation

34–47. a, b, c, d, f
p 643
multifetal pregnancy, management; β-mimetics; bed rest, multifetal pregnancy; tocolysis

34–48. a
pp 644–645
L/S rato, multifetal pregnancy; fetal lung maturity, multifetal pregnancy

34–49. premature labor; uterine dysfunction in labor; abnormal fetal presentation; umbilical cord prolapse; premature separation of a normally implanted placenta; immediate postpartum hemorrhage
p 645
multifetal pregnancy, complications; umbilical cord prolapse; postpartum hemorrhage; abnormal presentation

34–50. a, b, c, d, e
pp 645–646
anesthesia, multifetal pregnancy; analgesia, multifetal pregnancy

34–51. a, b, c, d, e
pp 646–647
ultrasonography; vaginal delivery, multifetal pregnancy; cesarean delivery, multifetal pregnancy

34–52. c
p 649
multifetal gestation; selective termination

35–1. b, c, d, e
p 653
hypertension, pregnancy

35–2. a diastolic blood pressure of 90 mm Hg or more or a rise in diastolic pressure of 15 mm Hg; a systolic blood pressure of 140 mm Hg or more or a rise in systolic pressure of 30 mm Hg; these blood pressures measured on two or more occasions at least 6 hours apart
p 653
hypertension, pregnancy; diastolic blood pressure, hypertension; systolic blood pressure, hypertension

35–3. d
p 653
chronic hypertensive disease, pregnancy

35–4. a
p 653
preeclampsia

35–5. c
p 653
superimposed preeclampsia

35–6. the occurrence of convulsions not caused by neurologic disease in women with preeclampsia
p 653
eclampsia; preeclampsia

35–7. b
p 653
preeclampsia; gestational hypertension

35–8. a, b, c, d, e, f, g, h
p 654
pregnancy-induced hypertension; preeclampsia

35–9. the presence of 300 mg or more of protein in a 24-hour urine collection or a protein concentration of at least 1 g/L in two random urine specimens collected 6 hours apart
p 654
proteinuria

35–10. e
p 654
preeclampsia; pregnancy-induced hypertension; edema, preeclampsia; proteinuria, preeclampsia

35–11. placental infarction; small placental size; placental abruption
p 655
placental infarction; placental abruption; uteroplacental insufficiency; perinatal mortality; pregnancy-induced hypertension; intrauterine growth retardation; fetal growth retardation

35–12. b
p 655
proteinuria; eclampsia

35–13. a
p 655
perinatal mortality, pregnancy-induced hypertension; pregnancy-induced hypertension

35–14. 1 = absent; 2 = present; 3 = absent; 4 = present; 5 = absent; 6 = present; 7 = absent; 8 = present; 9 = absent; 10 = present; 11 = absent; 12 = present; 13 = absent; 14 = present
p 655 (Table 35–2)
pregnancy-induced hypertension; abdominal pain, pregnancy; headache, pregnancy; thrombocytopenia, pregnancy; visual disturbance, pregnancy

35–15. b
p 655
intrauterine growth retardation, pregnancy-induced hypertension; intrauterine growth retardation, superimposed preeclampsia; fetal growth retardation

35–16. b
pp 655–656
eclampsia

35–17. a history of hypertension (>140/90) before pregnancy; the discovery of hypertension (>140/90) in a pregnant woman before the 20th week of gestation in the absence of hydatidiform mole or multifetal pregnancy
p 656
coincidental hypertension; chronic hypertension

35–18. a, c, d
p 656
chronic hypertension; intrauterine growth retardation; superimposed preeclampsia; fetal growth retardation

35–19. a, b, c, d
p 656
chronic hypertension; placental abruption; cerebrovascular accident

35–20. a
p 656
pregnancy-induced hypertension

35–21. a, b, c, d
p 657
pregnancy-induced hypertension, theories as to cause

35–22. a, b, e
p 657
preeclampsia; eclampsia; angiotensin II, pregnancy-induced hypertension

---

35–23. a
p 658
supine pressor response, pregnancy-induced hypertension

35–24. a, d
p 658
cardiac output, pregnancy; peripheral resistance, pregnancy

35–25. a, c
pp 659–660
cardiac output, pregnancy-induced hypertension; peripheral resistance, pregnancy-induced hypertension

35–26. a, b, c, d
p 660
cardiac function, assessment; preload, cardiac function; afterload, cardiac function; inotropic state of the myocardium; heart rate

35–27. c
p 660
afterload, cardiac function; α-adrenergic system

35–28. a
p 660
preload, cardiac function

35–29. hydralazine
p 661
hydralazine; preeclampsia, treatment; eclampsia, treatment; antihypertensive medication, pregnancy

35–30. a
pp 660–661
afterload, cardiac function

35–31. b
p 662
cardiac output, pregnancy-induced hypertension; peripheral resistance, pregnancy-induced hypertension

35–32. a, c, d
pp 662–663
preeclampsia, hematologic changes; eclampsia, hematologic changes; pregnancy, hypervolemia, pregnancy-induced hypertension

35–33. intravascular permeability causing excess accumulation of extracellular fluid (probably the most important cause); generalized vasoconstriction
pp 662–663
hemoconcentration; blood volume; preeclampsia, vascular changes

35–34. b
p 662
eclampsia, blood volume; intravascular volume, pregnancy-induced hypertension

35–35. a
p 662
eclampsia, blood volume; intravascular volume, pregnancy-induced hypertension

35–36. b, d
p 663
preeclampsia, coagulation changes; eclampsia, coagulation changes

35–37. a
pp 663–664
preeclampsia, coagulation changes; eclampsia, coagulation changes

35–38. b
p 665
preeclampsia, endocrine changes; renin

35–39. b
p 665
preeclampsia, endocrine changes; angiotensin II

35–40. b
p 665
preeclampsia, endocrine changes; aldosterone

35–41. c; sometimes **a**
p 665
preeclampsia, endocrine changes; deoxycorticosterone

35–42. b
p 665
preeclampsia, endocrine changes; edema, preeclampsia; deoxycorticosterone

35–43. b, d
p 666
proteinuria, renal cortical necrosis, diagnosis of preeclampsia

35–44. There is swelling of glomerular capillary endothelial cells and subendothelial deposition of proteinaceous material
p 666
preeclampsia, renal changes; pregnancy-induced hypertension, renal changes

35–45. tubular necrosis; renal cortical necrosis
p 666
pregnancy-induced hypertension, renal changes

35–46. b, c, d
pp 667–668
pregnancy-induced hypertension, hepatic effects

35–47. a
pp 667–668
pregnancy-induced hypertension, hepatic effects; subcapsular liver hemorrhage

35–48. None of these is abnormal in the brains of women with pregnancy-induced hypertension.
p 669
pregnancy-induced hypertension, brain

35–49. a
p 669
pregnancy-induced hypertension, brain; eclampsia, genetic determinant

35–50. **a, b, c, d, e**
p 669
pregnancy-induced hypertension, brain

35–51. **c**
p 671
placental perfusion; uteroplacental circulation

35–52. **b**
p 671
uteroplacental circulation, pregnancy-induced hypertension; intrauterine growth retardation; fetal growth retardation

35–53. **a, b, c, e**
p 667
uteroplacental circulation, pregnancy-induced hypertension; hydralazine; thiazide diuretics; dehydroisoandrostrone sulfate

35–54. **a, c**
p 672
preeclampsia; placental histologic changes

35–55. **a**
p 672
Doppler blood flow velocity; preeclampsia; growth retardation

35–56. **a**
p 657
pregnancy-induced hypertension, genetic determinant

35–57. **b**
p 672
preeclampsia; headache, pregnancy; visual disturbance, pregnancy; hypertension, pregnancy; proteinuria, pregnancy

35–58. **a, c**
p 672
preeclampsia, clinical aspects; diastolic blood pressure, preeclampsia

35–59. **a, d**
p 672
preeclampsia; proteinuria, pregnancy; headache, pregnancy; visual disturbance, pregnancy; epigastric pain, pregnancy; weight gain, preeclampsia

35–60. **b**
p 672
pregnancy-induced hypertension, prognosis

35–61. nulliparity; family history of preeclampsia–eclampsia; diabetes; chronic vascular disease; renal disease; hydatidiform mole; fetal hydrops; multifetal pregnancy
p 672
preeclampsia, predisposing factors; nulliparity; multifetal pregnancy; diabetes; hydatidiform mole; fetal hydrops

35–62. **a, b, c, d**
p 672
pregnancy-induced hypertension, detection

35–63. **b**
p 672
pregnancy-induced hypertension, weight gain

35–64. **b, c, d**
p 673
pregnancy-induced hypertension, diuretics; thiazide diuretics

35–65. **a**
p 673
prevention of preeclampsia

35–66. None of these statements about the treatment of pregnancy-induced hypertension is correct.
pp 673–674
pregnancy-induced hypertension, treatment

35–67. **a, b, c, e, f, g, h**
pp 673–674
antepartum care, pregnancy-induced hypertension; preeclampsia, mild

35–68. severity of the preeclampsia; gestational age of the fetus; condition of the cervix
pp 673–674
preeclampsia, management

35–69. **a, b, c**
pp 673–674
treatment of pregnancy-induced hypertension

35–70. **a, b, c, d, e**
pp 673–674
preeclampsia, management; hydralazine; magnesium sulfate; oliguria

35–71. **a, b, c**
p 675
preeclampsia, management; eclampsia, management; glucocorticosteroids, pregnancy-induced hypertension

35–72. None of these provides information that is otherwise unavailable.
p 675
pregnancy-induced hypertension, management

35–73. **a**
pp 675–676
intrauterine growth; retardation, pregnancy-induced hypertension; fetal growth retardation

35–74. **a, b**
p 676
pregnancy-induced hypertension, postpartum period

35–75. **b, c**
pp 676–677
management of preeclampsia

35–76. **b, d, e**
p 677
eclampsia, convulsions; eclampsia

35–77. a, c
pp 677–678
eclampsia, prognosis; pulmonary edema, eclampsia; fever, eclampsia

35–78. Intercurrent eclampsia is the uncommon situation where the woman returns to a completely oriented state after an eclamptic seizure and coma, occasionally with the disappearance of all evidence of preeclampsia–eclampsia.
p 678
eclampsia, intercurrent

35–79. The likelihood of chronic vascular or renal disease increases as the duration of postpartum hypertension increases.
p 677
chronic hypertension; postpartum hypertension

35–80. a, b, c, d, e, f, g
p 678
eclampsia, differential diagnosis

35–81. a
p 678
eclampsia, differential diagnosis

35–82. control of convulsions; correction of hypoxia and acidosis; lowering of blood pressure as needed; delivery once the mother is free of convulsions
p 679
eclampsia, treatment

35–83. None of these changes tends to be permanent.
p 679
eclampsia

35–84. control convulsions with magnesium sulfate; intermittent intravenous administration of hydralazine whenever diastolic pressure is >110 mm Hg; avoid diuretics and hyperosmotic agents; limit fluid intake except when fluid loss is excessive; effect delivery
p 679
eclampsia, treatment

35–85. a, b, c, d, e
pp 679–680
magnesium sulfate; eclampsia, treatment

35–86. c
p 681
magnesium sulfate, respiratory depression

35–87. b
pp 681–682
magnesium sulfate

35–88. a
pp 681–682
magnesium sulfate

35–89. calcium gluconate
p 682
magnesium sulfate, respiratory depression; calcium gluconate

35–90. a
p 683
hydralazine; hemorrhage, intracranial; preeclampsia, treatment; eclampsia, treatment

35–91. b
p 684
sodium nitroprusside, side effects

35–92. a
p 684
diazoxide, side effects

35–93. a
p 684
diazoxide, side effects

35–94. b
p 684
sodium nitroprusside, side effects

35–95. a, b, c, d, e
p 684
eclampsia, diuretics

35–96. b, d, e
p 684
eclampsia, fluid; hematocrit, eclampsia

35–97. b
p 685
preeclampsia; hemodynamic monitoring

35–98. e
p 686
delivery, eclampsia; anesthesia, eclampsia

35–99. a, b, c, d
p 686
anesthesia, eclampsia; delivery, eclampsia

35–100. a, c
p 686
magnesium sulfate; myometrial contractility

35–101. c
pp 686–687
eclampsia, treatment

35–102. a
pp 687–688
eclampsia, recurrence

35–103. b
pp 687–688
eclampsia, multifetal pregnancy

35–104. a
pp 687–688
preeclampsia, residual hypertension

35–105. a, b, c, d
p 688
chronic hypertension

35–106. e
p 690
chronic hypertension; superimposed preeclampsia; antihypertensive medication

35–107. There is a sudden rise in blood pressure which is almost always complicated by substantial proteinuria; in neglected cases oliguria, convulsions, and coma are likely. The frequencies of fetal growth retardation and prematurity are increased.
p 690
pregnancy-aggravated hypertension

36–1. Whole blood components are not immediately available.
p 695
obstetric hemorrhage; maternal mortality

36–2. a
p 695
obstetric hemorrhage; perinatal mortality; premature delivery; antepartum bleeding

36–3. a, d
p 695
blood loss, delivery; postpartum hemorrhage

36–4. 1000 to 2000 ml
p 695
pregnancy-induced hypervolemia; blood volume, pregnancy

36–5. b
p 695
obstetric hemorrhage

36–6. placenta previa; placental abruption; placenta accreta; ectopic pregnancy; midtrimester abortion; hydatidiform mole
p 695
obstetric hemorrhage, etiology; abnormal placental implantation

36–7. vaginal delivery other than spontaneous or outlet forceps; cesarean section or cesarean hysterectomy; uterine rupture
pp 695–696
obstetric hemorrhage, etiology; delivery, trauma

36–8. overdistended uterus; exhausted myometrium; anesthesia; previous atony
pp 696–697
obstetric hemorrhage, etiology; uterine atony

36–9. small woman; pregnancy hypervolemia not yet maximal; pregnancy hypervolemia obtunded
p 696
obstetric hemorrhage, etiology; small blood volume

36–10. placental abruption; prolonged retention of dead fetus; amnionic fluid embolism; induced abortion; sepsis; gross intravascular hemolysis; massive hemorrhage treated with packed red cells plus electrolyte solution or old whole blood; eclampsia or severe preeclampsia; abnormalities of coagulation coincidental to pregnancy
p 696
obstetric hemorrhage, etiology; coagulation defects

36–11. b
p 696
obstetric hemorrhage; third trimester bleeding

36–12. b, c, d
p 696
obstetric hemorrhage, etiology; placental site; uterine atony

36–13. a
p 697
obstetric hemorrhage, etiology; genital tract lacerations

36–14. a
p 697
obstetric hemorrhage, management; oxytocics; uterine massage

36–15. uterine atony; retained placental fragments; trauma to genital tract
pp 696–697
obstetric hemorrhage, etiology; uterine atony; placental fragments; genital tract, trauma

36–16. a, b, c, d
p 697
obstetric hemorrhage, management

36–17. None; all of the techniques are imprecise when used alone.
pp 697–698
obstetric hemorrhage, diagnosis; tilt test

36–18. a
pp 697–698
obstetric hemorrhage; tilt test; blood loss

36–19. venodilatation (reducing venous return); renal diarrhea (loss of fluids and electrolytes)
p 697
obstetric hemorrhage; diuretics, side effects

36–20. b
p 698
obstetric hemorrhage; oxytocics

36–21. a, b, c
pp 698–699
obstetric hemorrhage; blood volume measurements

36–22. a, c, d
  p 699
  obstetric hemorrhage; fluid replacement

36–23. Platelets in stored blood soon lose their functional capacity.
  p 699
  blood replacement; hypovolemia, management

36–24. b, c, d
  pp 699–700
  blood replacement; obstetric hemorrhage; coagulation defects; thrombocytopenia

36–25. a
  p 701
  thrombocytopenia; blood replacement

36–26. b
  p 700
  blood replacement; Factor V; Factor VIII

36–27. a, c, d, e, f
  p 700
  coagulation factors, pregnancy

36–28. d
  p 700
  coagulation, activation

36–29. b
  p 700
  coagulation, activation

36–30. a
  p 700
  coagulation, activation

36–31. c
  p 700
  coagulation, activation

36–32. delaying fibrin polymerization (prolonged thrombin time); causing defective fibrin clot structure (impaired clot retraction and stability)
  p 700
  coagulation, mechanism; fibrin degradation products

36–33. b
  pp 700–701
  consumptive coagulopathy; DIC; heparin; fibrinogen; epsilon-amino caproic acid

36–34. b
  p 700
  consumptive coagulopathy

36–35. b
  p 701
  hemostasis, defective

36–36. a
  p 701
  clinical and laboratory evidence of defective hemostasis; thrombin time

36–37. a, b, c, e
  p 701
  placental abruption; placenta previa; vasa previa; uterine bleeding; antepartum bleeding

36–38. a, b, c, d
  pp 701–702
  placental abruption

36–39. a
  p 702
  placental abruption; external hemorrhage

36–40. b
  pp 701, 704 (Fig. 36–4)
  placental abruption; concealed hemorrhage

36–41. b
  pp 701, 704 (Fig. 36–4)
  placental abruption; concealed hemorrhage

36–42. a, b, f
  p 702
  placental abruption, frequency; neonatal mortality; maternal mortality

36–43. a, b, c, d, e, f, g, h, i
  p 703
  placental abruption; hypertension, pregnancy associated; multifetal pregnancy; preeclampsia; eclampsia; uterine decompression; short cord syndrome

36–44. a
  p 703
  placental abruption; hypertension

36–45. a
  p 703
  placental abruption, recurrent

36–46. None of these serves to reliably identify imminent placental abruption.
  p 703
  placental abruption

36–47. a, c
  p 703
  placental abruption, pathology; spiral artery (arteriole) rupture

36–48. a, b, c, d
  p 704
  placental abruption; concealed hemorrhage

36–49. hemorrhage with retroplacental hematoma formation that is arrested without delivery occurring
  p 704
  placental abruption, chronic

36–50. b
p 704
placental abruption; fetal to maternal hemorrhage

36–51. d
p 705
placental abruption

36–52. b
p 705
placental abruption; ultrasonography

36–53. b, d, f
p 705 (Table 36–4)
placental abruption, signs; placental abruption, symptoms; premature labor; fetal distress; vaginal bleeding, third trimester

36–54. a
p 706
placental abruption; placenta previa

36–55. b
p 706
placental abruption

36–56. placental abruption
p 706
placental abruption; consumptive coagulopathy

36–57. a, b
p 706
comsumptive coagulopathy; placental abruption

36–58. b, c, d
p 706
renal failure; placental abruption

36–59. There is widespread extravasation of blood into the uterine musculature and beneath the uterine serosa.
pp 706–707
Couvelaire uterus

36–60. b
pp 706–707
Couvelaire uterus

36–61. a, c
p 707
placental abruption, management; third trimester bleeding, management

36–62. b
p 707
placental abruption, management; third trimester bleeding, management

36–63. c, perhaps also (**a**) depending on the cause of the distress
p 707
placental abruption, management; third trimester bleeding, management

36–64. b
p 707
ultrasonography; placental abruption, diagnosis

36–65. placental separation; maternal hemorrhage; fetal hemorrhage; uterine hypertonus
pp 707–708 (Figs. 36–8 and 36–9)
fetal distress; placental abruption

36–66. None of these is recommended for the treatment of uterine hypertonicity associated with fetal distress and placental abruption.
pp 707–708
placental abruption, management; fetal distress; tocolysis

36–67. a
p 708
placental abruption; cesarean delivery

36–68. a, b, c, d
p 708
vaginal delivery; placental abruption; fetal death; cesarean delivery; post-partum hemorrhage

36–69. b
pp 708–709
placental abruption; amniotomy

36–70. a, b, d
p 709
placental abruption, labor

36–71. b
p 709
placental abruption, delivery

36–72. None; the basic techniques for the management of obstetric hemorrhage apply in the case of placental abruption.
p 709
placental abruption; obstetric hemorrhage; hypovolemia

36–73. a, d, e, f
pp 709–710
coagulation defects, hemorrhage; thrombocytopenia; consumptive coagulopathy; obstetric hemorrhage; placental abruption

36–74. hepatitis
p 710
hypofibrinogenemia, management

36–75. b
pp 710–711
placental abruption; coagulation defects, management

36–76. a, b, c, d, e
p 712
consumptive coagulopathy, newborn

36–77. The placenta is over or very near the internal os instead of being implanted in the body of the uterus.
p 712
placenta previa

36–78. c
p 712
placenta previa, marginal

36–79. b
p 712
placenta previa, partial

36–80. d
p 712
placenta previa, low-lying

36–81. a
p 712
placenta previa, total

36–82. b
p 712
placenta previa, degree; cervix, dilation

36–83. c
p 712
placenta previa; placental abruption

36–84. a, b, c
pp 712–713
abortion; placenta previa; implantation

36–85. c
p 712
placenta previa, incidence; placental abruption, incidence

36–86. a, b, c, d, e, f, g
p 712
placenta previa, associated factors; multifetal pregnancy; erythroblastosis; placenta accreta

36–87. Painless hemorrhage that does not usually appear until the end of the second trimester or after
p 713
placenta previa

36–88. c, d
p 714
placenta previa; coagulation defects; obstetric hemorrhage

36–89. a, b, c, d, e
pp 714–715
placenta previa; ultrasonography; vaginal examination, placenta previa

36–90. b
p 715
placenta previa, management

36–91. The placenta may migrate away from the cervix.
p 714
placenta previa, management

36–92. a
p 715
placenta previa, management; cesarean delivery, placenta previa

36–93. b
p 716
placenta previa, management; vaginal delivery, placenta previa

36–94. a
p 716
placenta previa, management; vaginal delivery, placenta previa

36–95. a, b
pp 715–716
placenta previa; cesarean delivery, placenta previa; placenta accreta

36–96. simple rupture of the membranes
p 716
vaginal delivery, placenta previa; tamponade

36–97. a, b, c, d, e
p 716
placenta previa, prognosis; perinatal mortality; cesarean delivery

36–98. b
p 716
intrauterine fetal demise, management

36–99. a, b, c
p 716
intrauterine fetal demise; coagulation defects; labor, induction

36–100. d
p 716
intrauterine fetal demise

36–101. a, b
p 716
consumptive coagulopathy; intrauterine fetal demise

36–102. a
pp 717–718
intrauterine fetal demise; consumptive coagulopathy; heparin

36–103. b
p 718
intrauterine fetal demise; intrauterine pregnancy; consumptive coagulopathy; multifetal pregnancy

36–104. d, e
p 718
intrauterine fetal demise; consumptive coagulopathy

36–105. a, b, d
p 718
intrauterine fetal demise; pregnancy termination; consumptive coagulopathy; laminaria; prostaglandin E_2; oxytocin

36–106. c
pp 718–719
pregancy termination; prostaglandin E_2

36–107. a
pp 718–719
pregnancy termination; oxytocin

36–108. b
p 718
pregnancy termination; laminaria

36–109. d
p 719
pregnancy termination; hypertonic saline

36–110. A rent through the amnion and chorion; opened uterine or endocervical veins; a pressure gradient sufficient to force the amnionic fluid into the venous circulation
p 719
amnionic fluid embolism

36–111. a, b, c, d
p 721
amnionic fluid embolism

36–112. a, b, c
p 721
amnionic fluid embolism, diagnosis; amnionic fluid embolism, management

36–113. a, b, c, d, e
p 722
consumptive coagulopathy; abortion

36–114. a, b, c
p 723
consumptive coagulopathy; thromboplastin

36–115. b
p 723
septic abortion; consumptive coagulopathy

36–116. a
p 723
consumptive coagulopathy, etiology; obstetric hemorrhage

36–117. a, d
pp 722–723
preeclampsia; eclampsia; consumptive coagulopathy

37–1. a
p 727
Bartholin glands; Bartholin glands, infection

37–2. b
p 727
Bartholin duct cyst

37–3. None of these should be surgically excised during pregnancy.
p 727
urethral diverticula; periurethral abscess; periurethral cyst

37–4. a, b
p 727
condylomas

37–5. a
p 727
vulvar varices

37–6. vaginal delivery of a large infant without episiotomy and with tearing of the lower genital tract
p 727
cystocele; retocele

37–7. b, c
p 727
cystocele; rectocele

37–8. b
p 727
stress incontinence, pregnancy

37–9. Gartner or müllerian duct remnants
p 728
vaginal cysts, origin; Gartner duct; müllerian duct

37–10. b
p 728
vaginal cysts, management

37–11. b, d, e
p 728
cervical neoplasia, pregnancy, colposcopy

37–12. a, b, c, d
p 728
cervical dysplasia; conization

37–13. b
p 728
cervical dysplasia; endocervical curettage

37–14. c
p 728
cervical dysplasia

37–15. a
pp 728–729
cervical carcinoma, pregnancy; staging, cervical carcinoma

37–16. a, b, c, d
pp 728–729
cervical carcinoma, invasive; staging, cervical carcinoma

37–17. a
p 728
cervical dysplasia, management

37–18. a
p 728
carcinoma in situ, management

37–19. e
pp 728–729
cervical carcinoma, management

37–20. c
pp 728–729
cervical carcinoma, management

37–21. b
p 729
uterine myoma, pregnancy; tumors, pregnancy

37–22. lack of or faulty fusion of the müllerian ducts; unilateral maturation of the müllerian duct with incomplete or absent development on the opposite side; defective canalization of the vagina
p 729
reproductive tract, developmental abnormalities; müllerian duct

37–23. d
p 729
reproductive tract, developmental abnormalities; double uterus

37–24. c
p 729
reproductive tract, developmental abnormalities; bicornuate uterus

37–25. b
p 729
reproductive tract, developmental abnormalities; septate uterus

37–26. a
p 729
reproductive tract, developmental abnormalities; single uterus

37–27. single (normal cervix); septate (single muscular ring partitioned by a septum); double (two distinct cervices); single hemicervix
p 730
cervix, developmental abnormalities

37–28. 1 = there is faulty longitudinal fusion of the müllerian anlage; 2 = the united müllerian anlage does not canalize normally
p 730
vagina, longitudinally septate; vagina, transversely septate; reproductive tract, developmental abnormalities

37–29. c
p 730
reproductive tract, developmental abnormalities

37–30. a, b, c, d, e
p 730
reproductive tract, developmental abnormalities; hemiuterus, obstetric significance; uterine abnormalities, obstetric significance

37–31. a
p 730
uterine abnormalities; obstetric significance

37–32. b
p 730
anatomic abnormalities, diagnosis

37–33. urinary tract
p 733
reproductive tract, developmental abnormalities; urinary tract, developmental abnormalities

37–34. a, b, c, d
p 733
uterine abnormalities, obstetric significance; cesarean delivery; abortion

37–35. c
pp 734–735
anatomic abnormalities, treatment; metroplasty

37–36. a synthetic, nonsteroidal estrogen
p 736
stilbestrol

37–37. b, c
p 736
stilbestrol, reproductive tract abnormalities; clear cell adenocarcinoma

37–38. b, c, d, e
p 737
uterus, retroversion; uterus, anteflexion; sacculation; uterine incarceration

37–39. extensive dilation of the lower portion of the body of the uterus
p 737
uterus, sacculation

37–40. a, b, c, d
p 738
uterus, prolapse; prolapsed uterus, management

37–41. a
p 738
cystocele; rectocele

37–42. Early in the second trimester, the chorion fuses with the decidua to completely obliterate the uterine cavity.
p 739
salpingitis, pregnancy

37–43. hydrorrhea gravidarum
p 739
hydrorrhea gravidarum; rupture of the membranes

37–44. none of these
p 739
endometriosis

38–1. the accurate determination of gestational age
p 741
gestational age; fetal growth, appropriate

38–2. b, c
p 742
preterm fetus; premature fetus

38-3. a
p 742
term fetus

38-4. d
p 742
postterm fetus

38-5. c
p 742
preterm fetus

38-6. a
p 742
preterm fetus; fetal growth retardation; intrauterine growth retardation

38-7. b
p 742
fetal growth retardation; intrauterine growth retardation

38-8. 1 = 10th; 2 = 90th
p 742
fetal weight; gestational age; intrauterine growth retardation; fetal growth retardation

38-9. b
p 742
fetal weight; gestational age

38-10. a
pp 742–743
fetal growth retardation, prematurity; prematurity; intrauterine growth retardation

38-11. a, b, c
p 744
fetal weight, term pregnancy

38-12. 1 = 3,335; 2 = 3,280 to 3,400 g
p 744
fetal weight, term pregnancy

38-13. c
p 742 (Fig. 37-2)
fetal growth rate

38-14. a
p 745
high-risk pregnancy

38-15. b
pp 741–745
fetal distress, definition

38-16. a, e, f
p 746
neonatal care; neonatal mortality rate; fetal weight

38-17. a
p 747
survival rates by birthweight

38-18. Is further intrauterine stay likely to be of benefit or harm to the fetus?
p 750
preterm birth; intrauterine environment

38-19. b
pp 745–747
intrauterine environment; preterm birth; fetal growth retardation; intrauterine growth retardation

38-20. b
p 749
rupture of the membranes, premature

38-21. a
p 749
rupture of the membranes, preterm

38-22. a
p 749
labor; rupture of the membranes, premature

38-23. Perform one sterile speculum examination to document rupture of the membranes to determine effacement and dilation, presentation, and to rule out umbilical cord prolapse. If the gestational age is 33 weeks or less and if there are no maternal or fetal indications for delivery, use close observation without the administration of prophylactic antibiotics. If the gestational age is 33 weeks or greater, deliver either by induction, if possible, or by cesarean section. Labor and delivery should be managed to minimize maternal hypotension, fetal hypoxia, and infection.
p 749
rupture of the membranes, preterm; labor, induction; cesarean delivery; infection, intrapartum

38-24. membranes ruptured for more than 24 hours
p 750
rupture of the membranes, prolonged

38-25. b
pp 750–751
neonatal mortality; rupture of the membranes, prolonged; rupture of the membranes, premature

38-26. a, b, c, d, e, f
pp 750–751
surfactant; fetal lung maturation; chronic maternal disease; heroin addiction; sickle cell disease; hyperthyroidism; chorionamnionitis; placental infarction

38-27. b
pp 751–752
rupture of the membranes, preterm; fetal lung maturation

38-28. b, c, d, e
p 752
glucocorticosterioids, fetal lung maturation; rupture of the membranes, preterm; surfactant; fetal lung maturation

38–29. c, d, e, f
pp 750–752
preterm labor; incompetent cervix; rupture of the membranes; hydramnios; multifetal pregnancy

38–30. b
p 753
preterm labor

38–31. uterine contractions occurring at least every 10 minutes and lasting for 30 seconds or more; progressive dilation of the cervix
pp 755–756
preterm labor; cervix, dilation; labor

38–32. b
p 755
preterm labor; labor, inhibition; tocolysis

38–33. a, c, e
pp 755–756
preterm labor; episiotomy; neonatal morbidity, prematurity

38–34. a
p 764
fetal growth retardation; neonatal mortality; intrauterine growth retardation

38–35. None of these statements about the management of preterm labor is correct.
pp 756–758
preterm labor, management; bed rest, preterm labor; tocolysis; progesterone, preterm labor; ethanol, preterm labor

38–36. a, b, d
p 756
preterm labor, management; magnesium sulfate; patellar reflex, magnesium sulfate; tocolysis

38–37. a
pp 756–757
β-adrenergic receptors

38–38. b
pp 756–757
β-adrenergic receptors

38–39. b, c, d
pp 756–757
preterm labor, management; β-adrenergic receptors, stimulants; β-adrenergic receptors, agonists; epinephrine, myometrium; tocolysis

38–40. b
pp 756–757
preterm labor, management; β-adrenergic receptors, agonists; ritodrine; tocolysis

38–41. b, c
pp 756–757
preterm labor, management; β-adrenergic receptors, agonists; ritodrine; terbutaline; tocolysis, complications

38–42. a, b
pp 756–757
preterm labor, management; β-adrenergic receptors, agonists; isoxsuprine; ritodrine; tocolysis, complications

38–43. b, e
pp 756–757
preterm labor, management; β-adrenergic receptors, agonists; ritodrine; fenoterol; tocolysis, complications

38–44. b, c
p 757
preterm labor; antiprostaglandins; ductus arteriosus; diazoxide; tocolysis; tocolysis, complications

38–45. b
p 758
postterm pregnancy

38–46. errors in the reported gestational age
p 759
postterm pregnancy; gestation age

38–47. a, b, d, e
p 759
postterm pregnancy; anencephaly, postterm pregnancy; ectopic pregnancy, postterm pregnancy; placental sulfatase activity, postterm pregnancy

38–48. a, b, c, d
p 759 (Table 38–11)
postterm pregnancy; fetal distress; meconium, aspiration

38–49. *Postterm and favorable for induction:* attempt induction of labor; if induction is unsuccessful and there is no sign of fetal distress, wait and repeat induction in 1 week. *Postterm and unfavorable for induction:* if at 42 or 43 weeks and there is no maternal indication for intervention, no history of decreased fetal movement, and no oligohydramnios, wait 1 week and reevaluate; if undelivered by 44 weeks, induce, if possible, or deliver by cesarean. *Possible postterm:* if there is no evidence of complications or oligohydramnios, evalute the patient weekly.
pp 759, 762–763
postterm pregnancy, management

38–50. at the onset of labor; at delivery
pp 759–760
postterm pregnancy

38–51. a
pp 759, 762–763
postterm pregnancy; meconium, aspiration; cesarean delivery

38–52. a
p 761
postterm pregnancy; contraction stress test, postterm pregnancy; nonstress test, postterm pregnancy

38–53. a
p 761
postterm pregnancy, oligohydramnios; fetal distress

38–54. a, c, e, f, g, i, j
pp 765–766
fetal growth retardation; chronic maternal disease; cyanotic heart disease; smoking; alcoholism; cytomegalic inclusion disease; rubella; intrauterine growth retardation

38–55. a
p 766
fetal growth retardation; placental abruption, focal; intrauterine growth retardation

38–56. a
p 766
fetal growth retardation; placental infarction; intrauterine growth retardation

38–57. b
p 766
fetal growth retardation; placenta previa; intrauterine growth retardation

38–58. a
p 766
fetal growth retardation; chorangioma; intrauterine growth retardation

38–59. b
p 766
fetal growth retardation; circumvallate placenta; intrauterine growth retardation

38–60. b
p 767
fetal growth retardation; intrauterine growth retardation

38–61. a, b, c, d
pp 767–768
fetal growth retardation; multifetal pregnancy, fetal growth retardation; fetal infection, fetal growth retardation; prolonged pregnancy, fetal growth retardation; ectopic pregnancy, fetal growth retardation; intrauterine growth retardation

38–62. a
p 767
fundal height; fetal growth retardation; intrauterine growth retardation

38–63. b, c
p 766
screening and diagnosis of fetal growth retardation; identification after delivery

38–64. a
p 771
fetal growth retardation; delivery, fetal growth retardation; intrauterine growth retardation

38–65. d
p 771
fetal lung maturity; preterm labor, management; bed rest, preterm labor

38–66. b, c, d
pp 772–773
management of fetal growth retardation; labor and delivery

38–67. a
p 773
subsequent development and growth of the growth retarded fetus

38–68. a, b, c, d
pp 772–773
fetal growth retardation; cesarean delivery, fetal growth retardation; uteroplacental insufficiency, fetal growth retardation; hypothermia; hypoglycemia, neonatal; intrauterine growth retardation

38–69. b
p 771
fetal growth retardation, symmetrical; fetal growth retardation, sequelae; intrauterine growth retardation

38–70. a
p 771
fetal growth retardation, asymmetrical; fetal growth retardation, sequelae; intrauterine growth retardation

38–71. a
p 773
fetal length; fetal growth retardation, sequelae; intrauterine growth retardation

38–72. b
p 773
fetal growth retardation, sequelae; intrauterine growth retardation

38–73. a, b, d
p 771
ultrasonography; fetal growth retardation, symmetric; fetal growth retardation, asymmetric; intrauterine growth retardation

39–1. a, b, c, d
p 779
medical disease, pregnancy

39–2. a, b, c, d
p 780
anemia

39–3. a, b, c
p 780
anemia; anemia, pregnancy; anemia, puerperium

39–4. a
p 780
anemia; plasma expansion, pregnancy; red cell volume, pregnancy

39–5. a, b, d
pp 780–781
anemia, pregnancy; iron supplementation, pregnancy; red cell volume, pregnancy

39–6. iron deficiency and blood loss
p 781
anemia, pregnancy; iron deficiency, pregnancy; blood loss, vaginal delivery

39–7. d
p 781
iron, pregnancy

39–8. b
p 781
iron, pregnancy

39–9. c
p 781
iron, pregnancy

39–10. a
p 781
iron, pregnancy

39–11. a
pp 781–782
iron deficiency anemia; anemia, pregnancy

39–12. c, e, f
pp 781–782
iron deficiency anemia; erythropoiesis, pregnancy; Plummer-Vinson syndrome

39–13. a, b, c, d, e, f
p 782
anemia, pregnancy; CBC, pregnancy; sickle cell preparation; ferritin

39–14. c
p 782
iron deficiency anemia, treatment; iron replacement, pregnancy

39–15. a, e
p 782
iron deficiency anemia, treatment; iron supplementation, pregnancy; ferrous sulfate

39–16. exchange transfusion
p 782
anemia; exchange transfusion

39–17. a, b, c, d
p 782
acute blood loss anemia; obstetric hemorrhage; anemia, acute blood loss; blood loss, vaginal delivery

39–18. a, c, d
p 782
anemia, chronic disease; anemia, pregnancy; iron supplementation, pregnancy

39–19. b, d, e, g
p 783
megaloblastic anemia; folic acid, deficiency; vitamin B₁₂, deficiency; anemia, pregnancy

39–20. a, b, c
p 783
folic acid, deficiency; anemia, pregnancy

39–21. a, b
p 783
pernicious anemia

39–22. a
p 783
vitamin B₁₂, deficiency; breast feeding; megaloblastic anemia, neonatal

39–23. a, b, c, d, e
p 783
hemolytic anemia, acquired; pregnancy-induced hypertension; hemolytic anemia, autoimmune; anemia, pregnancy; Coombs' test; Clostridium perfringens exotoxin

39–24. b
p 784
paroxysmal nocturnal hemoglobinuria

39–25. a
p 784
hemolytic anemia, drug-induced; glucose-6-phosphate dehydrogenase

39–26. a, b, c, f, g
p 785
aplastic anemia; leukopenia, pregnancy; anemia, pregnancy; thrombocytopenia, pregnancy

39–27. hemorrhage and infection
p 785
aplastic anemia; infection, aplastic anemia; hemorrhage, aplastic anemia; anemia, pregnancy

39–28. sickle cell anemia; sickle cell-hemoglobin C disease; sickle cell-β-thalassemia
p 786
sickle cell anemia; sickle cell-hemoglobin C disease; sickle cell-β-thalassemia; hemoglobinopathies, pregnancy

39–29. a, b, c
p 786
sickle cell anemia; neonatal mortality, sickle cell anemia; maternal mortality, sickle cell anemia; folic acid, supplementation; anemia, pregnancy

39–30. a, b
pp 786–787
contraception, sickle cell anemia; sickle cell disease, contraception; oral contraception, sickle cell disease; intrauterine device, sickle cell disease

39–31. b, c, e, f
p 786
sickle cell-hemoglobin C disease; iron supplementation; folic acid supplementation; exchange transfusion, maternal; pulmonary dysfunction, hemoglobinopathies

39–32. 1 = b; 2 = a
p 786
sickle cell-β-thalassemia; perinatal mortality, sickle cell hemoglobinopathies; anemia, pregnancy; perinatal morbidity, sickle cell hemoglobinopathies

39–33. b
p 786
sickle cell hemoglobinopathy, pregnancy; exchange transfusion, sickle cell hemoglobinopathy

39–34. b, c, d
p 786
sickle cell trait; bacteriuria, asymptomatic

39–35. a
p 787
hemoglobin C

39–36. a, b
p 787
hemoglobin C; hemoglobin E

39–37. a, b
p 787
hemoglobin C; hemoglobin E; iron supplementation; folic acid supplementation

39–38. a, b
p 787
hemoglobin C; hemoglobin E

39–39. b
p 787
hemolytic anemia, sickle cell anemia; hemolytic anemia, sickle cell-hemoglobin C disease

39–40. 1 = c; 2 = c
p 787
hemoglobinopathy, genetic inheritance

39–41. a, b, c
p 788
sickle cell anemia; fetoscopy; amniocentesis, genetic; chorionic villus biopsy

39–42. a, b, d
pp 790–791
hereditary spherocytosis

39–43. genetic disorders that are characterized by impaired production of one or more globin peptide chains
pp 789–790
thalassemias

39–44. a
pp 789–790
α-thalassemia; hemoglobin Bart disease

39–45. b
p 790
α-thalassemia; hemoglobin H disease

39–46. c
p 790
α-thalassemia; α-thalassemia minor

39–47. c
p 790
α-thalassemia; α-thalassemia minor

39–48. d
p 790
α-thalassemia; α-thalassemia, carrier state

39–49. a, b, d
p 790
α-thalassemia; hemoglobin Bart disease; α-thalassemia minor; sickle cell anemia, α-thalassemia; hydrops fetalis, nonimmune; anemia, pregnancy

39–50. c, d
p 790
β-thalassemia; β-thalassemia, minor; β-thalassemia, intermedia; infertility

39–51. a, b, c, d, e, f, g
p 791
thrombocytopenia; aplastic anemia; hemolytic anemia, acquired; eclampsia, consumptive coagulopathy; lupus erythematosus; megablastic anemia

39–52. a, c, e
p 791
immune idiopathic thrombocytopenia

39–53. c
p 792
immune idiopathic thrombocytopenia

39–54. None of the listed treatments is an effective treatment for immune idiopathic thrombocytopenia.
p 792
immune idiopathic thrombocytopenia

39–55. fever; neurologic abnormalities; thrombocytopenia; renal impairment; hemolytic anemia
p 793
thrombotic thrombocytopenic purpura

39–56. a
p 793
thrombotic microangiopathies

39–57. a, c, e
pp 793–794
thrombotic thrombocytopenic purpura; plasmapheresis, exchange transfusion, maternal

39–58. b
p 795
obstetrical hemorrhage

39–59. a, b, c, e
p 795
hemophilia A; coagulation disorders, pregnancy

39-60. a
p 795
obstetrical hemorrhage; Factor VIII, coagulation factors; coagulation disorders, pregnancy

39-61. b
p 795
hemophilia B; Factor IX, coagulation factors; coagulation disorders, pregnancy

39-62. c, d, e
p 795
von Willebrand's disease; Factor VIII, coagulation factors; coagulation disorders, pregnancy

39-63. d
p 795
coagulation disorders, pregnancy

39-64. a, c
p 796
rheumatic heart disease; congenital heart disease; cardiac disease, pregnancy

39-65. d
pp 795–796
cardiac disease, pregnancy

39-66. a, b, c, d
p 796
cardiac disease, pregnancy

39-67. a, b, c, d, e
p 796
cardiac disease, pregnancy

39-68. c
p 797
cardiac disease, class III; cardiac disease, N.Y. Heart Association classification

39-69. d
p 797
cardiac disease, class IV; cardiac disease, N.Y. Heart Association classification

39-70. a
p 797
cardiac disease, class I; cardiac disease, N.Y. Heart Association classification

39-71. b
p 797
cardiac disease, class II; cardiac disease, N.Y. Heart Association classification

39-72. a, b, c, d, e
p 797
cardiac disease, pregnancy

39-73. a, b, c
p 797
cardiac disease, class I; cardiac disease, class II; infection, cardiac failure

39-74. b, c, d, e
p 798
cardiac disease, pregnancy; heart failure

39-75. maternal hypotension
p 798
cardiac disease, delivery, anesthesia, conduction; anesthesia, cardiac disease; hypotension, cardiac disease

39-76. a, d
p 798
cardiac disease; delivery, cardiac disease; anesthesia, cardiac disease

39-77. b
p 798
cardiac failure, labor

39-78. a, b, e
p 798
cardiac failure, pregnancy

39-79. a, b, d
pp 797–802
cardiac failure; cardiac decompensation; antepartum care, cardiac disease; furosemide

39-80. a, b, c
p 798
cardiac disease, class III; cardiac decompensation

39-81. cardiac decompensation must be corrected
p 798
cardiac failure; abortion, cardiac failure

39-82. d
p 800
specific heart disease; rheumatic heart disease

39-83. a
p 799
prematurity; intrauterine death; hypoxia, maternal; abortion

39-84. b, c, d, e
pp 799–800
cardiac disease, pregnancy; artificial heart valves, pregnancy; anticoagulation, pregnancy; heparin; abortion, spontaneous; low birthweight

39-85. just before delivery
pp 799–800
heparin; artificial heart valves; anticoagulation, pregnancy; delivery, anticoagulation

39-86. a reverse of blood flow from the pulmonary artery to the aorta with the development of cyanosis
p 800
patent ductus arteriosus; congenital heart defects; pulmonary hypertension

39–87. a
pp 800–801
polycythemia, spontaneous abortion; abortion, spontaneous

39–88. c
p 801
pulmonary hypertension

39–89. a, b
p 801
ischemic heart disease; coarctation of the aorta; cardiomyopathy; mitral valve prolapse

39–90. a, b, c
pp 803–804
infective endocarditis; antimicrobial prophylaxis

39–91. a, b, c, d
p 804
kyphosclerotic heart disease; kyphosis; abortion, therapeutic

39–92. None of the cardiac arrhythmias is incompatible with a normal pregnancy outcome.
pp 804–805
cardiac arrhythmias, pregnancy

39–93. a
p 805
pulmonary function, pregnancy; transverse thoracic diameter

39–94. b
p 805
pulmonary function, pregnancy; vertical chest diameter

39–95. b
p 805
pulmonary function, pregnancy; residual volume

39–96. a
p 805
pulmonary function, pregnancy; respiratory rate

39–97. a
p 805
pulmonary function, pregnancy; tidal volume

39–98. b
p 805
pulmonary function, pregnancy; plasma carbon dioxide, pregnancy

39–99. a
p 805
pulmonary function, pregnancy; oxygen consumption, pregnancy

39–100. a, b, c, d
p 805
pneumonia, pregnancy; infection, pregnancy; pulmonary function, pregnancy

39–101. a
p 806
throboembolism; pulmonary infarction

39–102. a, d, e
p 806
asthma; goiter, fetal

39–103. a, b, c, d
p 806
asthma

39–104. b, d
pp 806–807
tuberculosis

39–105. Pyridoxine should be administered to avoid neurotoxicity in the fetus.
pp 806–807
tuberculosis; isoniazid; pyridoxine

39–106. b
p 807
adult respiratory distress syndrome

39–107. b
p 807
sarcoidosis

39–108. a, c, d, e
pp 807–808
cystic fibrosis; infertility

39–109. c, d, e
pp 860–861
leukemia; Hodgkin disease; polycythemia; erythropoietin

39–110. a
p 810
urinary tract diseases, pregnancy

39–111. d, e
p 811
urinary tract diseases, pregnancy cystitis; pyelonephritis; acute bacteria

39–112. a, b, c, e
p 808
cystitis

39–113. d
p 808
urethritis; Chlamydia

39–114. e
pp 809–810
pyelonephritis, acute

39–115. a, b, c, d
p 810
pyelonephritis, acute; labor; placental abruption; appendicitis; myomata, infarction

39-116. Compression of the ureter by the enlarged uterus and ovarian veins results in a progressive dilation of the renal calyces, pelves and ureters, accompanied by a decrease in tone and peristaltic action. These changes lead to urinary stasis, which increases the susceptibility to renal infection.
p 810
pyelonephritis, acute; bacteriuria; urinary tract, pregnancy changes

39-117. a, b, c, d, e
p 810
pyelonephritis, acute; anesthesia, effects; bladder overdistension; oxytocin, antidiuretic effect; catheterization, bladder

39-118. persistent, actively multiplying bacteria within the urinary tract without the symptoms of a urinary tract infection
p 581
bacteriuria, asymptomatic

39-119. a, d
p 808
bacteriuria, asymptomatic; sickle cell trait; urinary tract infection, pregnancy

39-120. a
pp 808–809
bacteriuria, asymptomatic; prematurity; low birthweight

39-121. c
p 809
bacteriuria, asymptomatic

39-122. a, b, e
pp 809–810
pyelonephritis, chronic; pyelonephritis, acute

39-123. c, d
p 810
urinary tract infection, pregnancy; pylonephritis, acute

39-124. e
p 810
gentamicin; ototoxicity; urinary tract infection, pregnancy

39-125. b
p 810
nitrofurantoin; hemolysis, maternal; urinary tract infection, pregnancy

39-126. c
p 810
tetracycline; jaundice, maternal; urinary tract infection, pregnancy

39-127. c
p 810
tetracycline; tooth discoloration, neonatal; urinary tract infection, pregnancy

39-128. a
p 810
sulfonamide; kernicterus; urinary tract infection, pregnancy

39-129. e
p 810
gentamicin; nephrotoxicity; urinary tract infection, pregnancy

39-130. d
p 810
chloramphenicol; aplastic anemia; urinary tract infection, pregnancy

39-131. e
p 810
urinary tract infection, pregnancy; ampicillin; gentamicin

39-132. b
p 810
urinary tract infection, pregnancy; pyuria

39-133. b
pp 810–811
renal tuberculosis

39-134. b, d
p 811
urinary calculi; hyperparathyroidism; urinary tract infection, pregnancy

39-135. a, b, c, d
p 812
glomerulonephritis, acute; preeclampsia

39-136. a, c, d, e
p 812
glomerulonephritis, chronic; preeclampsia

39-137. a, b, c, d
p 812
nephrosis (nephrotic syndrome)

39-138. c
p 812
nephrotic syndrome

39-139. a
p 813
nephrotic syndrome

39-140. c
p 813
acute renal failure

39-141. a, b
p 814
acute tubular necrosis; eclampsia; preeclampsia; septic shock

39-142. a, b, c
p 814
acute tubular necrosis; eclampsia, preeclampsia; blood replacement; septic shock

39-143. b, e
p 814
renal cortical necrosis; placental abruption; pregnancy-induced hypertension; preeclampsia; eclampsia; septic shock

39–144. **a, b, d, e**
p 814
hemolytic uremic syndrome, postpartum; thrombocytopenia

39–145. **a, b, c, d, e**
p 815
renal transplantation; polycystic kidney; orthostatic proteinuria, nephrectomy; hemodialysis

39–146. **a, c**
p 816
diabetes mellitus

39–147. **a, b**
pp 816–817
diabetes

39–148. **a, b, c, d**
pp 818–819
diabetes; macrosomia; stillbirth

39–149. **b**
pp 818–819
glucose tolerance test; diabetes in pregnancy

39–150. **a, b, c, d**
p 817
diabetes; glucose tolerance test

39–151. **a, b, c, d**
p 817
diabetes; insulin, pregnancy; placental lactogen; estrogen; progesterone; placental insulinase

39–152. **a, b, c**
p 817
diabetes, pregnancy

39–153. **a, b, c, d, e, f**
p 817
diabetes, pregnancy; cesarean delivery; pregnancy-induced hypertension; infection; macrosomia; hydramnios; postpartum hemorrhage; preeclampsia

39–154. **a, b, c, d, e, f, g**
p 817
diabetes, fetal effects; perinatal death rate; birth injury; respiratory distress; congenital anomalies

39–155. **a, b, c, d**
p 818
diabetes

39–156. **a, c, e**
p 818
diabetes, class A; diabetes, overt

39–157. **b, c, d**
p 819
diabetes, congenital anomalies

39–158. **a, b, c, d, e**
pp 819, 820
diabetes; gestational age

39–159. **b**
pp 819, 820
diabetes; glucosuria; insulin, diabetes management

39–160. Acetonuria usually indicates a need to increase the insulin dose.
p 819
diabetes; acetonuria; insulin, diabetes, management

39–161. **a**
p 823
hemoglobin A1c

39–162. **c**
p 822
diabetes; fetal well-being; nonstress test

39–163. **a, b, c, d, e, f**
pp 821–822
diabetes; induction of labor, diabetes

39–164. **a, c, e**
p 822
diabetes; delivery, diabetes; insulin, diabetes management

39–165. **a, c, d, e**
p 822
diabetes; perinatal morbidity, diabetes; respiratory distress; hypoglycemia, neonatal; hypocalcemia, neonatal; hyperbilirubinemia

39–166. **b**
p 822
diabetes; fetal development, diabetes

39–167. **c**
p 822
diabetes; contraception, diabetes; barrier methods

39–168. **a, b, d**
p 822
thyroid disease; endocrine system, changes in pregnancy

39–169. **a, b, c, d, e**
p 823
hyperthyroidism

39–170. **a, b**
p 823
hyperthyroidism

39–171. **b**
p 824
hyperthyroidism; propylthiouracil; propranolol; iodine; goiter, fetal

39–172. The dose is increased until the woman appears clinically to be only minimally thyrotoxic and the level of thyroxine in the blood is in the upper range of normal for pregnancy.
p 824
hyperthyroidism; propylthiouracil

39–173. a, b, c, d, e
p 824
propranolol; hyperthyroidism; fetal growth retardation; fetal distress; hypoglycemia, neonatal; hyperbilirubinemia, neonatal

39–174. a
p 824
hyperthyroidism; thyroidectomy

39–175. b
p 824
hyperthyroidism in pregnancy; propothiouracil

39–176. Maternal thyroid–stimulating immunoglobulins cross the placenta to cause hyperthyroidism in the fetus and newborn.
p 824
hyperthyroidism, neonatal; Grave disease; thyroid-stimulating hormone; placental transfer

39–177. a
p 824
hyperthyroidism, neonatal; propylthiouracil

39–178. b
p 824
thyroid storm

39–179. a, b, c
p 824
hyperthyroidism, neonatal; cretinism; infertility; abortion, spontaneous

39–180. a, b
p 824
hyperparathyroidism; hypoparathyroidism; tetany, neonatal

39–181. a, c, e
p 824
adrenal dysfunction; Addison disease; Cushing disease; aldosteronism; pheochromocytoma

39–182. a
pp 826–827
pituitary disease; diabetes insipidus; pituitary microadenomas; bromocriptine

39–183. a, c, d, e, f
p 827
liver disease; palmar erythema; spider angiomata; albumin, serum

39–184. intrahepatic cholestasis; hepatocellular damage due to pregnancy-induced hypertension; acute fatty liver; hepatic dysfunction due to hyperemesis gravidarum
p 827
liver disease; intrahepatic cholestasis; pregnancy-induced hypertension; acute fatty liver; hyperemesis gravidarum

39–185. a, b, c, d
p 827
intrahepatic cholestasis

39–186. icterus, pruritis
p 827
intrahepatic cholestasis

39–187. b, c, d
p 827
intrahepatic cholestasis

39–188. a, b, c, d
p 827
acute fatty liver

39–189. a, d
pp 827–828
acute fatty liver; Reye syndrome

39–190. epigastric or right upper quadrant pain
p 828
liver disease; preeclampsia

39–191. a, b, c, d
p 828
hyperemesis gravidarum; hepatitis; pyelonephritis; gasteroenteritis; cholestasis; peptic ulcer; jaundice, maternal

39–192. a, b, c, d, e
p 828
hyperemesis gravidarum

39–193. a, b, c, d, e
p 830
hepatitis A

39–194. b
p 830
hepatitis A; gamma globulin

39–195. a, b, c, d, e, f
p 830
hepatitis B; immune globulin, hepatitis B

39–196. a, b,
p 830
hepatitis A; hepatitis B

39–197. a, b
p 830
hepatitis A; hepatitis B

39–198. b
p 830
hepatitis B

39–199. It is an indication of the infectious state. It correlates with the number of circulating virus particles. It also relates to the vertical transmission (mother to fetus) of hepatitis.
p 830
hepatitis B

39–200. a, b, c, d
p 831
hepatitis in pregnancy; delta hepatitis

39–201. a
p 831
non-A-non-B hepatitis; immune globulin

39–202. a, b
p 831
chronic active hepatitis

39–203. a
p 831
cirrhosis

39–204. a, b
pp 831–832
gallbladder disease; cholelithiases

39–205. the common occurrence of anorexia, nausea, and vomiting during pregnancy; the displacement of the appendix by the enlarging uterus; the occurrence of leukocytosis during pregnancy; presence of other diseases during pregnancy that may be confused with appendicitis (e.g., pyelonephritis, placental abruption)
p 832
appendicitis

39–206. c, d, f
p 832
appendicitis

39–207. a, b, c
pp 833–834
peptic ulcer; preeclampsia; pancreatitis; abdominal pain, pregnancy

39–208. d
p 833
ulcerative colitis; regional enteritis

39–209. a, b, c, d
p 835
parenteral nutrition

39–210. b
p 835
obesity; weight reduction, pregnancy

39–211. a
p 835
obesity; gastric bypass; jejunoileal bypass

39–212. malar rash; discoid rash; photosensitivity; oral ulcers; arthritis; serositis; renal disorders; neurologic disorders; hematologic disorders; immunologic disorders; antinuclear antibody
p 836
systemic lupus erythematosus

39–213. b
p 836
systemic lupus erythematosus

39–214. a, b, c, d
p 838
systemic lupus erythematosus; azathioprine

39–215. c, d, e
p 837
systemic lupus erythematosus

39–216. neuropathy; convulsions; thrombocytopenia
p 838
systemic lupus erythematosus; preeclampsia; eclampsia

39–217. a, b, c, d, e, f, g
p 838
systemic lupus erythematosus, fetal effects; fetal growth retardation; heart block; stillbirth

39–218. b, c, d
p 838
systemic lupus erythematosus; contraception, systemic lupus erythematosus

39–219. It is an IgM or IgG immunoglobin. It can be associated with lupus or exist in patients without lupus. It incites thrombosis, and may be associated with recurrent fetal loss.
p 839
systemic lupus erythematosus; lupus anticoagulant

39–220. a, b, d
pp 841–842
diseases of the skin

39–221. b, c
p 843
epilepsy; phenytoin

39–222. a, b, c, d, e, f
p 844
phenytoin, fetal anomalies; mental retardation; craniofacial anomalies; distal limb dysmorphosis; cleft lip; cleft palate; congenital heart disease; hemorrhagic disease, newborn

39–223. b
p 844
valproic acid; craniofacial anomalies

39–224. a
   p 844
   carbamazepine (Tegretol); microcephalus

39–225. b
   p 844
   valproic acid; neural tube defects

39–226. b
   p 844
   valproic acid; skeletal anomalies

39–227. b
   p 844
   epilepsy; anticonvulsant medications, pregnancy

39–228. megaloblastic anemia, due to a deficiency of folic acid
   p 844
   megaloblastic anemia; epilepsy; folic acid

39–229. a, b, d
   p 245
   cerebrovascular disease in pregnancy

39–230. a, c
   p 845
   intracranial hemorrhage; therapeutic abortion, intracranial hemorrhage

39–231. h. Now that a DNA probe has been identified for the prenatal diagnosis of their dread disease, management can be more accurately provided.
   p 846
   therapeutic abortion; Huntington chorea

39–232. a, b, c, d, e
   p 846
   spinal cord lesion, pregnancy; labor, second stage; fetopelvic disproportion; urinary tract infection; autonomic hyperreflexia

39–233. a
   p 846
   multiple sclerosis

39–234. b, c, d, f
   p 846
   myasthenia gravis; labor, second stage; myasthenia gravis, newborn

39–235. a, b, c, d
   p 846
   myasthenia gravis, newborn

39–236. a, b, c, d
   p 846
   myasthenia gravis; quinine; magnesium sulfate; kanamycin; gentamicin

39–237. b, d
   pp 846–847
   psychosis; lithium; cardiac defects, neonatal; breast feeding

39–238. b, c, d, e, f
   pp 847–848
   varicella; varicella pneumonia; acyclovir; immune globulin

39–239. a, b
   p 848
   mumps; abortion; prematurity

39–240. a, b, d
   p 849
   rubeola; abortion; prematurity

39–241. c, e
   p 848
   influenza; pneumonia

39–242. e, f
   p 849
   common cold

39–243. c, f
   p 849
   poliomyelitis

39–244. a, b, c
   p 849
   typhoid fever; abortion; prematurity

39–245. a, b
   p 850
   malaria; abortion; prematurity

39–246. None of these is an indication for therapeutic abortion.
   pp 848–849
   abortion, therapeutic

39–247. b
   p 850
   sexually transmitted diseases

39–248. a, d, e
   p 851
   syphilis

39–249. condyloma latum
   p 851
   syphilis; condyloma latum

39–250. a
   p 851
   syphilis, congenital; stillbirth; syphilis

39–251. a, c, d
   p 851
   syphilis; VDRL

39–252. a, d, e
   p 851
   syphilis, treatment; benzathine penicillin G; erythromycin; tetracycline

39–253. a, d, e
   p 851
   syphilis, treatment; gonorrhea, treatment; benzathine penicillin G; erythromycin; tetracycline

39–254. d
   p 851
   erythromycin; syphilis, treatment

39–255. a
   p 851
   benzathine penicillin G; syphilis, treatment

39–256. b
   p 851
   benzathine penicillin G; syphilis, treatment

39–257. b
   p 851
   benzathine penicillin G; syphilis, treatment

39–258. c
   p 851
   crystalline penicillin G; benzathine penicillin G; syphilis, treatment

39–259. at least every 6 months for 3 years
   p 852
   syphilis

39–260. a, b, e
   p 852
   syphilis

39–261. a, d
   p 852
   syphilis, congenital

39–262. The chorion laeve has fused with the decidua parietalis; this obliterates the endometrial cavity and prevents disease transmission up into the oviducts.
   p 852
   gonorrhea; chorion laeve; decidua parietalis; salpingitis

39–263. a, b, c, d
   p 852
   gonorrhea; cervix; urethra; Bartholin's; glands; paraurethral glands

39–264. infection of the sexual partner; gonococcal arthritis; gonococcal endocarditis; gonococcal ophthalmia of the newborn; postpartum pelvic infection
   p 852
   gonorrhea; ophthalmia neonatorum

39–265. a
   p 852
   gonorrhea

39–266. a
   p 853
   gonorrhea; procaine penicillin, aqueous

39–267. b
   p 853
   gonorrhea, penicillin resistant; spectinomycin

39–268. a, f
   p 853
   gonorrhea; erythromycin; procaine penicillin, aqueous; Chlamydia

39–269. c, d
   p 853
   gonorrhea, disseminated infection; crystalline penicillin; ampicillin

39–270. c
   p 853
   crystalline penicillin; gonorrhea, neonatal

39–271. spectinomycin; cefoxitin; cefotaxime
   p 853
   gonorrhea, penicillin resistant; spectinomycin; cefoxitin; cefotaxime

39–272. The infant should be isolated and treated for 24 hours with IV penicillin. Eye care by an experienced practitioner is also important.
   p 853
   gonorrhea, neonatal; gonococca; ophthalmia

39–273. a
   p 854
   Chlamydia; lymphogranuloma venereum

39–274. b, c, d
   p 854
   preterm birth and low-birthweight infants; puerperal infection; lymphogranuloma venereum

39–275. type II
   p 854
   herpes, genital

39–276. b, c, d, e
   p 855
   herpes, genital; cervix

39–277. b
   p 855
   herpes, genital; acyclovir

39–278. a, b, c
   p 855
   herpes, genital; cervical neoplasia

39–279. d, e
   p 855
   herpes, neonatal

39–280. the threat of fetal infection with transvaginal delivery and the attendant increase in perinatal morbidity and mortality
   p 855
   herpes, delivery; cesarean delivery, herpes; perinatal morbidity; perinatal mortality

39–281. c
p 856
herpes; cesarean delivery; neonatal care, herpes; breast feeding, herpes

39–282. a, b, c, d
p 857
acquired immunodeficiency syndrome

39–283. a
p 857
acquired immunodeficiency syndrome

39–284. a
p 858
acquired immunodeficiency syndrome; prevention of transmission

39–285. a, b
p 859
human papilloma virus

39–286. a
p 859
chancroid

39–287. b
p 859
granuloma inguinale

39–288. a
p 859
chancroid

39–289. b
p 859
granuloma inguinale

39–290. a
p 859
chancroid

39–291. a
p 859
chancroid

39–292. b
p 859
granuloma inguinale; Donovan bodies

39–293. None of the statements are true concerning breast cancer in pregnancy.
pp 859–860
breast carcinoma

39–294. a, b, c, d
p 860
Hodgkin disease

39–295. b
p 860
leukemia

39–296. a, c, d
p 861
melanoma

40–1. c
p 871
vulva, anatomy

40–2. a, b, c, d
p 871
vulva, anatomy

40–3. a, d, e
p 871
vulva; labia majora; perineum

40–4. a, b, d
p 871
vulva, anatomy; labia majora

40–5. b, d, e
pp 871–872
vulva, anatomy; labia minora

40–6. b, c, d, e
pp 872–873
vulva, anatomy; clitoris

40–7. a
pp 872–873
vulva; clitoris

40–8. b, c, d
p 873
vestibule

40–9. a, b, d, e
p 874
vulva; Bartholin glands

40–10. c
pp 874–875
vulva, innervation; hymen; innervation, genitals

40–11. b
p 874
vulva; hymen

40–12. b
p 874
hymen; virginity

40–13. myrtiform caruncles
p 874
hymen; myrtiform caruncles

40–14. a
pp 873–874 (Fig. 40–1)
vulva; clitoris

40–15. k
p 871 (Fig. 40–1)
vulva; labia majora

40–16. d
p 874 (Fig. 40–1)
vulva; hymen

40–17. f
p 874 (Fig. 40–1)
vulva; perineal body

40–18. b, l
p 874 (Fig. 40–1)
vulva; frenulum; prepuce

40–19. a, b, d
pp 874–875
vagina

40–20. a, b, c, e
pp 874–875
vagina, anatomy; vagina, embryology; parturition

40–21. pouch (cul-de-sac) of Douglas
pp 874–875
vagina; cul-de-sac of Douglas

40–22. b
p 874
vagina, anatomy

40–23. b, c, d
p 874
vagina, anatomy

40–24. c, d
p 877
vagina; exfoliative cytology, vagina

40–25. c
p 877
vagina, vasculature

40–26. a
p 877
vagina, vasculature

40–27. b, d
p 877
vagina, vasculature

40–28. a, b, d
pp 871–872, 877
vulva; vaginal delivery; genitalia, venous system; hematoma, parturition

40–29. hypogastric (internal iliac)
p 877
vagina, vasculature

40–30. a
p 877
vagina, lymphatics; vulva, lymphatics; inguinal nodes

40–31. b
p 877
vagina, innervation

40–32. b, c
p 877
perineum; urogenital diaphragm

40–33. a, d
pp 877, 878
perineum; urogenital diaphragm

40–34. a, b, c
p 877
perineum; perineal body

40–35. b
pp 877–879
uterus, anatomy

40–36. d
pp 877–879
uterus, anatomy; uterus, corpus

40–37. b
pp 878–879
cervix

40–38. a
p 878
uterus, anatomy; uterus, cornu

40–39. c
pp 877–878
uterus, anatomy; uterus, fundus

40–40. b
p 879
uterus

40–41. b
p 878
uterus, anatomy; uterus, isthmus; lower uterine segment

40–42. b, c
pp 878–879
cervix, anatomy

40–43. a
p 878
cervix; external cervical os

40–44. a
p 879
cervix; incompetent cervix

40–45. c, d
p 880
cervix, anatomy; Nabothian cysts

40–46. just above the bladder and at the lateral margins
p 880
uterus, anatomy

40–47. a, c,
p 880
endometrium

40–48. a, b
p 881
uterus, vasculature; uterine artery; ovarian artery

40–49. a, b, c
p 881
uterus, blood supply; endometrium; coiled arterioles; basal arteries

40–50. b
p 881
myometrium

40–51. a, b, c
pp 881–882
broad ligament; uterus, ligaments; mesosalpinx; infundibulopelvic ligament; cardinal ligament

40–52. b
pp 881–882
cardinal ligament; uterus, ligaments

40–53. a
p 881
infundibulopelvic ligament; uterus, ligaments; ovarian artery; ovarian vein

40–54. c
pp 882
round ligaments; uterus, ligaments

40–55. d
pp 882
uterosacral ligament; uterus, ligaments

40–56. d
p 882 (Fig. 40–14)
cervix, position

40–57. i
p 882 (Fig. 40–14)
round ligament

40–58. j
pp 882–884 (Fig. 40–14)
ovarian artery; ovarian vein

40–59. g
p 882 (Fig. 40–14)
urethra

40–60. b
p 882 (Fig. 40–14)
utero-ovarian ligament

40–61. a, b, c
p 882
uterus, position

40–62. hypogastric (internal iliac) artery
pp 882–883
uterus, vasculature; hypogastric artery; uterine artery

40–63. a, b, c, d
p 883
uterus, vasculature; uterine artery

40–64. c
p 883
uterine artery; ureter

40–65. There is the possibility of surgical injury to the ureter when clamping and ligating uterine vessels.
p 883
uterine artery; ureter

40–66. b, c, d
pp 883–884
uterus, vasculature; ovarian artery; infundibulopelvic ligament; uterine artery

40–67. a, b, d
p 885
uterus, vasculature; uterus, veins; ovarian vein; pampiniform plexus

40–68. a
p 885
cervix, lymphatics; hypogastric nodes; pudendal nerve

40–69. a, b
p 885
uterus, lymphatics; hypogastric nodes; periaortic nodes

40–70. a, b, c, d
pp 885–887
reproductive tract, innervation

40–71. b
p 886
oviduct

40–72. a, b, d
p 887
oviduct

40–73. a
p 887
oviduct

40–74. a
p 887
oviduct

40–75. Diverticula
p 887
oviduct; ectopic pregnancy

40–76. a, b, c, e
p 887
oviduct, embryonic development; uterus, embryonic development

40–77. a, b, e
pp 887–888
ovary, anatomy; ovary, vascular supply; infundibulopelvic ligament

40–78. a
p 888
ovary, cortex

40–79. a, b
p 888
ovary, cortex; ovary, medulla

40–80. a
p 888
ovary, cortex

40–81. a
p 888
ovary, cortex

40–82. b
p 888
ovary, medulla

40–83. b
p 888
ovary, medulla

40–84. b
p 888
ovary

40–85. The ventral surface of the embryonic kidney at 4 weeks.
p 888
ovary, embryonic development

40–86. b
p 888
ovary, embryonic development; primordial germ cells

40–87. a, b, c, d
p 888
testis, embryonic development; mesonephros

40–88. a, e
pp 888–889
ovary, embryonic development; oogenesis

40–89. mesovarium
pp 888–889
ovary, embryonic development; mesovarium

40–90. a
pp 889–890
ovary, cortex; primordial follicles

40–91. a
p 891
mesonephric duct, embryonic remnants; Gartner duct

40–92. b
p 891
mesonephric tubules, embryonic remnants; paroophoron

40–93. a
p 891
mesonephric duct, embryonic remnants; parovarium

41–1. a
p 893
overview of reproductive success

41–2. a, b
p 893
overview of reproductive success

41–3. c
p 893
reproduction in women

41–4. b
p 893
rate of relative infertility

41–5. a
p 893
success rate of in vitro fertilization

41–6. b
p 895
human reproduction in perspective

41–7. 1 = 24; 2 = 2 hours
p 895
predictions of success and failure in human reproduction

41–8. b
p 896 (Fig. 41–1)
reproductive success and failure

41–9. a, b
p 897
fecundability

41–10. Estimates vary anywhere from 67 to 80 percent.
p 898
early loss of conceptus

41–11. 1. age of puberty; 2. extent of embryonic and fetal death; 3. perinatal mortality; 4. the duration of lactational amenorrhea
p 894
human reproduction in perspective

41–12. ovulation
p 900
ovulation; menses

41–13. a
p 901
ovary, embryology

41–14. a
p 901
ovary, embryology

41–15. b
p 901
ovary, embryology; oogonia

41–16. b
p 901
oogonia

41–17. d
p 901
oogonia

41–18. c
p 901
oogonia

41–19. a
p 901
oogonia

41–20. b
p 902
graafian follicle, histology

41–21. e
p 904
graafian follicle, histology

41–22. f
p 904
graafian follicle, histology

41–23. d
p 904
graafian follicle, histology

41–24. c
p 904
graafian follicle, histology

41–25. a
p 904
graafian follicle, histology

41–26. a
p 904
graafian follicle

41–27. b
p 904
graafian follicle

41–28. b
p 904
graafian follicle

41–29. d
p 906
oocyte, maturation

41–30. a, b
p 906
oocyte, maturation

41–31. a, b, c, d
p 906
FSH

41–32. meiosis
p 906
meiosis

41–33. d
p 907
gametogenesis; germ cells; autosomes

41–34. b
p 907
gametogenesis; germ cells

41–35. b
p 908
meiosis; mitosis

41–36. b
p 908
meiosis, prophase

41–37. c
p 908
meiosis, prophase

41–38. a
p 908
meiosis, prophase

41–39. d
p 908
meiosis, prophase

41–40. zona pellucida
p 908
follicle; zona pellucida

41–41. b, c, d
p 908
oogenesis; meiosis

41–42. a
  p 908
  oogenesis

41–43. c
  p 908
  gametogenesis, meiosis; meiosis

41–44. c
  p 908
  oogenesis

41–45. b
  p 908
  meiosis

41–46. b
  p 908
  cybernin; oocyte maturation inhibitor

41–47. e
  p 910
  fertilization; sperm migration

41–48. b
  p 910
  fertilization; sperm migration

41–49. a
  pp 910–911
  fertilization

41–50. c
  p 913
  progesterone, synthesis; cholesterol

41–51. a, b, c
  pp 913–914
  ovulation

41–52. a
  p 914
  ovulation, timing; luteal phase

41–53. c
  p 914
  ovulation, timing; menstrual cycle

41–54. c
  p 915
  ovulation; progesterone, actions

41–55. None
  p 915
  ovulation; progesterone, actions

41–56. a, b, c
  pp 915–917
  corpus luteum

41–57. a, c, d
  p 918
  corpus luteum

41–58. b
  p 918
  corpus luteum, pregnancy

41–59. d
  pp 918–919
  corpus luteum, pregnancy

41–60. corpora albicantes (corpus albicans)
  p 919
  corpora albicantes; corpus luteum

41–61. a, b, c
  p 919
  follicle, atresia

41–62. a–f are causes of infertility.
  p 920
  infertility

42–1. d
  p 921
  contraception; fertility

42–2. a
  p 921
  family planning; commonly employed contraceptive techniques

42–3. a, b, c
  p 921
  contraception; ovulation; amenorrhea; menopause

42–4. 1 = 2; 2 = 5; 3 = 10; 4 = 10–20; 5 = 19; 6 = 24
  p 922 (Table 42–1)
  contraception; failure rates, contraceptives; oral contraceptives, failure rate; intrauterine device, failure rate; condom, failure rate; diaphragm, failure rate; rhythm method, failure rate

42–5. a
  p 924
  contraceptives, failure rate

42–6. a, c, d
  pp 923–924
  oral contraceptives; estrogen-progestin contraceptives; ethinyl estradiol; progestin, oral contraceptives

42–7. a, b, c
  pp 923–924
  oral contraceptives; estrogen-progestin contraceptives; withdrawal bleeding

42–8. b
  pp 923–924
  oral contraceptives; estrogen-progestin contraceptives

42-9. b
pp 923–924
estrogen–progestin contraceptives; oral contraceptives; ethinyl estradiol; mestranol

42-10. b
pp 923–924
estrogen-progestin contraceptives; oral contraceptives; progestin

42-11. a, c, d, e, f
p 924
estrogen–progestin contraceptives; oral contraceptives; endometrial carcinoma; ovarian carcinoma; rheumatoid arthritis; menstruation; blood loss, menstruation

42-12. a
p 924
estrogen-progestin contraceptives; oral contraceptives; oral contraceptives, side effects

42-13. a
pp 924–925
estrogen-progestin contraceptives; oral contraceptives

42-14. b
p 925
estrogen-progestin contraceptives; oral contraceptives; hepatitis

42-15. a, c
p 925
estrogen–progestin contraceptives; oral contraceptives; oral contraceptives, side effects; hepatic focal nodular hyperplasia

42-16. 1 = b; 2 = b
p 925
estrogen-progestin contraceptives; oral contraceptives; blood loss, menstrual; dysmenorrhea

42-17. a, d, e, f
p 925
estrogen–progestin contraceptives; oral contraceptives; stroke, oral contraceptives; hypertension, oral contraceptives; myocardial infarction, oral contraceptives; thromboembolic disease, oral contraceptives

42-18. thromboembolism, current or past; cerebrovascular accident, current or past; coronary artery disease; impaired liver functions; liver adenoma, current or past; breast cancer; hypertension; diabetes; gallbladder disease; cholestatic jaundice during pregnancy; sickle cell hemoglobinopathy; surgery completed within 4 weeks; major surgery on or immobilization of a lower extremity; patient over 40 years of age; smoking
p 925
estrogen–progestin contraceptives; oral contraceptives, contraindications; thromboembolism; cerebrovascular accident; coronary artery disease; liver function, impaired; liver adenoma; breast cancer; hypertension; diabetes; gallbladder disease; cholestatic jaundice; sickle cell hemoglobinopathy; smoking

42-19. a
p 928
estrogen–progestin contraceptives; oral contraceptives; ovulation

42-20. a, b, c, d
p 928
estrogen–progestin contraceptives; oral contraceptives; cervical mucorrhea; myomas, uterine; vulvovaginitis

42-21. b
pp 928–929
breast feeding; estrogen–progestin oral contraceptives; oral contraceptives

42-22. higher incidence of irregular bleeding; higher pregnancy rate
p 929
oral contraceptives; progestin contraceptives

42-23. a, b, c, d, e
p 929
progestins, injectable; lactation; amenorrhea; anovulation

42-24. stilbestrol
p 929
oral contraceptives; stilbestrol

42-25. inserted only once; complete protection against pregnancy; not spontaneously expelled; no adverse effects that necessitate removal; after removal, it would have induced no changes detrimental to pregnancy
p 930
intrauterine device

42-26. chemically inert device made of nonabsorbable (radioopaque) material; device from which there is a continuous elution of a chemically active substance
pp 930–931
intrauterine device

42-27. Neither of the devices has achieved all the ''ideal'' criteria.
p 930
intrauterine device; contraception

42-28. d
pp 930–931
Progestasert; intrauterine device; contraception

42-29. The precise mechanism of action is not known. The primary action seems to be interference with successful implantation. Effectiveness increases with size and extent of contact with the endometrium.
p 931
intrauterine device, action; contraception

42-30. b
p 931
intrauterine device, action; contraception; copper; Cu7

42-31. a
p 931
intrauterine device, complications; contraception

42–32. b, c, d
p 931
intrauterine device, complications; contraception; pelvic inflammatory disease

42–33. a, c
p 931
intrauterine device, complications; contraception

42–34. b
p 931
intrauterine device; actinomyces, intrauterine device; contraception

42–35. b, c
pp 931–932
intrauterine device, lost device; ultrasonography; intrauterine device, extrauterine; contraception

42–36. a
p 932
intrauterine device; pregnancy, intrauterine device

42–37. a, b, c, e
p 932
intrauterine device; pregnancy, intrauterine device

42–38. 1 = b; 2 = c
p 932
intrauterine device; abortion, intrauterine device; pregnancy, intrauterine device

42–39. b
pp 932–933
intrauterine device; ectopic pregnancy; contraception

42–40. a, c, e
p 932
intrauterine device, insertion; abortion, intrauterine device; puerperium, intrauterine device

42–41. a, b, c, d, e, f, g
p 932
intrauterine device, contraindications; gonorrhea; cervical stenosis; dysmenorrhea; contraception

42–42. b, a, d, c, e, g, f
p 933
intrauterine device, insertion; contraception

42–43. a, c
p 933
intrauterine device, expulsion; contraception

42–44. d
p 934
Lippes Loop; intrauterine device; contraception

42–45. b
p 934
Cu7; intrauterine device; contraception

42–46. b
p 934
Copper T; intrauterine device; contraception

42–47. a
p 934
Progestasert; intrauterine device; contraception

42–48. b, c
p 934
condoms; contraception, barrier

42–49. b, c, e, f
p 934
contraceptives, intravaginal

42–50. b
p 934
contraceptives, intravaginal; congenital malformations, contraceptive use

42–51. to the superior surface along the rim and centrally
pp 934–935
contraceptives, barrier; diaphragm; spermicide

42–52. a, b
pp 934–935
contraceptives, barrier; diaphragm

42–53. b
p 935
contraceptives, sponge

42–54. a, c
p 935
contraceptives, breast feeding; breast feeding

42–55. calendar; temperature; cervical mucus (Billings)
pp 935–936
contraception; rhythm method, contraception; cervical mucus

42–56. c, d
p 936
contraception, surgical; tubal sterilization

42–57. a
p 936
Irving procedure, tubal sterilization; tubal sterilization

42–58. b
p 936
Pomeroy procedure, tubal sterilization; tubal sterilization

42–59. c
pp 936–937
Parkland procedure, tubal sterilization; tubal sterilization

42–60. d
p 937
Madlener procedure, tubal sterilization; tubal sterilization

42–61. e
p 937
fimbriectomy; tubal sterilization

42–62. a
p 936
Irving procedure, tubal sterilization; tubal sterilization

42–63. b
p 936
Pomeroy procedure, tubal sterilization; tubal sterilization

42–64. c
pp 937–938
sterilization, surgical; postoperative care, surgical sterilization

42–65. The three principal surgical techniques are ligation and resection; application of rings/clips; and electrocoagulation.
p 938
sterilization, surgical; sterilization, nonpuerperal

42–66. a, b, c, d
pp 938–939
tubal sterilization, complications

42–67. general anesthesia without endotracheal intubation
pp 938–939
tubal sterilization, complications; mortality, tubal sterilization; anesthesia

42–68. a, b, c, d, e
p 939
tubal sterilization; morbidity, tubal sterilization

42–69. b
p 940
tubal sterilization; posttubal ligation syndrome

42–70. b
p 940
tubal sterilization, reversal

42–71. a, b, c, d
p 940
hysterectomy, sterilization

42–72. b
p 940
sterilization, surgical; tubal sterilization; hysterectomy, sterilization

42–73. a, b
pp 940–941
vasectomy; sterilization

42–74. microsurgical technique; length of time after vasectomy; presence of sperm granulomas
p 940
vasectomy, reversal

42–75. d
p 940
contraception, male

Topics Index

The numbers following each entry indicate chapter and question numbers.

The numbers following each entry indicate chapter and question numbers.

The numbers following each entry indicate chapter and question numbers.

The numbers following each entry indicate chapter and question numbers.

The numbers following each entry indicate chapter and question numbers.

The numbers following each entry indicate chapter and question numbers.

Prostaglandins (*cont.*)
  actions, 6–48, 10–26
  cervical softening, 29–61
  labor, 10–14
  synthesis, 4–34, 10–27
Prostaglandin E₂, 36–105, 36–106
Prostaglandin synthesis, 10–15
Prostaglandin synthetase inhibitors, 6–48
Protamine sulfate, 28–17
Protein metabolism, 7–36
  pregnancy, 7–35
Protein requirements, pregnancy, 14–37
Proteinuria, 35–9, 35–12, 35–43
  preeclampsia, 35–10
  pregnancy, 7–105, 35–57, 35–59
Protracted labor, 18–33 (*See also* Labor)
  active phase, 18–7
  disorders, labor, 18–15, 18–16
Pseudocyesis, spurious pregnancy, 2–59
Pseudomembranous colitis, 27–21
Psychoprophylaxis, 16–1
Psychosis, 39–237
Psychotropic drugs, 32–28
Puberty, 3–35, 3–37
Pudenal block, 17–28 through 17–30
Pudenal nerve, 17–24, 17–25, 40–68
Puerpera, 14–6
Puerperal diuresis, 13–29, 13–30
Puerperal fever, 28–33
Puerperal infection, 27–1, 27–2, 27–4 through 27–9, 27–13, 27–15
    through 27–20, 27–24, 27–25, 27–31, 28–36, 39–274
Puerperal morbidity, 27–2, 27–3
Puerperium, 7–58, 13–2 through 13–8, 13–26, 13–20 through
    13–31, 13–33, 13–41 through 13–43
  abdominal wall, 13–36
  bladder, 13–39
  bladder function, 13–39
  breast care, 13–40
  constipation, 13–35, 13–40
  definition, 13–1
  disorder, 28–20
  diet, 13–37
  diuresis, 7–34
  early ambulation, 13–35
  fever, 27–3, 27–24
  intrauterine device, 42–40
  morbidity, 27–24
  oxytocics, 13–38
  regeneration of endometrium, 13–13
  weight loss, 7–34, 13–32
Pulmonary dysfunction, hemoglobinopathies, 39–31
Pulmonary edema, eclampsia, 35–77
Pulmonary embolism, 27–13, 27–15, 28–7, 28–19, 28–21 through
    28–23
  recurrent, 28–24
Pulmonary function, pregnancy, 7–93 through 7–99, 39–93
    through 39–100
Pulmonary hypertension, 39–86, 39–88
  neonatal 33–8
Pulmonary hypoplasia, fetal, 31–105
Pulmonary infarction, 39–101
Purine, 32–64
Pushing, 10–54, 18–31 (*See also* Voluntary expulsive forces)

Pyelonephritis, 5–52, 21–16, 39–111, 39–191
  acute, 39–114 through 39–117, 39–122, 39–123
  chronic, 39–122
Pyopagus, 34–22
Pyridoxine, 39–105
Pyrimidine, 32–64
Pyuria, 39–132

Quick one-stage prothrombin time, 7–69
Quinine, 39–236

Radiation, pregnancy, 32–32, 32–33
Radiation therapy, 31–87
Radiography, 2–34, 15–43 (*See also* X-ray pelvimetry)
Radioimmunoassay, 2–45
Rectocele, 23–1, 37–6, 37–7, 37–41
Rectum, tumors, 21–20
Red cell volume, pregnancy, 39–4, 39–5
Regional anesthesia, 17–26
Regional enteritis, 39–208
Relaxin, 4–54
  pregnancy, 7–15
Renal agenesis, 6–87
Renal cortical necrosis, 35–43, 39–143
Renal failure, 29–82, 36–58
Renal function, pregnancy, 7–101
Renal function tests, pregnancy, 7–102, 7–103
Renal transplantation, 39–145
Renal tuberculosis, 39–133
Renin, 7–124, 35–38
Repeat cesarean delivery, timing, 26–9, 26–10
Reproduction, women, 41–3
Reproductive function in women, 2–5
Reproductive mortality, definition, 1–16
Reproductive success, overview, 41–1, 41–2
Reproductive success and failure, 41–8
Reproductive tract, innervation, 40–70
  developmental abnormalities, 37–22 through 37–26, 27–28
    through 37–30, 37–33
Residual volume, 39–95
Respiration
  fetal, 12–1
  initiation, 12–14
  newborn, 12–1 through 12–3, 12–6, 12–7
Respiratory depression, 12–29
  newborn, 17–16
Respiratory distress, 39–154, 39–165
Respiratory distress syndrome, 6–91, 6–96, 6–97, 12–5, 15–10
    through 15–13, 33–1 through 33–3, 33–5, 33–7, 33–56,
    33–102
Respiratory function, pregnancy, 7–41, 7–92
Respiratory rate, 39–96
Respiratory system
  fetus, 6–89, 6–99
  pregnancy, 7–94 through 7–100
Respiratory tract pregnancy, 7–93
Restriction endonuclease, 32–71
Restriction fragment length polymorphisms, 32–67
Resuscitation, neonate, 12–19 through 12–21, 12–23, 12–24, 12–28
    through 12–33, 33–15
Retained placenta, 24–5, 24–6, 31–18

The numbers following each entry indicate chapter and question numbers.

The numbers following each entry indicate chapter and question numbers.